Cancer Drug Discovery and Development

Series editor:

Beverly A. Teicher
Bethesda, MD, USA

The Cancer Drug Discovery and Development series (Beverly A Teicher, series editor) is the definitive book series in cancer research and oncology, providing comprehensive coverage of specific topics and the field. Volumes cover the process of drug discovery, preclinical models in cancer research, specific drug target groups and experimental and approved therapeutic agents. The volumes are current and timely, anticipating areas where experimental agents are reaching FDA approval. Each volume is edited by an expert in the field covered and chapters are authored by renowned scientists and physicians in their fields of interest.

More information about this series at http://www.springer.com/series/7625

Shay Soker • Aleksander Skardal

Editors

Tumor Organoids

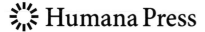 Humana Press

Editors
Shay Soker
Institute for Regenerative Medicine
Wake Forest School of Medicine
Winston-Salem, NC, USA

Aleksander Skardal
Institute for Regenerative Medicine
Wake Forest School of Medicine
Winston-Salem, NC, USA

ISSN 2196-9906   ISSN 2196-9914   (electronic)
Cancer Drug Discovery and Development
ISBN 978-3-319-86874-5   ISBN 978-3-319-60511-1   (eBook)
DOI 10.1007/978-3-319-60511-1

Printed on acid-free paper

This Humana Press imprint is published by Springer Nature
The registered company is Springer International Publishing AG
The registered company address is: Gewerbestrasse 11, 6330 Cham, Switzerland

I want to dedicate this book to my family, and especially to my wife, who has supported me throughout my career, and to all the students and research fellows who have worked hard to advance the science for the benefit of all patients.

Shay Soker

Contents

Contributors

Manuel Almeida Digestive Pathology Research Group, Instituto de Investigación Sanitaria de Aragón (IIS Aragón), Zaragoza, Spain

Pedro M. Baptista Digestive Pathology Research Group, Instituto de Investigación Sanitaria de Aragón (IIS Aragón), Zaragoza, Spain

Instituto de Investigación Sanitaria de la Fundación Jiménez Díaz, Madrid, Spain

Departamento de Bioingeniería, Universidad Carlos III de Madrid, Madrid, Spain

CIBERehd, Madrid, Spain

María Inés Diaz Bessone, PhD Instituto de Nanosistemas, Universidad Nacional de San Martín, Buenos Aires, Argentina

Rosemary Clare Burke Virginia Tech-Wake Forest School of Biomedical Engineering and Sciences, Wake Forest University School of Medicine, Winston-Salem, NC, USA

Department of Biomedical Engineering, University of Texas Austin, Austin, TX, USA

Aaron E. Chiou Nancy E. and Peter C. Meinig School of Biomedical Engineering, Cornell University, Ithaca, NY, USA

Melissa L. Fender Pashayan Department of Physics, Wake Forest University, 100 Olin Physical Laboratory, Wake Forest University, Winston-Salem, NC, USA

Claudia Fischbach Nancy E. and Peter C. Meinig School of Biomedical Engineering, Cornell University, Ithaca, NY, USA

Kavli Institute at Cornell for Nanoscale Science, Cornell University, Ithaca, NY, USA

Manasa Gadde Department of Biomedical Engineering, The University of Texas at Austin, Austin, TX, USA

Steven C. George Department of Biomedical Engineering, Washington University in St. Louis, St. Louis, MO, USA

Manuel M. Gomez Department of Physics, Wake Forest University, 100 Olin Physical Laboratory, Wake Forest University, Winston-Salem, NC, USA

Adam R. Hall Virginia Tech-Wake Forest School of Biomedical Engineering and Sciences, Wake Forest University School of Medicine, Winston-Salem, NC, USA

Comprehensive Cancer Center, Wake Forest University School of Medicine, Winston-Salem, NC, USA

Parker Hambright Virginia Tech-Wake Forest School of Biomedical Engineering and Sciences, Wake Forest University School of Medicine, Winston-Salem, NC, USA

Department of Biology, Wake Forest University, Winston-Salem, NC, USA

Priscilla Y. Hwang Department of Biomedical Engineering, Washington University in St. Louis, St. Louis, MO, USA

Kimberly Jen Unit for Laboratory Animal Medicine (ULAM), University of Michigan, Ann Arbor, USA

Aleksandra Karolak Integrated Mathematical Oncology Department, H. Lee Moffitt Cancer Center & Research Institute, Tampa, FL, USA

Sandra F. Lam Department of Biomedical Engineering, Washington University in St. Louis, St. Louis, MO, USA

Alberto Lue Digestive Pathology Research Group, Instituto de Investigación Sanitaria de Aragón (IIS Aragón), Zaragoza, Spain

Gastroenterology Department, University Hospital Lozano Blesa, Zaragoza, Spain

Jed C. Macosko Department of Physics, Wake Forest University, 100 Olin Physical Laboratory, Wake Forest University, Winston-Salem, NC, USA

Dan Marrinan Department of Mechanical Engineering, The University of Texas at Austin, Austin, TX, USA

Andrea Mazzocchi Wake Forest Institute for Regenerative Medicine, Wake Forest School of Medicine, Medical Center Boulevard, Winston-Salem, NC, USA

Virginia Tech-Wake Forest School of Biomedical Engineering and Sciences, Wake Forest School of Medicine, Medical Center Boulevard, Winston-Salem, NC, USA

Rhys J. Michna Department of Mechanical Engineering, The University of Texas at Austin, Austin, TX, USA

Iris Pla-Palacín Digestive Pathology Research Group, Instituto de Investigación Sanitaria de Aragón (IIS Aragón), Zaragoza, Spain

Shiny Amala Priya Rajan Virginia Tech-Wake Forest School of Biomedical Engineering and Sciences, Wake Forest University School of Medicine, Winston-Salem, NC, USA

Sol Recouvreux, MSc Instituto de Oncología "Angel H. Roffo", Ciudad de Buenos Aires, Argentina

Katarzyna A. Rejniak Integrated Mathematical Oncology Department, H. Lee Moffitt Cancer Center & Research Institute, Tampa, FL, USA

Department of Oncologic Sciences, College of Medicine, University of South Florida, Tampa, FL, USA

Marissa Nichole Rylander Department of Biomedical Engineering, The University of Texas at Austin, Austin, TX, USA

Department of Mechanical Engineering, The University of Texas at Austin, Austin, TX, USA

Pilar Sainz-Arnal Digestive Pathology Research Group, Instituto de Investigación Sanitaria de Aragón (IIS Aragón), Zaragoza, Spain

Instituto Aragonés de Ciencias de la Salud (IACS), Zaragoza, Spain

Rocío Sampayo, PhD Instituto de Nanosistemas, Universidad Nacional de San Martín San Martín, Buenos Aires, Argentina

Trinidad Serrano Digestive Pathology Research Group, Instituto de Investigación Sanitaria de Aragón (IIS Aragón), Zaragoza, Spain

Gastroenterology Department, University Hospital Lozano Blesa, Zaragoza, Spain

Instituto de Investigación Sanitaria de la Fundación Jiménez Díaz, Madrid, Spain

CIBERehd, Madrid, Spain

Mary Kathryn Sewell-Loftin Department of Biomedical Engineering, Washington University in St. Louis, St. Louis, MO, USA

Venktesh S. Shirure Department of Biomedical Engineering, Washington University in St. Louis, St. Louis, MO, USA

Marina Simian, PhD Instituto de Nanosistemas, Universidad Nacional de San Martín, Buenos Aires, Argentina

Aleksander Skardal Wake Forest Institute for Regenerative Medicine, Wake Forest School of Medicine, Medical Center Boulevard, Winston-Salem, NC, USA

Virginia Tech-Wake Forest School of Biomedical Engineering and Sciences, Wake Forest School of Medicine, Medical Center Boulevard, Winston-Salem, NC, USA

Department of Cancer Biology, Wake Forest School of Medicine, Medical Center Boulevard, Winston-Salem, NC, USA

Comprehensive Cancer Center at Wake Forest Baptist, Wake Forest Baptist Health Sciences, Medical Center Boulevard, Winston-Salem, NC, USA

Amanda M. Smelser Department of Cancer Biology, Wake Forest Baptist Medical Center, Medical Center Boulevard, Winston-Salem, NC, USA

Scott Smyre Department of Physics, Wake Forest University, 100 Olin Physical Laboratory, Wake Forest University, Winston-Salem, NC, USA

Shay Soker Wake Forest Institute for Regenerative Medicine, Wake Forest School of Medicine Medical Center Boulevard, Winston-Salem, NC, USA

Virginia Tech-Wake Forest School of Biomedical Engineering and Sciences, Wake Forest School of Medicine, Medical Center Boulevard, Winston-Salem, NC, USA

Department of Cancer Biology, Wake Forest School of Medicine, Medical Center Boulevard, Winston-Salem, NC, USA

Comprehensive Cancer Center at Wake Forest Baptist, Wake Forest Baptist Health Sciences, Medical Center Boulevard, Winston-Salem, NC, USA

Estela Solanas Digestive Pathology Research Group, Instituto de Investigación Sanitaria de Aragón (IIS Aragón), Zaragoza, Spain

Shuichi Takayama Department of Biomedical Engineering, Macromolecular Science and Engineering, Biointerfaces Institute, MCIRCC, University of Michigan, Ann Arbor, MI, USA

Tyson D. Todd Department of Biomedical Engineering, Washington University in St. Louis, St. Louis, MO, USA

Cameron Yamanishi Department of Biomedical Engineering, University of Michigan, Ann Arbor, USA

Introduction

Major challenges in cancer therapy are to determine if a local disease will progress to a malignant phenotype, and how to best "match" treatments to the type and stage of the disease. It is now well accepted that for many cancers they are no longer a single type of disease but a constellation of cancer types, pathologically classified by histology, which respond differently to drugs. For many years, basic cancer research and anticancer drug development utilized primary cancer cells and cell lines cultured in vitro on tissue culture plastic dishes. Although this approach yielded many of the anticancer medications used today, recent investigation has found this approach a poor analogue of tumor growth in vivo. For the most part, two-dimensional (2D) culture, like that in culture dishes, does not replicate the microenvironment of a tumor, a complex space typified by stromal cells, extracellular matrix (ECM) components, and a cocktail of signaling factors (Kunz-Schughart et al. 2004, Bhattacharya et al. 2011). For example, drug diffusion kinetics vary dramatically, drug doses effective in 2D are often ineffective when scaled to patients, and cell-cell/cell-matrix interactions are inaccurate (Ho et al. 2010, Drewitz et al. 2011). Tissue culture dishes have three major differences from the tissue where the tumor was isolated: surface topography, surface stiffness, and a 2D rather than 3D architecture. As a consequence, 2D culture places a selective pressure on cells that could substantially alter their molecular and phenotypic properties (Arnold et al. 2015, Li and Kilian 2015). These differences between laboratory cell culture and the native tissue have resulted in many drugs that were initially effective in the laboratory but were unexpectedly ineffective and/or toxic when tested in patients.

Instead, newly developed bioengineered tissue platforms, such as three-dimensional (3D) organoids, open new opportunities for tumor modeling, especially incorporating the complex cellular and physical tumor microenvironment (TME) that are known to drive cancer cells in a specific manner. There is a growing body of literature that illustrates the importance of tumor-stroma related effects (Luca et al. 2013, Catalano et al. 2013, Pietras and Ostman 2010). For example, the tumor stroma can activate or inactivate cancer-related pathways, alter ECM components, thereby making migration more or less difficult, as well as secrete signaling factors that guide cancer cells in a multitude of ways. Studies have demonstrated that placing normal epithelial cells into an activated stroma can produce cancerous growth from these healthy cells; and conversely, placing malignant cancer cells in a healthy stroma can cause a reversion from a cancerous state towards a normal phenotype (Cichon, Radisky, and Radisky 2011).

The chapters included in this book aim to provide a comprehensive overview on recent development in the generation of healthy and pathologic (mostly cancerous) small tissue construct (organoids). The tumor organoid platform incorporates other biofabrication methods such as innovative and smart biomaterials and microfabrication techniques. These models can be used to investigate tissue development and disease and serve as in vitro platforms for drug screening and testing. In the new era of personalized medicine there is a specific need for systems that incorporate patients' genetic information to serve as guidance for treatment selection. On the other hand, the tumor organoid technology opens a new window for researching the basic mechanisms of the initiation and progression of a disease such as cancer, and to develop therapeutic approaches. Mathematical modeling of disease progression and identification of specific factors that impact its dynamics is far easier in a fully controlled in vitro system.

Yamanishi and colleagues describe in their chapter on "Techniques to Produce and Culture Lung Tumor Organoids" several methods to generate functional lung organoids. Each method addresses physiologic and practical aspects of the lung organoids. Solana and colleagues discuss the need for alternative culture methods for primary hepatocytes. In their chapter "Tissue Organoids; Liver" they describe the liver organoids as a novel method to maintain function and viability of primary hepatocytes at higher levels for longer time. In the chapter "Mammary Gland Organoids," Sampayo and colleagues provide a historical perspective on 3D culture systems of primary mammary organoids. These systems have provided a platform to study the cell biology aspects of mammary gland development and function in physiologically relevant settings.

Mazzocchi and colleagues describe several biofabrication methods to create tumor organoids in their chapter "Tumor Organoids Biofabrication." Several matrix systems, built on various hydrogel platforms, allow for robust environmental manipulation in order to investigate a variety of biological mechanisms. The hydrogel biofabrication system is tunable, both in terms of stiffness and fiber alignment, allowing formation of discrete zones of different cell populations and physical parameters. These models are viable for long periods of time, develop functional properties similar to native tissues, and recapitulate the dynamic cell–cell, cell–ECM interactions in the tumor. Gadde and colleagues describe the development of a microfluidic technology combined with microfabrication techniques to yield a physiologically representative tumor environment, while allowing for dynamic monitoring and simultaneous control of multiple biochemical and mechanical factors such as cellular and extracellular matrix composition, fluid velocity, and wall shear stress. Their chapter "Evolution of Three Dimensional In Vitro Tumor Platforms for Cancer Discovery" implies that these systems are capable of serving, investigating various key stages in cancer evolution including angiogenesis and metastasis. Chiou and Fischbach use breast tumor organoids to demonstrate metastasis-associated changes to the bone microenvironment and current approaches to study bone metastasis in their chapter "Tissue-Engineered Models for Studies of Bone Metastasis." They discuss tissue-engineered model systems of bone metastasis as a promising alternative and describe specific design parameters to investigate the functional contribution of the microenvironment to the development, progression, and therapy response of bone metastasis. Shirur and colleagues, in their chapter "Organoid Systems to Investigate Angiogenesis," review the process of blood vessel growth, specifically blood vessels within the cancer microenvironment, and discuss the most recent advances to mimic blood vessel growth in the tumor microenvironment using 3D in vitro culture methods. They discuss several important factors that control blood vessel growth including hypoxia, cellular metabolism, and tissue mechanics.

Priya Rajan and colleagues describe in their chapter "Microfluidics in Cell and Tissue Studies" recent technological advances to investigate numerous, interdependent variables in discrete samples and the analysis of outcomes. They discuss microfluidic approaches that enable the study of cancer cells in tumor organoids. Smelser and colleagues address the effect of stiffness, or elasticity, on tumor cell behavior and describe a matrix that provides the integrin binding sites that are found in stroma in their chapter "Stiffness-Tuned Matrices for Tumor Cell Studies." They use cross-linking of collagen I to increase collagen's elasticity while controlling for binding site density and demonstrate that breast cancer cells survived and migrated on these matrices. Karolak and Rejniak describe in their chapter "Mathematical Modeling of Tumor Organoids; Towards Personalized Medicine" three different approaches to building in silico organoids, together with methods for integration with experimental or clinical data. One model is used to determine the mechanisms of development of breast tumor acini, based on their in vitro morphology. The other is used to predict conditions for the most effective cellular uptake of therapies targeting pancreatic cancers, incorporating intravital microscopy data. The last one provides a procedure for assessing patients' response to chemotherapeutic treatments, based on the biopsy data. These models can help biologists to generate testable hypotheses or predictions and they can also assist clinicians in assessing cancer patients' response to a given therapy and their risk of tumor recurrence.

References

1. Arnold, M., H. E. Karim-Kos, J. W. Coebergh, G. Byrnes, A. Antilla, J. Ferlay, A. G. Renehan, D. Forman, and I. Soerjomataram (2015). "Recent trends in incidence of five common cancers in 26 European countries since 1988: Analysis of the European Cancer Observatory." *Eur J Cancer* 51(9):1164–87. doi: 10.1016/j.ejca.2013.09.002
2. Bhattacharya, S., Q. Zhang, P. L. Carmichael, K. Boekelheide, and M. E. Andersen (2011). "Toxicity testing in the 21 century: defining new risk assessment approaches based on perturbation of intracellular toxicity pathways." *PLoS One* 6(6):e20887. doi: 10.1371/journal.pone.0020887

3. Catalano, V., A. Turdo, S. Di Franco, F. Dieli, M. Todaro, and G. Stassi (2013). "Tumor and its microenvironment: a synergistic interplay." *Semin Cancer Biol* 23(6 Pt B):522–32. doi: 10.1016/j.semcancer.2013.08.007

4. Cichon, M. A., E. S. Radisky, and D. C. Radisky (2011). "Identifying the stroma as a critical player in radiation-induced mammary tumor development." *Cancer Cell* 19(5):571–2. doi: 10.1016/j.ccr.2011.05.001

5. Drewitz, M., M. Helbling, N. Fried, M. Bieri, W. Moritz, J. Lichtenberg, and J. M. Kelm (2011). "Towards automated production and drug sensitivity testing using scaffold-free spherical tumor microtissues." *Biotechnol J* 6(12):1488–96. doi: 10.1002/biot.201100290

6. Ho, W. J., E. A. Pham, J. W. Kim, C. W. Ng, J. H. Kim, D. T. Kamei, and B. M. Wu (2010). "Incorporation of multicellular spheroids into 3-D polymeric scaffolds provides an improved tumor model for screening anticancer drugs." *Cancer Sci* 101(12):2637–43. doi: 10.1111/j.1349-7006.2010.01723.x

7. Kunz-Schughart, L. A., J. P. Freyer, F. Hofstaedter, and R. Ebner (2004). "The use of 3-D cultures for high-throughput screening: the multicellular spheroid model." *J Biomol Screen* 9(4):273–85. doi: 10.1177/1087057104265040

8. Li, Y., and K. A. Kilian (2015). "Bridging the Gap: From 2D Cell Culture to 3D Microengineered Extracellular Matrices." *Adv Healthc Mater* 4(18):2780–96. doi: 10.1002/adhm.201500427

9. Luca, A. C., S. Mersch, R. Deenen, S. Schmidt, I. Messner, K. L. Schafer, S. E. Baldus, W. Huckenbeck, R. P. Piekorz, W. T. Knoefel, A. Krieg, and N. H. Stoecklein (2013). "Impact of the 3D microenvironment on phenotype, gene expression, and EGFR inhibition of colorectal cancer cell lines." *PLoS One* 8(3):e59689. doi: 10.1371/journal.pone.0059689

10. Pietras, K., and A. Ostman (2010). "Hallmarks of cancer: interactions with the tumor stroma." *Exp Cell Res* 316(8):1324–31. doi: 10.1016/j.yexcr.2010.02.045

Techniques to Produce and Culture Lung Tumor Organoids

Cameron Yamanishi, Kimberly Jen, and Shuichi Takayama

Abstract Three-dimensional cell culture formats have been gaining popularity due to their ability to more closely mimic human physiology compared to conventional, two-dimensional culture. These 3D cultures exhibit in vivo-like behaviors, such as cell-cell adhesion, extracellular matrix secretion, and resilience against bacterial, chemical, and radiation insults. Various techniques for 3D organoid culture have been developed to recreate aspects of the lung microenvironment. This chapter examines the history and current applications of 3D lung tumor organoid culture, including Matrigel, hanging drop, magnetic levitation, rotating wall vessels, and non-adherent culture techniques. Each technique provides unique benefits for physiologic behavior, organoid access, and convenience. However, further work is required to advance the development of these systems for future biological discovery and high-throughput drug screening.

Keywords Lung organoid • Hanging drop • Rotating wall vessel • Non-adherent culture

C. Yamanishi
Department of Biomedical Engineering, University of Michigan, Ann Arbor, USA
e-mail: yamacam@umich.edu

K. Jen
Unit for Laboratory Animal Medicine (ULAM), University of Michigan, Ann Arbor, USA
e-mail: kyjen@med.umich.edu

S. Takayama (✉)
Department of Biomedical Engineering, Macromolecular Science and Engineering,
Biointerfaces Institute, MCIRCC, University of Michigan,
2800 Plymouth Rd, Ann Arbor, MI, USA
e-mail: takayama@umich.edu

© Springer International Publishing AG 2018
S. Soker, A. Skardal (eds.), *Tumor Organoids*, Cancer Drug Discovery
and Development, DOI 10.1007/978-3-319-60511-1_1

1   Introduction

Manipulation of cell culture was born out of a necessity to test model living systems in a controlled and replicable manner. Since their inception in 1907 [1], two-dimensional (2D) cultures enabled researchers to observe and manipulate cells outside of the mammalian body. 2D cultures have been critical in many landmark biological discoveries. However, 2D cultures fail to recapitulate the complex microenvironments within the body. While some cell behaviors are conserved, subtle differences can mask downstream cell behavior. For example, discrepancies between focal adhesion complexes in 2D vs three-dimensional (3D) culture [2] can alter metastatic behavior that relies on focal adhesion kinase signaling [3]. Discrepancies between conventional 2D cultures and whole organism behavior have led to the pursuit of more physiological in vitro cell cultures to strike a balance between whole organism complexity and in vitro accessibility. In recent years, these efforts have yielded a plethora of 3D culture techniques, which typically utilize in vitro or ex vivo multicellular tissue models. In many of these systems, cells self-organize into tissue-like structures with distinct cell layers and a hollow lumen. 3D tumor models made from these techniques exhibit greater resistance to chemical and radiation treatment, which more closely resembles behavior seen in vivo [4]. 3D cultures strive to recapitulate both structural and functional properties of the original tissue [5, 6]. Achieving 3D behavior requires control of many culture conditions, including growth factors, matrices, and culture chambers to coax cells into organized structures composed of several hundred cells to several thousand cells [7].

This chapter discusses current lung tumor organoid culture techniques, with organoids narrowly defined as 3D cultures without attachment of cells to a flat substrate, notably excluding decellularized and reseeded lung slices. Organoids are typically recognized as cell constructs that have self-organized to exhibit a 3D structure vaguely resembling the native organ. This chapter will cover simple cell spheroids, as well as more highly-organized organ-buds and acini. Conversely, this chapter will exclude microfluidic platforms, commonly referred to as organs-on-a-chip (OoC). These organotypic cell cultures utilize 2D cell culture systems on porous membrane supports to form distinct layers of cells. OoC systems have the additional advantage of exposing cells to controlled fluid flow, which mimics recirculation and mechanical stresses [8]. Those microfluidic systems, however, are often less 3D in cellular structure due to the rigid artificial substrates supporting cells. Furthermore, there are numerous recent reviews that focus solely on lungs-on-a-chip and they will not be discussed in this chapter. Compared to the microfluidic systems, the organoid culture techniques covered in this chapter are generally more amenable to high-throughput assays and drug discovery.

The progress in 3D organoid cultures to this point is largely driven by innovative culturing methods. However, successful creation and culture of lung organoids still pose several challenges: creating organ-specific architecture and morphology, maintaining stable cultures preferably within an air-liquid interface (ALI), integration of correct cell types including epithelial cells, fibroblasts, and goblet cells, and inclusion of proper extracellular matrix (ECM). This chapter summarizes culture techniques developed to overcome these challenges which include Matrigel culture, hanging drop culture, magnetic levitation (maglev), rotating wall vessels, and non-adherent attachment plates (Fig. 1), which have created various architectures, including hollowed out acinar structures resembling alveolar acini or filled spheroids.

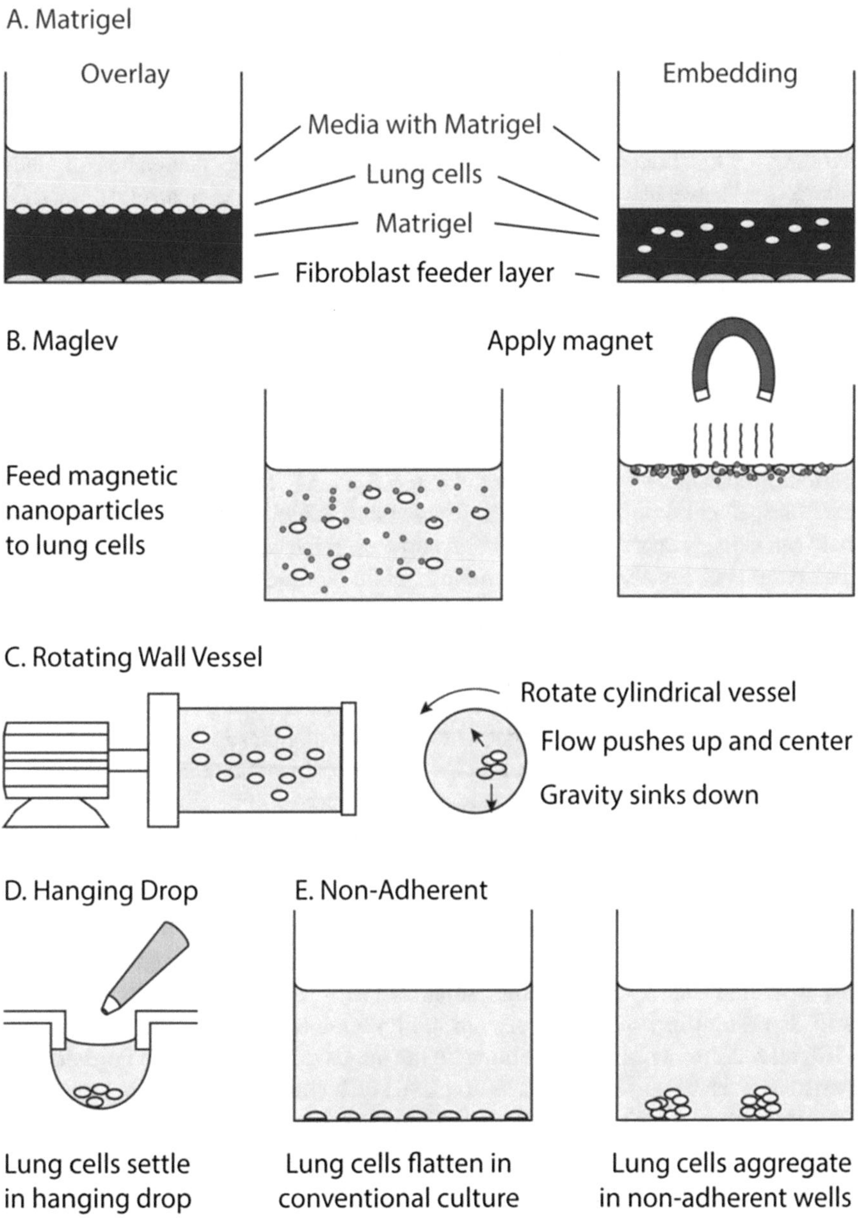

Fig. 1 Schematics of lung organoid culture techniques. (**a**) In Matrigel-overlay culture, lung cells are seeded on top of solid Matrigel above a feeder layer of fibroblasts, and covered with media containing low-concentration Matrigel. (**b**) In Maglev culture, lung cells are fed magnetic nanparticles and pulled to the top surface of the media by a permanent magnet. (**c**) In rotating wall vessel culture, lung cells are suspended in culture by the competition between circulating flow and gravity-induced sedimentation. (**d**) In hanging drop culture, lung cells sediment to the bottom, air-liquid interface of a media droplet. (**e**) In non-adherent culture, lung cells sediment to the bottom of a dish, where surface coatings inhibit cell attachment to the dish

2 Techniques

2.1 Matrigel

Working at the Laboratory of Developmental Biology and Anomalies to study interactions between cells and extracellular matrix, Hynda Kleinman and coworkers developed methods to extract ECM from Englebreth-Holm-Swarm mouse sarcomas [9]. In a 1986 Biochemistry report, the group described the composition and mechanical properties of the extract [10], later termed Matrigel. Their previous attempts to form physiologic ECM had used mixtures of known ECM components: purified laminin, collagen, and heparin sulfate proteoglycan [11]. While these components interacted to formed fiber-like precipitates, the precipitates lacked mechanical strength, unlike the more complete ECM from the tumor extracts, which interacted to form gels under physiologic conditions [10]. Subsequent reports from various groups in 1988 described cellular aggregation [12] and gland formation [13] in Matrigel culture. These cellular aggregates exhibited junctional complexes between cells, primarily on outer, basal surfaces, rather than inner, apical surfaces. The basal surfaces also contained more laminin-binding moieties, consistent with the laminin composition of Matrigel. Eventually, the NIH licensed the Matrigel technology for commercial distribution [9].

Lung cells grown in Matrigel conditions were soon observed to form hollow aggregates. In 1987, John Shannon examined the differentiation of type II alveolar epithelial cells (AEC2s) in Sprague-Dawley rats using plastic dishes and Matrigel [14]. Initially cultured in plastic, AEC2s quickly lost features that defined them as AEC2s, namely low DNA synthesis and the presence of intracellular lamellar bodies [15]. However, when seeded on top of gelated Matrigel, AEC2s retained their characteristic features for several days [15]. Rather than forming a flattened monolayer in plastic culture, Matrigel-seeded AEC2s aggregated and retained a low cuboidal morphology similar to their innate morphology in alveoli [14]. Matrigel-seeded AEC2s also continued to express surfactant proteins, although at lower levels than immediately after initial isolation [16]. These organoid aggregates of AEC2s on Matrigel were hollow with multiple lamellar bodies within the lumen [16], resembling surfactant secretion into the lumen of alveoli in vivo. Further comparisons of Matrigel-seeded AEC2s to plastic dish cultures have demonstrated that Matrigel cultured cells had more physiologic cytokeratin specification [17], intracellular adhesion molecule expression [18], and lipid composition [19]. Cytokeratin analysis of fetal rat AEC2s also showed that Matrigel culture aided in their maturation, thus inducing expression of cytokeratin 19, a marker of fully developed AEC2s [17]. In addition to growing organoids, Matrigel has commonly been used for in vitro cancer invasion assays [20, 21] and in co-injection to tumor cell injection in mice [22].

Several groups have recently reported using Matrigel to culture lung organoids from sources such as embryonic stem cells [23], induced pluripotent stem cells (iPSC) [24], immortalized bronchial epithelial cells [25, 26], and various mixtures of primary cells. In one version of this technique, cells are embedded in the Matrigel solution before gelation, whereas the alternative involves growing cells on a gelated layer of Matrigel covered by a layer of dilute Matrigel on top of the cells. Pluripotent lung stem cells are often cultured in these formats and require growth factor addition techniques to differentiate stem cells in Matrigel culture, which have been recently reviewed elsewhere [7]. However, with the ability to generate pluripotent stem cells from somatic cells, creating disease-specific cells that differentiate into disease-relevant cell types does allow for more targeted therapeutic approaches. Pluripotent stem cells in Matrigel have been induced to form the endoderm, one of the three fetal germ layers, which ultimately gives rise to lung and liver during embryogenesis. Dye *et al.* have successfully activated specific developmental pathways to form endoderm and subsequently, lung tissue [24]. Cells were cultured in Matrigel, where the resultant lung organoid consisted of both type I and type II alveolar epithelial cells. These proximal airway-like structures both resembled and expressed cell types found in the human fetal lung and gene expression analysis further confirmed the fetal lung phenotype.

In addition to iPSCs, immortalized human bronchial epithelial cells have also been shown to have stem-like properties in Matrigel. Human bronchial epithelial cells immortalized by expression of cyclin-dependent kinase 4 and human telomerase reverse transcriptase were overlaid onto Matrigel to form tubular organoids and retained p63 expression, a marker of stem/progenitor cells.

A variety of lung tumor models have been explored using Matrigel. In contrast to healthy epithelial cultures that formed acinar structures and contained either hollow lumens [27] or branching structures [28], cancer cells tended to form compact spheroids via the Matrigel overlay technique [29]. Healthy bronchial epithelial cells cultured in Matrigel also demonstrated increased resistance to DNA damage and transformation under gamma radiation, thus making in situ cancer induction difficult [28].

Overall, Matrigel culture offers a complex microenvironment with a plethora of growth factors and extracellular matrix components, making it a valuable and versatile hydrogel growth technique. However, Matrigel suffers disadvantages due to its mouse-derived origin and its undefined nature [30], wherein the inherent composition, such as growth factors, is not currently fully elucidated. Furthermore, it can suffer from minor lot-to-lot variability. This variability and undefined nature can then complicate the interpretation of experimental results. Other disadvantages of Matrigel include the known sequestration of cytokines and other secreted proteins, making assays such as ELISA difficult to interpret [31, 32]. Due to the hydrogel properties of Matrigel, it presents a physical barrier that inhibits the efficiency of standard techniques such as transfection or DNA/RNA extraction, however, recent microfluidic techniques have been applied to form Matrigel microgels, which could address some of the nutrient transport concerns [33].

2.2   Maglev

Recently, magnetic forces have been manipulated to facilitate 3D tissue engineering of keratinocyte epidermal sheets [34]. Originally, this method fed magnetite cationic liposomes to human keratinocytes, which were then seeded into ultralow-attachment plates. A 4000 G magnet was then placed under the culture well to pull the cells downward. Due to the magnetic force applied, keratinocyte epidermal sheets not only formed stratified layers, but also grew detached from the bottom of the plates within the culture medium, making collection relatively easy.

In contrast to the downward force in the keratinocyte study, magnetic levitation (maglev) of cell cultures involves magnetic nanoparticle co-culture to levitate cells to the upper surface of media. Typically, low-magnitude magnetic fields in the range of 30–500 G are used to levitate cells, because stronger fields can influence cell behavior [35, 36]. Once collected at the top surface of the media, the cells can interact to form larger 3D structures. Maglev techniques are now typically performed by introducing a nanoparticle assembly of magnetic iron oxide and gold nanoparticles to render the cells magnetic [37]. Once magnetized, cells can be manipulated by external application of permanent magnets.

Human bronchiole co-cultures of pulmonary endothelial cells, bronchial epithelial cells and pulmonary fibroblasts in a magnetically levitated system were able to produce highly organized ECM, composed primarily of collagen type I similar to the native lung [38]. The maglev system was able to better facilitate ECM production, because collagen type I produced in 2D cultures can only localize around the cell in its structurally restrictive state [38]. Likewise, in white adipose tissue cultures, the autocrine ECM provided the scaffold within which cells adhered to form a 3D structure and negated the need for artificial scaffolds such as Matrigel [39]. Much like other forms of tumor spheroid culture methods, maglev cultures of human adenocarcinoma of alveolar basal epithelial cells and A549 cells not only form spheroids but also maintain epithelial phenotype and function as shown by immunohistochemical staining patterns [40].

Advantages of maglev cultures include ease of use, applicability to a variety of cell types, and low cost. The materials used in this application are nontoxic and do not induce an inflammatory response in cultured cells. They also allow for greater spatial control and the production of physiologic ECM structures. Conversely, iron oxide within the nanoparticle assembly can cause a brown discoloration within the culture, which can interfere with various imaging modalities such as brown IHC colorimetric markers and confocal imaging that requires long light path lengths through the microtissue. Incomplete nanoparticle incubation results in adherence to the plate rather than levitation and can limit the number of useable cells. However; the use of ultra-low attachment (ULA) plates can limit this effect. While maglev culture has high potential, the use of magnetic nanoparticles on cells adds an unknown that could subtly influence cell behavior.

2.3   Rotating Wall Vessel

In an effort to test cellular behavior in microgravity at NASA's Johnson Space Center, Goodwin et al. invented rotating wall vessel culture in 1992 [41]. In the rotating wall vessel format, cells are seeded in a media-filled chamber that rotates on a horizontal axis. The rotation keeps the cells in a state of constant falling, preventing interaction and adherence with the vessel walls. Goodwin and coworkers initially examined human colon adenocarcinoma cell lines, finding that the cells would aggregate and produce spheroids. More recent work using rotating wall vessels seeded cells onto microbeads, which are often functionalized alginate or Cytodex, transparent small diameter spheres. As beads tumble and collide with each other, cells adhere and contract to aggregate the beads together into a large, single organoid, with microbeads occupying the space between cells.

Lung adenocarcinoma A549 organoids, grown by adapting the rotating wall vessel format, exhibited stronger immunostaining of junctional proteins and indicators of polarity than 2D cultures [5]. Interestingly, these lung organoids were also more resistant to *Pseudomonas aeruginosa* invasion than their 2D culture counterparts and secreted more pro- and anti-inflammatory cytokines, which is indicative of the complex negative-feedback seen in vivo. For a more in vivo-like phenotype with transformed cells in a rotating wall vessel culture, Vertrees et al. developed cancer spheroids in rotating wall vessel culture with collagen type I-coated Cytodex beads and BZR-T33 cells (H-*ras* transfected BEAS-2B) [42]. Prior to adding the transformed cells, the vessel was inoculated with human mesenchymal bronchial-tracheal cells (HBTC), which are known to generate invasive tumors in vivo. The HBTC and BZR-T33 co-culture in rotating wall vessel culture formed spheroids that exhibited cell-cell junctions and secreted mucins, similar to the in-vivo phenotype.

In a subsequent study, Wilkinson et al. used functionalized alginate beads and a mixture of stem cells, including human fetal lung cells and iPSCs, to form organoids in rotating wall vessel cultures [43]. This study demonstrated that fibroblasts were critical for connecting the alginate beads. When the organoids were cultured without fibroblasts or with the myosin II heavy chain phosphorylation inhibitor, blebbistatin, the organoids only loosely aggregated and broke apart under continued flow. Immunostaining of the completed organoids were positive for markers of surfactant proteins, endothelial adhesion markers, and fibroblast markers, closely resembling the immunostaining of adult human lungs. In pulmonary fibrosis, a progressive disease leading to stiffening of the lung and respiratory dysfunction [44], fibroblasts differentiate into highly contractile myofibroblasts, inducing elevated expression of α-smooth muscle actin [45, 46]. Wilkinson et al. added a fluorescent reporter of α-smooth muscle actin into fibroblasts to measure contractility by tracking the cross-sectional area of the organoids [43]. The organoids responded as expected to the pro-fibrotic stimulus, TGF-β1, by expressing α-smooth muscle actin and contracting the organoid. Although this model resembles pulmonary fibrosis in many ways, a hypothesized mechanism of pulmonary fibrosis progression involves alveolar collapse, which was artificially prevented by the alginate beads used in the rotating wall vessel culture [46, 47]. Nonetheless, the rotating wall vessel culture provides a useful tool to examine complex in vitro lung tissue. To examine the potential use of these organoids as a drug screening tool, organoids have been formed in a 96-well format by rotating the entire plate. Although organoids formed in each well, variability across the plate in distance from the axis generated differences in centrifugal acceleration of a factor of 9.3, hampering its use in high-throughput studies.

Despite its shortcomings, rotating wall vessel culture presents intriguing possibilities where it can bridge some of the benefits of Matrigel culture and hanging drop culture by using soft microbeads in non-adherent culture. In lung specific tissue cultures, the alginate beads occupy spaces corresponding to respiratory channels such as alveolar or bronchiolar spaces, thus forcing the organoid to approximate native lung structure. Furthermore, flexibility in choice of microbeads and their surface chemistry makes this culture format adaptable to diverse tissue types. Although diffusion of nutrients to the center of these organoids may be slow for large organoids (mm scale) as in Wilkinson et al. [43], the surrounding space consists of media, making cytokine measurements more feasible than gel-embedded cultures. Engineering approaches to scale up the throughput of rotating wall vessel culture will be critical for future large-scale adoption.

2.4 Hanging Drop

The properties of a hanging drop have been used over many decades in cell culture-applications, such as bacterial motility assays originating from the early 1900s, which hold a hanging drop in a concavity on a glass slide [48]. Other applications of the hanging drop include detection of microorganisms [49] and characterization of sickle cell anemia [50]. Hanging drop cultures of mammalian tissues of the 1900s and of current day cell culture are relatively simple and utilize the natural disposition of adherent cells to aggregate. Using various cell types, Kelm et al. first found that consistent and uniform spheroids could be created by dispensing cells and media onto a MicroWell MiniTray (Nunc) and inverting the tray to generate hanging drops, which clung to the top surface by surface tension [51]. The method also requires no specialized equipment and is adaptable to various cells types.

Hanging drop culture facilitates organoid formation in the absence of exogenous cellular attachment surfaces. In this format, single-cell suspensions are pipetted into small ~15–50 μL droplets on the lid of a dish. After inverting the lid, the drops cling to the bottom of the lid by surface tension. Recently, several labs and companies have designed custom microplates with through-holes (InSphero AG and 3D Biomatrix) to facilitate easier plate handling [52, 53]. Using the InSphero system, Amann et al. have co-cultured non-small cell lung cancer cell lines with lung fibroblasts to develop a cancer organoid model [54]. In their model, the co-culture self-assembled into a solid spheroid, with fibroblasts occupying the core and epithelial cells forming the outer layer. The hanging drop format enabled longer-term fibroblast culture without adherence to the dish. A comparison between monoculture and fibroblast co-culture found that the co-culture spheroids developed a more compact morphology and a corresponding decrease in cell viability. The reduction in viability was attributed to a lack of nutrient transportation through the compact spheroid.

In comparison to Matrigel-embedded techniques, hanging drop culture is more appropriate for studies of secretion into the supernatant, and it allows for applications utilizing the air-liquid interface, created by the proximity of organoids to the bottom of the droplet, which has yet to be fully utilized. The commercialization of hanging drop microplates also enables high-throughput organoid culture. However, hanging drop cultures can be delicate and require care to handle as droplets can fall from the well if the plate is bumped or shaken [55]. The location of organoids at the bottom of the droplet facilitates imaging by inverted microscopy. However, due to the high surface area to volume ratio of hanging drops, evaporation can also become problematic, particularly during imaging where light sources and lasers produce heat. Some new products, such as the multiple pore type plate from Elplasia, have recently been developed to address this issue. This microplate forms droplets at 500 μm pores, which are sufficiently small to withstand hydrostatic pressure from moderately large media reservoirs above the pores. The larger volumes can buffer against the harmful effects of evaporation. However, the small pore size may prevent formation of large organoids and these dishes have not yet been used for lung culture.

2.5   Non-adherent Cultures

In non-adherent culture methods, culture plates are often coated with non-adherent materials, such as agarose, to prevent cells from attaching to the dish, enabling the cells to naturally form 3D structures. Agar or agarose-coated plates have been used to induce tumor spheroid formation [56], sometimes with the aid of Matrigel [57]. Other commercially available ultra-low attachment (ULA) plates are coated with hydrophilic, neutrally charged surface moieties that force cells into a suspended state and enable the formation of 3D structures.

A comparison of agar-coated plates and ULA plates in the formation of spheroids using 40 different cell lines, including lung adenocarcinoma (NCl-H23), found that ULA plates were more advantageous for generating robust spheroids [56]. Spheroids grown in ULA systems were larger, showed a more compact structure, and were also more suited for image analysis due to the variability in thickness of agarose-coated plates [56]. Recent studies of novel materials, such as the NanoCulture plates with nanoscale rectangular grid patterns that prevent cell adhesion, found that some cell lines form tight spheroids, while others only loosely aggregate [58]. Thus, choice of cell line can also contribute to spheroid-forming ability, as is the case with many culture methods.

In another examination of multidrug treatments, two human non-small cell lung cancer cell lines (INER-37 & INER-51) were seeded onto agarose-coated wells [59]. These cells formed compact spheroids. INER-37 spheroids were small and tightly packed, while INER-51 spheroids had a tightly packed outer ring of cells and loose cells on the inside. However, both cell lines displayed strong resistance to multiple chemotherapeutics in 3D culture. Overall, non-adherent materials have thus far proven useful in the application of 3-D tumor spheroid models resembling in vivo tumors.

3 Discussion

Lung organoid cultures are promising techniques that may make in vitro testing more predictive of in vivo behavior. In contrast to in vivo models, they also allow for the use of human tissues, rather than only animal tissues. In these 3D environments, lung cells have been shown to exhibit aspects of physiologic behavior, such as organogenesis, inflammatory response, and fibrosis (Table 1). The various techniques presented in this chapter each provide specific advantages and limitations. Lung organoids have been formed in hydrogels and in suspension culture formats, with reports from both techniques showing hollow acinar morphology and lung-relevant protein expression. Hydrogel culture, such as Matrigel, provides extracellular matrix and tunable mechanical stiffness, but suffers from low diffusivity and a lack of air-liquid interface. In contrast, suspension cultures, such as hanging drop, magnetic levitation, and rotating wall vessel, trade mechanical control for modularity and improved nutrient transport. Likewise, microbead cultures provide intermediates. Many of these techniques are readily replicated without specialized equipment and can be modified to utilize various tumorigenic cell lines, including those found in the respiratory tract.

Tumor organoids have been touted as having applications both in preclinical drug discovery as well as having potential to have applications in point-of-care testing. Recently, Henry et al. [61] generated lung spheroids from healthy human donors in ULA culture plates. Pulmonary fibrosis was induced with bleomycin in severe combined immunodeficient (SCID) mice, which were then intravenously injected with the previously generated human lung spheroids as therapeutic lung progenitor cells. Spheroid treated mice showed an inhibition of fibrosis, tissue infiltration, and cell apoptosis, but promoted angiogenesis compared to controls. Both grossly and histologically, spheroid treated mouse lungs indicated an amelioration of the fibrotic effects of bleomycin [61]. Applications in cancer research are vast and such studies can build on the concepts of Henry et al. to lead to the development of personalized therapeutic treatments.

To date, lung organoid culture has produced insights into developmental biology [6, 7], but many fields could benefit from further investigation with lung organoids. Following reports of physiologic behavior, lung organoids have been developed

Table 1 Techniques for lung tumor organoid culture

Method	Cell type	Structure	References
Matrigel	Multiple – Differentiated from pluripotent stem cells & fetal human lung fibroblasts	Cyst-like spheroids	[23]
	Human bronchiole epithelial cells (HBEC3)	Branching with overlay; hollow lumen with embedded	[25]
	Human bronchial epithelial cell line; human lung epithelial adenocarcinoma (A549); human umbilical vein endothelial cells (HUVEC)	Spheroids with vasculogenesis branching	[26]
	Human embryonic; induced pluripotent stem cells (iPSC)	Immature alveolar airway like structures	[24]
Maglev	Human pulmonary microvascular endothelial cells; human bronchial epithelial cells; human pulmonary fibroblasts; human tracheal smooth muscle cells	Layered spheroid	[38]
	A549	Layered spheroid	[40]
	Human prostate cancer epithelial; human lung fibroblast (HLF-1)	Spheroid	[37]
Hanging drop	A549	Spheroids	[60]
	A549, human lymph node (Colo699); human lung fibroblast (SV-80)	Layered spheroids	[54]
Rotating wall vessel	A549	Multi-luminal aggregate	[5]
	Bronchiole epithelial, transformed (BZR-T33)	Spheroid	[42]
	Human fetal lung 18- to 20-week old; adult lung-derived iPSC	Multi-luminal aggregate	[43]
Non-adherent	Human non-small cell lung cancer (INER-37 & INER -51)	Spheroid	[59]
	Lung adenocarcinoma (NCI-H23) 40 various tumor cells lines	Spheroid	[56]

with specific built-in assays, such as the fibrosis model with contraction and gene transcription reporting [43]. Moreover, typical assayable endpoints for lung organoid culture include sublethal endpoints, including DNA damage and cytokine secretion [60]. Other measurable outputs which have been used in microfluidic or organoid cultures and applied to organoid cultures include barrier integrity characterization, such as immunostaining of tight-junction proteins occludin, ZO-1 and ZO-2 [62]; cell markers MUC5AC, E-cadherin and cytokeratin [24]; or various imaging modalities. Presently, confocal laser microscopy, multi-photon microscopy, transmission electron microscopy and scanning election microscopy have been applied to organoid imaging with varying techniques for resolving the architecture of 3D constructs [8]. Further work is needed to expand this repertoire of measurements, address current limitations of each technique, increase throughput and reproducibility, and finally to implement lung organoid culture for biological and pharmaceutical investigation.

References

1. Harrison RG, Greenman MJ, Mall FP, Jackson CM (1907) Observations of the living developing nerve fiber. Anat Rec 1(5):116–128
2. Cukierman E, Pankov R, Stevens DR, Yamada KM (2001) Taking cell-matrix adhesions to the third dimension. Science 294(5547):1708–1712. doi:10.1126/science.1064829
3. Shibue T, Weinberg RA (2009) Integrin beta1-focal adhesion kinase signaling directs the proliferation of metastatic cancer cells disseminated in the lungs. Proc Natl Acad Sci U S A 106(25):10290–10295. doi:10.1073/pnas.0904227106
4. Eke I, Cordes N (2011) Radiobiology goes 3D: how ECM and cell morphology impact on cell survival after irradiation. Radiother Oncol 99(3):271–278. doi:10.1016/j.radonc.2011.06.007
5. Carterson AJ, Honer zu Bentrup K, Ott CM, Clarke MS, Pierson DL, Vanderburg CR, Buchanan KL, Nickerson CA, Schurr MJ (2005) A549 lung epithelial cells grown as three-dimensional aggregates: alternative tissue culture model for Pseudomonas Aeruginosa pathogenesis. Infect Immun 73(2):1129–1140. doi:10.1128/IAI.73.2.1129-1140.2005
6. Shamir ER, Ewald AJ (2014) Three-dimensional organotypic culture: experimental models of mammalian biology and disease. Nat Rev Mol Cell Biol 15(10):647–664. doi:10.1038/nrm3873
7. Nadkarni RR, Abed S, Draper JS (2016) Organoids as a model system for studying human lung development and disease. Biochem Biophys Res Commun 473(3):675–682. doi:10.1016/j.bbrc.2015.12.091
8. Konar D, Devarasetty M, Yildiz DV, Atala A, Murphy SV (2016) Lung-on-a-chip technologies for disease modeling and drug development. Biomed Eng Comput Biol 7(Suppl 1):17–27. doi:10.4137/BECB.S34252
9. Kleinman HK, Martin GR (2005) Matrigel: basement membrane matrix with biological activity. Semin Cancer Biol 15(5):378–386. doi:10.1016/j.semcancer.2005.05.004
10. Kleinman HK, McGarvey ML, Hassell JR, Star VL, Cannon FB, Laurie GW, Martin GR (1986) Basement membrane complexes with biological activity. Biochemistry 25(2):312–318
11. Kleinman HK, McGarvey ML, Hassell JR, Martin GR (1983) Formation of a supramolecular complex is involved in the reconstitution of basement membrane components. Biochemistry 22(21):4969–4974
12. Tung PS, Choi AH, Fritz IB (1988) Topography and behavior of Sertoli cells in sparse culture during the transitional remodeling phase. Anat Rec 220(1):11–21. doi:10.1002/ar.1092200103
13. Rinehart CA Jr, Lyn-Cook BD, Kaufman DG (1988) Gland formation from human endometrial epithelial cells in vitro. In Vitro Cell Dev Biol 24(10):1037–1041
14. Shannon JM, Mason RJ, Jennings SD (1987) Functional differentiation of alveolar type II epithelial cells in vitro: effects of cell shape, cell-matrix interactions and cell-cell interactions. Biochim Biophys Acta 931(2):143–156
15. Rannels SR, Rannels DE (1989) The type II pneumocyte as a model of lung cell interaction with the extracellular matrix. J Mol Cell Cardiol 21(Suppl 1):151–159
16. Shannon JM, Emrie PA, Fisher JH, Kuroki Y, Jennings SD, Mason RJ (1990) Effect of a reconstituted basement membrane on expression of surfactant apoproteins in cultured adult rat alveolar type II cells. Am J Respir Cell Mol Biol 2(2):183–192

17. Paine R, Ben-Ze'ev A, Farmer SR, Brody JS (1988) The pattern of cytokeratin synthesis is a marker of type 2 cell differentiation in adult and maturing fetal lung alveolar cells. Dev Biol 129(2):505–515

18. Paine R 3rd, Christensen P, Toews GB, Simon RH (1994) Regulation of alveolar epithelial cell ICAM-1 expression by cell shape and cell-cell interactions. Am J Phys 266(4 Pt 1):L476–L484

19. Kawada H, Shannon JM, Mason RJ (1990) Improved maintenance of adult rat alveolar type II cell differentiation in vitro: effect of serum-free, hormonally defined medium and a reconstituted basement membrane. Am J Respir Cell Mol Biol 3(1):33–43. doi:10.1165/ajrcmb/3.1.33

20. Saiki I, Murata J, Makabe T, Matsumoto Y, Ohdate Y, Kawase Y, Taguchi Y, Shimojo T, Kimizuka F, Kato I et al (1990) Inhibition of lung metastasis by synthetic and recombinant fragments of human fibronectin with functional domains. Jpn J Cancer Res 81(10):1003–1011

21. Thompson EW, Paik S, Brunner N, Sommers CL, Zugmaier G, Clarke R, Shima TB, Torri J, Donahue S, Lippman ME et al (1992) Association of increased basement membrane invasiveness with absence of estrogen receptor and expression of vimentin in human breast cancer cell lines. J Cell Physiol 150(3):534–544. doi:10.1002/jcp.1041500314

22. Fridman R, Benton G, Aranoutova I, Kleinman HK, Bonfil RD (2012) Increased initiation and growth of tumor cell lines, cancer stem cells and biopsy material in mice using basement membrane matrix protein (Cultrex or Matrigel) co-injection. Nat Protoc 7(6):1138–1144. doi:10.1038/nprot.2012.053

23. Gotoh S, Ito I, Nagasaki T, Yamamoto Y, Konishi S, Korogi Y, Matsumoto H, Muro S, Hirai T, Funato M, Mae S, Toyoda T, Sato-Otsubo A, Ogawa S, Osafune K, Mishima M (2014) Generation of alveolar epithelial spheroids via isolated progenitor cells from human pluripotent stem cells. Stem Cell Rep 3(3):394–403. doi:10.1016/j.stemcr.2014.07.005

24. Dye BR, Hill DR, Ferguson MA, Tsai YH, Nagy MS, Dyal R, Wells JM, Mayhew CN, Nattiv R, Klein OD, White ES, Deutsch GH, Spence JR (2015) In vitro generation of human pluripotent stem cell derived lung organoids. Elife 4. doi:10.7554/eLife.05098

25. Delgado O, Kaisani AA, Spinola M, Xie XJ, Batten KG, Minna JD, Wright WE, Shay JW (2011) Multipotent capacity of immortalized human bronchial epithelial cells. Plos One 6 (7). doi:ARTN e22023 10.1371/journal.pone.0022023

26. Franzdottir SR, Axelsson IT, Arason AJ, Baldursson O, Gudjonsson T, Magnusson MK (2010) Airway branching morphogenesis in three dimensional culture. Respir Res 11:162. doi:10.1186/1465-9921-11-162

27. Wu X, Peters-Hall JR, Bose S, Pena MT, Rose MC (2011) Human bronchial epithelial cells differentiate to 3D glandular acini on basement membrane matrix. Am J Respir Cell Mol Biol 44(6):914–921. doi:10.1165/rcmb.2009-0329OC

28. El-Ashmawy M, Coquelin M, Luitel K, Batten K, Shay JW (2016) Organotypic culture in three dimensions prevents radiation-induced transformation in human lung epithelial cells. Sci Rep 6:31669. doi:10.1038/srep31669

29. Fessart D, Begueret H, Delom F (2013) Three-dimensional culture model to distinguish normal from malignant human bronchial epithelial cells. Eur Respir J 42(5):1345–1356. doi:10.1183/09031936.00118812

30. Hughes CS, Postovit LM, Lajoie GA (2010) Matrigel: a complex protein mixture required for optimal growth of cell culture. Proteomics 10(9):1886–1890. doi:10.1002/pmic.200900758

31. Lortat-Jacob H, Kleinman HK, Grimaud JA (1991) High-affinity binding of interferon-gamma to a basement membrane complex (matrigel). J Clin Invest 87(3):878–883. doi:10.1172/JCI115093

32. Akashi T, Minami J, Ishige Y, Eishi Y, Takizawa T, Koike M, Yanagishita M (2005) Basement membrane matrix modifies cytokine interactions between lung cancer cells and fibroblasts. Pathobiology 72(5):250–259. doi:10.1159/000089419

33. Dolega ME, Abeille F, Picollet-D'hahan N, Gidrol X (2015) Controlled 3D culture in Matrigel microbeads to analyze clonal acinar development. Biomaterials 52:347–357. doi:10.1016/j.biomaterials.2015.02.042

34. Ito A, Hayashida M, Honda H, Hata K, Kagami H, Ueda M, Kobayashi T (2004) Construction and harvest of multilayered keratinocyte sheets using magnetite nanoparticles and magnetic force. Tissue Eng 10(5–6):873–880. doi:10.1089/1076327041348446

35. Wang Z, Yang P, Xu H, Qian A, Hu L, Shang P (2009) Inhibitory effects of a gradient static magnetic field on normal angiogenesis. Bioelectromagnetics 30(6):446–453. doi:10.1002/bem.20501

36. Koves TR, Li P, An J, Akimoto T, Slentz D, Ilkayeva O, Dohm GL, Yan Z, Newgard CB, Muoio DM (2005) Peroxisome proliferator-activated receptor-gamma co-activator 1alpha-mediated metabolic remodeling of skeletal myocytes mimics exercise training and reverses lipid-induced mitochondrial inefficiency. J Biol Chem 280(39):33588–33598. doi:10.1074/jbc.M507621200

37. Ghosh S, Kumar SR, Puri IK, Elankumaran S (2016) Magnetic assembly of 3D cell clusters: visualizing the formation of an engineered tissue. Cell Prolif 49(1):134–144. doi:10.1111/cpr.12234

38. Tseng H, Gage JA, Raphael RM, Moore RH, Killian TC, Grande-Allen KJ, Souza GR (2013) Assembly of a three-dimensional multitype bronchiole coculture model using magnetic levitation. Tissue Eng Part C Methods 19(9):665–675. doi:10.1089/ten.TEC.2012.0157

39. Daquinag AC, Souza GR, Kolonin MG (2013) Adipose tissue engineering in three-dimensional levitation tissue culture system based on magnetic nanoparticles. Tissue Eng Part C Methods 19(5):336–344. doi:10.1089/ten.TEC.2012.0198

40. Haisler WL, Timm DM, Gage JA, Tseng H, Killian TC, Souza GR (2013) Three-dimensional cell culturing by magnetic levitation. Nat Protoc 8(10):1940–1949. doi:10.1038/nprot.2013.125

41. Goodwin TJ, Jessup JM, Wolf DA (1992) Morphologic differentiation of colon carcinoma cell lines HT-29 and HT-29KM in rotating-wall vessels. In Vitro Cell Dev Biol 28A(1):47–60

42. Vertrees RA, McCarthy M, Solley T, Popov VL, Roaten J, Pauley M, Wen XD, Goodwin TJ (2009) Development of a three-dimensional model of lung cancer using cultured transformed lung cells. Cancer Biol Ther 8(4):356–365. doi:10.4161/cbt.8.4.7432

43. Wilkinson DC, Alva-Ornelas JA, Sucre JM, Vijayaraj P, Durra A, Richardson W, Jonas SJ, Paul MK, Karumbayaram S, Dunn B, Gomperts BN (2016) Development of a three-dimensional bioengineering technology to generate lung tissue for personalized disease modeling. Stem Cells Transl Med. doi:10.5966/sctm.2016-0192

44. Raghu G, Weycker D, Edelsberg J, Bradford WZ, Oster G (2006) Incidence and prevalence of idiopathic pulmonary fibrosis. Am J Respir Crit Care Med 174(7):810–816. doi:10.1164/rccm.200602-163OC

45. Selman M, King TE, Pardo A, American Thoracic Society, European Respiratory Society, American College of Chest Physicians (2001) Idiopathic pulmonary fibrosis: prevailing and evolving hypotheses about its pathogenesis and implications for therapy. Ann Intern Med 134(2):136–151

46. Todd NW, Atamas SP, Luzina IG, Galvin JR (2015) Permanent alveolar collapse is the predominant mechanism in idiopathic pulmonary fibrosis. Expert Rev Respir Med 9(4):411–418. doi:10.1586/17476348.2015.1067609

47. Katzenstein AL (1985) Pathogenesis of "fibrosis" in interstitial pneumonia: an electron microscopic study. Hum Pathol 16(10):1015–1024

48. Tittsler RP, Sandholzer LA (1936) The use of semi-solid agar for the detection of bacterial motility. J Bacteriol 31(6):575

49. Spring D (1931) Morphologic variation within the same species of dermatophyte as observed in hanging-drop cultures. Arch Dermatol Syphilol 23(6):1076–1086

50. Archibald RG (1926) A case of sickle cell anaemia in the Sudan. Trans R Soc Trop Med Hyg 19(7):389–393

51. Kelm JM, Timmins NE, Brown CJ, Fussenegger M, Nielsen LK (2003) Method for generation of homogeneous multicellular tumor spheroids applicable to a wide variety of cell types. Biotechnol Bioeng 83(2):173–180. doi:10.1002/bit.10655

52. Tung YC, Hsiao AY, Allen SG, Torisawa YS, Ho M, Takayama S (2011) High-throughput 3D spheroid culture and drug testing using a 384 hanging drop array. Analyst 136(3):473–478. doi:10.1039/c0an00609b
53. Drewitz M, Caminada D, Moritz W, Lichtenberg J, Kasper C, Kelm JM (2011) Verfahren zur automatisierten Tropfenbildung für die Massenproduktion von organotypischen Mikrogeweben novel production technology to automate the generation of hanging drops for mass production of organotypic microtissues. Chemie Ingenieur Technik 83(12):2170–2176. doi:10.1002/cite.201100063
54. Amann A, Zwierzina M, Gamerith G, Bitsche M, Huber JM, Vogel GF, Blumer M, Koeck S, Pechriggl EJ, Kelm JM, Hilbe W, Zwierzina H (2014) Development of an innovative 3D cell culture system to study tumour–stroma interactions in non-small cell lung cancer cells. PLoS One 9(3):e92511. doi:10.1371/journal.pone.0092511
55. Hsiao AY, Tung YC, Kuo CH, Mosadegh B, Bedenis R, Pienta KJ, Takayama S (2012) Micro-ring structures stabilize microdroplets to enable long term spheroid culture in 384 hanging drop array plates. Biomed Microdevices 14(2):313–323. doi:10.1007/s10544-011-9608-5
56. Vinci M, Gowan S, Boxall F, Patterson L, Zimmermann M, Court W, Lomas C, Mendiola M, Hardisson D, Eccles SA (2012) Advances in establishment and analysis of three-dimensional tumor spheroid-based functional assays for target validation and drug evaluation. BMC Biol 10. doi:Artn 29 10.1186/1741-7007-10-29
57. Li Q, Chen CY, Kapadia A, Zhou QO, Harper MK, Schaack J, Labarbera DV (2011) 3D models of epithelial-Mesenchymal transition in breast cancer metastasis: high-throughput screening assay development, validation, and pilot screen. J Biomol Screen 16(2):141–154. doi:10.1177/1087057110392995
58. Yoshii Y, Waki A, Yoshida K, Kakezuka A, Kobayashi M, Namiki H, Kuroda Y, Kiyono Y, Yoshii H, Furukawa T, Asai T, Okazawa H, Gelovani JG, Fujibayashi Y (2011) The use of nanoimprinted scaffolds as 3D culture models to facilitate spontaneous tumor cell migration and well-regulated spheroid formation. Biomaterials 32(26):6052–6058. doi:10.1016/j.biomaterials.2011.04.076
59. Barrera-Rodriguez R, Fuentes JM (2015) Multidrug resistance characterization in multicellular tumour spheroids from two human lung cancer cell lines. Cancer Cell Int 15. doi:ARTN 47 10.1186/s12935-015-0200-6
60. Liu FF, Peng C, Escher BI, Fantino E, Giles C, Were S, Duffy L, Ng JC (2013) Hanging drop: an in vitro air toxic exposure model using human lung cells in 2D and 3D structures. J Hazard Mater 261:701–710. doi:10.1016/j.jhazmat.2013.01.027
61. Henry E, Cores J, Hensley MT, Anthony S, Vandergriff A, de Andrade JB, Allen T, Caranasos TG, Lobo LJ, Cheng K (2015) Adult lung spheroid cells contain progenitor cells and mediate regeneration in rodents with Bleomycin-induced pulmonary fibrosis. Stem Cells Transl Med 4(11):1265–1274. doi:10.5966/sctm.2015-0062
62. Firth AL, Dargitz CT, Qualls SJ, Menon T, Wright R, Singer O, Gage FH, Khanna A, Verma IM (2014) Generation of multiciliated cells in functional airway epithelia from human induced pluripotent stem cells. Proc Natl Acad Sci U S A 111(17):E1723–E1730. doi:10.1073/pnas.1403470111

Tissue Organoids: Liver

Estela Solanas, Iris Pla-Palacín, Pilar Sainz-Arnal, Manuel Almeida, Alberto Lue, Trinidad Serrano, and Pedro M. Baptista

Abstract The development of novel and consistent biologic surrogates for drug discovery, toxicology, and cancer research is presently intense and involves a growing number of research groups and institutions around the world. The Twilight of the days of immortalized cell lines as the workhorse of most of our drug development and cancer research efforts seem now to be heading to their end with the introduction of body-on-a-chip platforms, bioengineered tissues and stem cell organoids. In this chapter, we describe the fundamental work and the different

E. Solanas • I. Pla-Palacín • M. Almeida
Digestive Pathology Research Group, Instituto de Investigación Sanitaria de Aragón (IIS Aragón), Zaragoza, Spain

P. Sainz-Arnal
Digestive Pathology Research Group, Instituto de Investigación Sanitaria de Aragón (IIS Aragón), Zaragoza, Spain

Instituto Aragonés de Ciencias de la Salud (IACS), Zaragoza, Spain

A. Lue
Digestive Pathology Research Group, Instituto de Investigación Sanitaria de Aragón (IIS Aragón), Zaragoza, Spain

Gastroenterology Department, University Hospital Lozano Blesa, Zaragoza, Spain

T. Serrano
Digestive Pathology Research Group, Instituto de Investigación Sanitaria de Aragón (IIS Aragón), Zaragoza, Spain

Gastroenterology Department, University Hospital Lozano Blesa, Zaragoza, Spain

Instituto de Investigación Sanitaria de la Fundación Jiménez Díaz, Madrid, Spain

CIBERehd, Madrid, Spain

P.M. Baptista (✉)
Digestive Pathology Research Group, Instituto de Investigación Sanitaria de Aragón (IIS Aragón), Zaragoza, Spain

Instituto de Investigación Sanitaria de la Fundación Jiménez Díaz, Madrid, Spain

Departamento de Bioingeniería, Universidad Carlos III de Madrid, Madrid, Spain

CIBERehd, Madrid, Spain
e-mail: pbaptista.iacs@aragon.es

© Springer International Publishing AG 2018
S. Soker, A. Skardal (eds.), *Tumor Organoids*, Cancer Drug Discovery and Development, DOI 10.1007/978-3-319-60511-1_2

strategies that lead to some of the breakthroughs in the generation of hepatic tissue ex vivo. Lastly, we define its increasing use and applications by pharmaceutical industry and research laboratories.

Keywords Liver tissue engineering • Drug discovery • Toxicology • Cancer • 3D cultures

1   Introduction

The necessity of reliable biologic surrogates for drug discovery, toxicology, including more basic biology disciplines – like cell biology, biochemistry, cancer, etc. – has been a constant source of research and concern [1]. From the early days of the first immortalized cell culture lines (including the world famous HeLa cells [2]) to body-on-a-chip platforms there are roughly 60 years of intense research and development (R&D) work.

In the particular case of the liver, it is one of the most important organs in metabolism and homeostasis, since it plays a critical role in these physiologic functions. It is responsible for the production of many proteins, vitamins, lipids, carbohydrates, carries on the detoxification of several metabolites and synthesizes substances necessary for homeostasis and digestion. Hence, since early on, the culture of primary hepatocytes became a priority, to capture liver's vital role in xenobiotic metabolism and human physiology in a petri dish. In this line of work, hepatocyte isolation started in the mid-1960s, when Howard *et al.* isolated rat hepatocytes developing a combined mechanical/enzymatic digestion technique, later improved by Berry and Friend [3, 4]. This method was additionally enhanced by Seglen to become the two-step collagenase perfusion technique, still widely used in today's laboratories [5].

Despite these advances in isolation and cell culture, culturing primary hepatocytes was never a trivial and easy task. In 2D cultures, they showed a natural propensity to suffer de-differentiation into fibroblastic-like cells and lose their liver-specific functions, since these types of cultures did not reproduce their physiologic niche.

It was not until 1989, that Dunn JC et al. finally published a reliable and secure method to extend their in vitro viability and function by culturing them in a collagen I gel sandwich, becoming the gold standard culture method still in use today [6]. Although, even by extending their viability in vitro, function decays rapidly with time, limiting their use in drug metabolism and toxicology to the initial days of the culture. These prompted researchers in the field to look into other culture configurations that could maintain function and viability at higher levels for a longer time.

2   Strategies for the Generation of Hepatic Tissue

2.1   *Hepatocyte Aggregates and Spheroids*

Spheroids are spontaneous non-adherent aggregations of cells that form a 3D tissue construct. Primary hepatocytes are capable of creating these structures called hepatospheres, where the majority of attachments among cells and extracellular matrix are preserved, being this essential to maintain both hepatic differentiation and functionality [1]. Studies in primary rat hepatocyte spheroids have demonstrated that they can recreate the liver's microanatomy [7].

However, size is an important aspect in the formation of spheroids that needs to be always kept in mind size [8]. Glickis et al. found that cell viability decline with increasing spheroid size. They created a mathematical model based on his group's observations that hepatocyte spheroids larger than 100 μm might block the diffusion of oxygen causing necrotic areas in their core [9].

In a first step, the spheroids originate small cell aggregates stimulated by integrin-ECM binding. These multiple multicellular aggregates give rise to a spheroid via cadherin-cadherin interactions. Hence, spheroid assembly represents the most energy efficient structure by minimizing their surface.

In 1961, Moscona et al. described how from individual embryonic cells it is possible to generate in vitro tissue-like constructions under standard controlled conditions [10]. The term *aggregation pattern* began being used to describe the capacity of different cell types in certain conditions to give rise to aggregates within 24 h. However, it was not until the 1980s when Landry et al. started to use the word spheroids to describe 3D cellular aggregates [11]. In this work, isolated rat liver cells re-aggregate and form structures very similar to those that we can find in vivo when prevented from attaching to a solid surface. This way, the cells produced their own ECM and hepatocytes can preserve their metabolic functions [11].

The key in the spheroids formation is to discover a reproducible protocol capable of rebuilding, in the case of the liver, the hepatic tissue. Presently, there are several techniques to achieve this, such as (1) non-adherent dishes under static conditions, (2) agitation cultures or (3) hanging drops.

The simplest way is to seed the hepatocytes in a low adherent well. After an initial attachment to the surface, the hepatocytes give rise to a monolayer that little by little separates from the dish forming spheroids. Also, different conditions like uncoated plates with a positive surface charge, coated dishes with albumin, or the single elimination of serum factors have been demonstrated to be useful in spheroid formation [12]. By contrast, coatings with collagens, fibronectin or laminin inhibit spheroid formation since they support hepatocyte adhesion.

Besides static conditions, agitation cultures such as rocked and rotary cultures in Petri dishes or bioreactors have been developed to improve spheroid formation. One example of this was the development of an innovative bioreactor in 2005 that rapidly gives rise to spheroids when loaded with porcine hepatocytes [12]. Compared with monolayer cultures, hepatocyte spheroids from this bioreactor showed less cell death and increased metabolic functions [12].

Though, recently it has been demonstrated that rocked cultures increase the spheroids formation due to an increment of the number of times hepatocytes clash compared with rotary cultures [13].

However, all techniques described above have several drawbacks, among them, we can distinguish the necessity of manually achieving a homogeneous population of aggregates since irregular geometry is typical. Kelm et al. described a universal method to form hanging drops applicable to a lot of cell lines [14]. This culture method consists of a few cells in suspension seeded upside down in the lid of a culture dish. The hepatospheres formed have high size reproducibility with less than 10% of variations.

A big challenge in tissue engineering is vascularization; therefore it is critical to constructing a functional vascular network. For this reason, the introduction of endothelial cells in the hepatocyte spheroids production has emerged as a possible solution [15]. Not only due to the intended need of angiogenesis but also to increase cell functionality by adding a non-parenchymal cell population.

Stellate cells also have an important role in revascularization after liver injury as they secrete laminin between hepatocytes, which will lay down a pathway that will give rise to the hepatic sinusoids. Hence, spheroids formed by hepatocytes and stellate cells are also an attractive in vitro system that has today great potential in drug discovery and many other applications [16]. The search for more biologically relevant systems is making scientists more aware of the importance of the hepatic non-parenchymal cell populations when assembling these cellular structures.

2.2 Liver Tissue Engineering

Up to date, only liver transplantation provides treatment for a huge variety of end-stage liver diseases. Due to the shortage of liver donors, hepatic tissue engineering has become a promising strategy for the treatment of different liver diseases. In this quest, a large effort has been dedicated to the development of suitable supporting biomaterials that mimic the liver extracellular matrix (ECM) and that allow steady cell growth, the maintenance of their differentiation and metabolic functions, and hepatic tissue organization with the mechanical and biological properties observed in vivo. As mentioned above, it is also fundamental to identify the most appropriate cells, to recapitulate in vitro the natural liver microarchitecture, comprised of multiple cell types. Under specific stimuli, these cells should interact with neighboring cells and the ECM and form liver parenchymal tissue, which could then be transplanted into patients to repair damaged tissue and increase liver function. From this point of view, this tissue engineered liver constructs are also excellent biological surrogates for the most multiple biomedical and pharmaceutical applications. Hence, we will provide a short review of some of the efforts in this area.

Briefly, different types of biomaterials have been used to date, and alginate scaffolds constitute one of the most widely used in tissue engineering due to its hydrophilic properties, porosity, weak adhesive properties and excellent tissue compatibility. Some studies suggest that alginate scaffolds loaded with hepatocytes or mesenchymal stem cells (MSC) increase the survival of animal models with 70–80% partial hepatectomy [17, 18]. Alginate scaffolds can also be used not for direct implantation, but for encapsulation of hepatocytes differentiated from bone marrow–derived MSC (BM-MSCs) [19]. This represents a new source of hepatic cells required for liver tissue engineering, as well as human embryonic (hES) or induced pluripotent stem cells (hiPS). These scaffolds are also used to induce hepatocyte differentiation in vitro [20]. Chitosan is another biomaterial used as a scaffold. It consists of linear amino heteropolysaccharide derived from chitin with unusual characteristics like low cytotoxicity, high biocompatibility, and high biodegradability. Its structure is very similar to the glycosaminoglycans (GAGs) present in the liver ECM. In this study [21], Shang et al. built a hybrid sponge made of galactosylated chitosan and hyaluronic acid to mimic the liver microenvironment and seeded hepatocytes and endothelial cells.

As mentioned above, type I collagen has also been used extensively for hepatocyte in vitro models. Because these cells lose their differentiated functions in 2D cultures, collagen sandwich consists of a matrix for cell attachment, allowing hepatic polarity and maintenance of their differentiated functions [22]. This is due to the capacity of sandwiches to mimic liver microenvironment, promoting cell-cell and cell-ECM interactions [23]. In other studies [24], like Melgar-Lesmes et al., people have used collagen constructs to seed endothelial cells. These matrices were then transplanted into living animals, showing liver damage reparation, suggesting that endothelial cells play a critical role in hepatic repair. Ranucci et al. bet on the utilization of void size collagen foams to induce rat hepatocyte differentiation, suggesting that pore sizes of the substrate (collagen I in this case) are quite relevant for particular cell morphogenesis [25]. Hyaluronic acid is another example. It consists of one of the main components of the ECM and plays a significant role in cell proliferation and migration. It is also commonly used for liver tissue engineering as a scaffold for cell growth [26, 27].

Not only naturally-derived materials have been used in liver tissue engineering efforts. Due to historical reasons, polyglycolic acid (PGA) scaffolds have been extensively used at the beginning of this field of science to generate hepatic tissue when seeded with primary hepatocytes, showing some albumin and urea secretion capability [28, 29].

More complex composite biomaterials have also been designed. The use of some of the compounds described above (chitosan, gelatin, type I collagen and hyaluronic acid) plus a conducting polymer: 3,4-ethylenedioxythiophene (PEDOT) [30]. The reason for the use of this polymer is to conduct charges to make local electrical fields inside of the scaffold, which would improve cell attachment, proliferation and protein expression of the seeded cells.

Recently, another innovative technique is to use acellular matrix derived from cells in culture. Kanninen et al. [31] demonstrated that after seeding hiPS in a

HepaRG-derived acellular matrix, this matrix induced hepatic commitment of the hiPS, suggesting the importance of HepaRG acellular matrix in hepatic differentiation and maturation. Tiwari et at. also used these type of acellular scaffold, in this case, to seed hematopoietic stem/progenitor cells for its expansion [32].

Hence, despite the different strategies chosen by the multiple authors described above, most of the generated hepatic tissues reported have shown some degree of functionality, either in transplantation or in vitro assays. However, the end goal of producing *bona fide* hepatic tissue in vitro with the complexity observed in vivo is still distant in most of the presented cases.

2.3 Liver Bioengineering and Liver Organoids

In the past years, organ bioengineering has flourished, and several techniques have proved to be suitable candidates for the job at hand. Most strategies have relied on scaffolds with increasing complexity to replicate the liver microarchitecture and niche better, but there is also some work done in scaffold-free organogenesis focused approaches.

Recently, there has been an alternative to the approaches mentioned above, in which instead of trying to produce liver tissue or hepatic niche cell cultures and co-cultures, researchers have been thinking of the more sophisticated alternative of whole bioengineering liver or physiologically relevant liver structures like liver lobes, liver buds, liver vasculature and ducts.

So far, the most widely described technique for liver bioengineering is the use of decellularized liver scaffolds for liver regeneration. In this technique, the rationale is that if the ECM remains in good condition after decellularization, then the different components of the ECM will serve as a guide for the cells and will aid not only in the attachment but also in the formation of the various structures that characterize hepatic tissue. This kind of approach is based on a two-step process, the decellularization step and the recellularization step.

For decellularization, since the objective is to remove all cells and cellular material, protocols are based on the combination of various cell-damaging factors such as freezing/thawing cycles, hypotonic stress, enzymes, shear stress and lipid surfactant action. The chemical action of detergent solutions is the most widely described method for dense non-hollow organs such as the liver. These solutions are perfused throughout the vasculature to detach the cellular material from the ECM so that only the structured ECM remains. As far as these solutions go, there is a tendency for the use of detergents such as Triton X-100 and SDS [33–37], but there have also been various other papers using solutions ranging from enzymes such as trypsin to chelating agents such as EDTA or EGTA [38, 39]. Additionally, there have been successful attempts while using as an inlet the vena cava, the portal vein, and the hepatic artery, as well as using fixed flow [35], fixed pressure [36] or even oscillating conditions [37].

After this step, again through perfusion, hepatocytes, stellate cells, endothelial cells and various other cell types can be used to repopulate the obtained scaffold. Some examples include the repopulation with mesenchymal and endothelial cell lines for vascular regeneration [40] or the repopulation with hepatic cell lines for metabolic, viability or functional assessments [34, 41].

A very similar approach to the one mentioned before relies on the substitution of the decellularized liver scaffold with an artificial biomimetic scaffold. By using an artificial scaffold, some issues pertaining the utilization of an animal-derived scaffold would be eliminated such as the possibility of transmission of zoonotic diseases and the vast ethical constraints associated with products of animal origin. As the objective is to create a structured microenvironment that resembles the natural liver ECM in which the cells can generate functional, structured and vascularized liver tissue, the artificial scaffold has to provide both support and a plethora of different cues to direct the cells towards the desired goal, liver organogenesis. So, to do just that, a biomimicry approach reliant on biofabrication techniques such as 3D printing, can be used. Either to generate an artificial scaffold, which can then be seeded with the desired cell types or to produce an already seeded scaffold/tissue if the cells are present in the printing solution (bioprinting) [42–46].

A different tactic, when compared to the previous ones, is to rely on the multipotency of progenitor cells and their ability of self-organizing into complex structures. In this way, through the study of developmental biology, protocols could be designed to mimic the natural conditions that lead to liver organogenesis. So far, the most relevant example is the liver bud experiment [47, 48], in which by controlling the set of conditions to which a 2D co-culture of iPS-derived hepatocytes, MSCs and hUVECs is exposed to, this culture contracts into a 3D budding structure reminiscent of a liver. It is worth mentioning that in this trial, the liver bud was able to form a non-functioning vascular network and rapidly emulated an adult liver when connected to a working vasculature (when transplanted). Additionally, it has been shown to be functional as it helped rescue drug-induced lethal liver failure models.

Other experiments related, pertain to the creation of hepatic/liver organoids from hepatic cell lines that even without having all of the defined organ structure, still show function and regenerative capabilities, such as the ability to generate new bile ducts or the actual organoid development from a single cell [49]. Liver organoids have also been obtained by using hydrogels in microfluidic settings [50], and similar results like the development of bile duct have also been achieved through encapsulation in alginate [51].

2.4   Future Perspectives

Regarding applications of liver bioengineering strategies, the most prominent (and most distant) one is transplantation. When considering this target, one must consider all of the safety concerns common for all medical applications and for that each different technique shows its strengths. When thinking of an off-the-shelf product for transplantation, the fastest option would be to have already a full liver ready for transplant, which is incompatible with an autologous and theoretically safer transplant. This fact leads to two routes, one being the production of sterile scaffolds ready to be seeded with the patient's cells to generate a functional, transplantable liver or the production of allogenic bioengineered livers. Regarding Immunogenicity, the primary concern is the cells since natural scaffolds do not seem to trigger an intense immune response and in the long term are completely substituted by the patient's own ECM (scaffolds are bioabsorbed completely in 90 days [52]). Artificial scaffolds meant for this aim will have to be designed and prepared so that they pass all quality controls for medical use.

Other more easily achieved, and just as critical applications, include disease modeling, and drug testing. For these requests, the liver buds appear to be excellent candidates as if the study is a disease that causes liver malformation. In these cases, development of the liver bud can be easily followed. Other diseases can also be observed and studied over time with this strategy. Drugs can also be tested in this system to study not only normal parameters such as efficacy/toxicity and drug metabolism but also the effect of drugs in liver organogenesis. Other liver bioengineering strategies like biofabrication [42, 53] and liver organoids [50] can also be used for this kind of applications.

3 Drug Development and Toxicology

3.1 Need of Engineered Liver Tissues for Drug Development

To launch a single drug into the market is a very hard (12–15 years) and costly ($3 – $5 billion) process [54]. After an initial screening, lead candidate compounds are characterized in vitro and in vivo for their ADME-Tox (absorption, distribution, metabolism, excretion and toxicity) properties before proceeding with clinical trials. However, most of the compounds (>90%) fail during these final stages. 43% of these failures occur due to a lack of efficacy and 33% due to the appearance of adverse effects [55], particularly in the liver, a phenomenon known as DILI (drug-induced liver injury) [56]. Taking into account that the liver is the organ where most drugs are metabolized and transformed to metabolites/active compounds, some of these substances by-products may result toxic to the own liver and the rest of the body. Hence, drug withdrawals at clinical stages in humans are mainly due to the use of inappropriate/inaccurate in vitro and in vivo liver models in the course of drug studies.

On the other hand, the liver is the target organ of some very common current diseases, such as infectious HBV, HCV [57], malaria [58], overnutrition-induced (type 2 diabetes, NAFLD, fibrosis, cirrhosis) [59–61] or tumoral diseases (hepatocellular carcinoma represents the 6th most common cancer worldwide) [62].

Considering all the above, liver models result necessarily for the development of novel drugs, not only for the study of xenobiotics metabolism and toxicity but also for the development of specific drugs for liver diseases. Hence, more realistic in vitro human liver models that resemble as closely as possible in vivo liver structure, physiology and pharmacological response are needed.

3.2   Limitations of Current In Vitro Liver Models to Test Drugs

As mentioned above, maintaining liver parenchymal function ex vivo results essential to generate stable systems for efficacy and toxicology drug studies, so fully functional hepatocytes are needed. For that, the 3D relationship of cells within the differential microenvironments of the liver (e.g. periportal versus pericentral), the regional hemodynamic flow patterns, and other physiological factors, such as oxygen tension and cytokine profiles have to be simulated in vitro. However, current cell-based models that are routinely used in drug testing are simple monoculture systems (typically standard microtiter plate formats) employed under static, non-physiologic conditions, that makes them suboptimal models for drug efficacy and safety testing, unable to mimic or predict more complex mechanisms of action [63].

Hepatocyte viability in suspension decreases significantly after 4 h [4]. Because of that, for years cryopreserved human hepatocytes in monolayer cultures have been the gold standard to test drug metabolism and toxicity [64]. However, cryopreservation also reduced hepatocyte viability, and function [65] and their culture in monolayer downregulate cell receptors involved in cell-cell and cell-extracellular matrix interactions, reducing drastically cell functionality over time [64]. The development of 2D cultures models, such as sandwich culture, allowed for increasing basal and induced drug-metabolizing enzyme activities and simulating in vivo biliary excretion rates [64, 66]. However, dedifferentiation of hepatocytes in long-term cultures and the lack of non-parenchymal cells that interact with hepatocytes continued being inherent disadvantages of these models [67]. The co-culture of hepatocytes with other liver cells, such as stellate cells, Kupffer cells, liver sinusoidal endothelial cells or liver epithelial cells diminishes to some extent these limitations, improving longevity/functionality of cells and producing higher expression of CYP and Phase II isoforms than in monotypic culture [68–71]. Nevertheless, co-cultures are usually based on the random mixing of different cell types and, thus, do not account for their particular anatomical relationship. More recently, looking for more relevant models, to emulate three-dimensional organization and morphology of hepatocytes within the liver, 3D cultures have been developed. 3D cultures range in complexity from monotypic or heterotypic spheroids [72, 73] to 3D scaffold systems [1] or more advanced models using microfluidic in vitro systems [1, 74]. Multiple commercial 3D co-culture platforms have been developed for drug screening and drug studies, such as the "Hepatopac" platform [75]; the 3D InSight™ Human Liver Microtissues of Insphero, the HepaChip® in vitro microfluidic system [76] or the HμreI® microliver platforms [77].

Today, despite the fact that some issues have been addressed for certain applications with the models mentioned above, others continue to be biologically and technically challenging [66, 78].

3.3 Organoids in Drug Development

Organoids represent more complex models that try to simulate three-dimensional cell-cell and cell-ECM relationships in more relevant physiological conditions which mimic liver microenvironments arrangement and result amenable to high-throughput screening of compounds and feasible enough to guarantee long-term studies.

The optimal liver role is not only dependent on the coordinated function of the parenchymal and non-parenchymal cells within the hepatic acinus but also dependent on hepatic blood microcirculation. Aspects of the microcirculation can be simulated in vitro, via perfusion models, to create a dynamic in vivo like environment. In the last years, different macroscopic perfused in vitro liver systems, initially developed as bioartificial liver devices, have been created [74], providing evidence that perfusion can improve longevity and function in sophisticated hepatic systems, and thus show a better in vivo mimicry. Although these models represent the most physiologically practical systems, their size makes them unfeasible to be used in drug testing studies, as they lack the throughput and analytical flexibility for drug screening. The use of these organoids in drug development involves their miniaturization to a microscopic level. This new class of in vitro tools, often called "on-a-chip" tissue models, can mimic the architecture of small tissue sections and individual characteristics of the dynamic in vivo flow environment, while also offering more precise spatial and temporal control of soluble factors. These models, apart from resulting amendable to high throughput screening approaches, can be engineered for a real-time monitoring of the state of cells and their extracellular environment, which is crucial for determining cellular mechanisms of action in drugs [74].

Several organoid systems have been developed for drug screening and testing. One of the best examples of these organoids rests on microfluidic systems. Already in 2006, Kane et al. developed a microfluidic co-culture system of hepatocytes and T3-J2 fibroblasts in an 8×8 well array, demonstrating stable albumin and urea excretion for 32 days. Some years later, Hμrel Corporation developed a similar microfluidic in vitro liver platform for drug screening with commercial purposes (Hμrelflow TM) [77]. This platform, formed by multiple fluidically interconnected microscale cell culture compartments, enables simulation of the interaction of test substrates with two or more organs which provide an enhanced prediction of human response. In fact, in vivo-like absorption, distribution, metabolism, bioaccumulation, and toxicity of naphthalene were demonstrated when lung, adipose, and liver cells were fluidically connected [77]. Furthermore, the size of the system enabled microscopic imaging, oxygen sensing, physiologically appropriate ratios of chamber sizes, hydrodynamic shear stress and less consumption of media and cells. Even so, some issues, such as sample removal, complexity to maintain recirculation, cell monolayers on chips and not physiological tissue constructs limit the model significantly. Some years later, Au et al. developed another microfluidic model, a microfluidic organoid for drug screening (MODS) platform [79]. The novelty of this system comparing with previously developed MODS, was the ability to evaluate different conditions simultaneously and the automation of time-consuming processes such as the generation of mixtures and the formation of serial dilution series, which can result in more efficient screening of lead drug candidates. Recently, Vernetti et al. have developed and characterized a sophisticated system for investigating drug safety and efficacy in liver models of disease. This system includes a human 3D microfluidic four-cell sequentially layered, self-assembly liver model (SQL-SAL), and furthermore, fluorescent protein biosensors for mechanistic readouts and a microphysiology system database (MPS-Db) to manage, analyze, and model data [80].

Hollow fiber reactors have also been adapted to drug testing. In 2010, Schelzer et al. developed a microscale prototype of a hollow-fiber reactor. In this model, the bioreactor consisted of four cell chambers each of which included four compartments, (one for cells, two for culture medium, and the last one for oxygen supply) connected to provide the cells with a physiologically-based environment [81]. The prototype allowed for small numbers of cells and limited reagent use, microscopic evaluation of the cells and monitoring of oxygen concentrations. Later, a similar system with co-culture of parenchymal and non-parenchymal liver cells was also developed for studies of pharmacokinetics and drug toxicity, showing maintained albumin synthesis and CYP activity for 2–3 weeks [82]. Nevertheless, some limitations also arise in this kind of systems, such as the lack of physiologic gradients typically seen in liver tissue, the complexity of many tubing lines or the limited throughput since only a few different conditions can be assessed simultaneously.

As also mentioned above, decellularization constitutes a novel approach in liver models [33, 83]. This macroscopic model that can be used to investigate the liver development and regeneration can also be miniaturized for high-throughput drug studies.

Apart from physiological models, in the last years, organotypic models of liver diseases are also being developed for drug testing. Drug metabolism, toxicity, and efficacy in diseased livers differ substantially comparing with healthy conditions, so accurate models of disease are required. In this sense, Skardal et al. developed liver-based cell organoids in a rotating wall vessel bioreactor that inoculated with colon carcinoma cells to generate liver-tumor organoids for in vitro modeling of liver metastasis [84]. Recently, Leite et al. have developed hepatic organoids with fibrotic features, such as hepatic stellate cell activation and collagen secretion and deposition, for the study of drug-induced liver fibrosis [85]. Similarly, Lee et al. have generated a reversible- and irreversible-injured alcoholic liver disease model in spheroid-based microfluidic chips where rat primary hepatocytes and hepatic stellate cells (HSCs) are co-cultured [86].

Although enormous advances have been made in the last years to developed more realistic and predictive in vitro liver models for drug testing, the field is still dawning. There are critical issues that should be solved for the field to move forward. Standardizing model/platform characterization for drug-based studies (viability, secretory capacity, enzymatic and toxicology activities and drug transporter activity should be established for each model). Building specificity and sensitivity of the systems, recreating more accurately parenchyma zonation, developing better detection systems and better materials [74], or finding new unlimited fully functional cell sources [87] are some of the challenges to face today in the development of in vitro liver models for drug studies.

3.4 Cancer Research

Liver cancer leads to a considerable number of cancer-related deaths worldwide. Primary liver cancer, hepatocellular carcinoma (HCC), is the 5th most frequent cancer and the 3rd leading cause of cancer death. Approximately 700,000 people die because HCC every year [88]. Moreover, metastasis to the liver is a common occurrence in patients with cancer affecting other organs, usually by hematologic dissemination. The presence of liver metastasis changes dramatically patient's survival, leading to the 2nd highest number of cancer-related deaths in the U.S [89].

In the majority of in vitro models of carcinogenesis tumor growth and metastasis are not optimal. The 2D models cannot represent the complexity of in vivo cancer architecture and the interactions between the healthy tissue and cancer cells. Liver organoids, as described above, are 3D in vitro cultures that can replicate much better the microenvironment of in vivo tissue. For this reason, organoids can be useful to evaluate better the cellular changes that lead to tumorigenesis and cancer progression [90, 91]. Further, organoids 3D culture could serve as a model to test cancer response to a drug. Drug diffusion kinetics and metabolism change dramatically in 3D culture. Probably because in this context it is also possible to reproduce the interactions between cells and matrix, that are not well recreated in 2D models. This hypothesis could explain why drugs that are effective in 2D models are often ineffective when tested in patient [90, 91].

Primary organoid culture including epithelial and mesenchymal cells has been successfully used in pancreatic, gastric and colorectal cancers [90, 91]. Nowadays, unlike other cancers, there is a lack of evidence and data published about utilization of liver organoids in primary liver cancer research, such as HCC and intrahepatic cholangiocarcinoma. Only one study released by Kosaka et al. has evaluated the application for cytotoxicity assay of alcohols of spheroid cultures of human hepatoblastoma cells (HuH-6 line) [92].

Recently liver organoids have been used for in vitro modeling of liver metastasis of colorectal adenocarcinoma [84]. Skardal et al. have evaluated the role of liver tumor organoids for modeling tumor growth and drug response in vitro. In this work, the authors created a liver-based cell organoid in a rotating wall vessel bioreactor that then was inoculated with colon carcinoma cells (CCC). The authors observed that there was a clear phenotypic difference between CCC cultivated in 2D and those inoculated in the liver organoids. In particular, inoculated CCC present a transition from an epithelial to a mesenchymal phenotype showing weak expression of ZO-1, E-cadherin, and vinculin, cytoplasmic expression of beta-catenin and expression of N-cadherin and MMP-9. All these changes suggest a switch to a mesenchymal, mobile and metastatic phenotype, similar to those of the metastatic CCC in vivo. CCC cells in the 2D culture did not present these changes and showed an epithelial phenotype. Another aim of the study was to evaluate the potential role of organoids as a model for drug screening studies. The authors were able to demonstrate that modification of WNT signal pathway through its activation or inhibition could modify the response to 5-fluorouracil [84].

The results of this study are an example of the potential of liver organoids in cancer research. 3D culture models offer a more accurate environment for the study of tumorigenesis and progression. The greater advantage versus 2D models is that organoids seem to be a more precise model of the architecture of the tissue in vivo. Recently, the introduction of novel biomaterials and biofabrication techniques also allowed for a more accurately evaluation of the interaction between cells and ECM.

Finally, the field which liver cell-based organoids seem to have more application is the advanced personalized medicine. Liver malignancies affect a considerable number of patients and are a leading cause of cancer-related death worldwide. In patients with primary liver cancer or liver metastasis future studies may use host-tissue based organoids to screen pharmacologic agents for activity against tumors and toxicity in the normal tissues.

4   Conclusions

Liver tissue engineering and bioengineering of whole livers are shaping the present and potentially the future of regenerative medicine. Nevertheless, the use of these lab created hepatic tissues is exploding in multiple biomedical and pharmaceutical applications. Most of the organoids, tissues and whole organs described above might not be ready for prime time at the bedside, but they already represent very accurate liver models to spur a new age of drug testing and discovery. When compared to the classic 2D models, their higher metabolic function and *bona fide* physiology are an assurance that we might have finally the tools to change the decades' old models of 2D hepatocyte culture. To the field of toxicological and pharmaceutical research, maybe the time to modify the model used in the past two decades as come, hopefully changing with it the trend of drug development attrition rates.

References

1. Godoy P et al (2013) Recent advances in 2D and 3D in vitro systems using primary hepato-cytes, alternative hepatocyte sources and non-parenchymal liver cells and their use in investigating mechanisms of hepatotoxicity, cell signaling and ADME. Arch Toxicol 87:1315–1530
2. Scherer WF, Syverton JT, Gey GO (1953) Studies on the propagation in vitro of poliomyelitis viruses. IV. Viral multiplication in a stable strain of human malignant epithelial cells (strain HeLa) derived from an epidermoid carcinoma of the cervix. J Exp Med 97:695–710
3. Howard RB, Christensen AK, Gibbs FA, Pesch LA (1967) The enzymatic preparation of isolated intact parenchymal cells from rat liver. J Cell Biol 35:675–684
4. Berry MN, Friend DS (1969) High-yield preparation of isolated rat liver parenchymal cells: a biochemical and fine structural study. J Cell Biol 43:506–520
5. Seglen PO (1976) Preparation of isolated rat liver cells. Methods Cell Biol 13:29–83
6. Dunn JC, Yarmush ML, Koebe HG, Tompkins RG (1989) Hepatocyte function and extracellular matrix geometry: long-term culture in a sandwich configuration. FASEB J: official publication of the Federation of American Societies for Experimental Biology 3:174–177
7. Abu-Absi SF, Friend JR, Hansen LK, Hu WS (2002) Structural polarity and functional bile canaliculi in rat hepatocyte spheroids. Exp Cell Res 274:56–67
8. Lin RZ, Chang HY (2008) Recent advances in three-dimensional multicellular spheroid culture for biomedical research. Biotechnol J 3:1172–1184
9. Glicklis R, Merchuk JC, Cohen S (2004) Modeling mass transfer in hepatocyte spheroids via cell viability, spheroid size, and hepatocellular functions. Biotechnol Bioeng 86:672–680
10. Moscona A (1961) Rotation-mediated histogenetic aggregation of dissociated cells A quantifiable approach to cell interactions in vitro. Exp Cell Res 22:455–475
11. Landry J, Bernier D, Ouellet C, Goyette R, Marceau N (1985) Spheroidal aggregate culture of rat liver cells: histotypic reorganization, biomatrix deposition, and maintenance of functional activities. J Cell Biol 101:914–923
12. Koide N et al (1990) Formation of multicellular spheroids composed of adult rat hepatocytes in dishes with positively charged surfaces and under other nonadherent environments. Exp Cell Res 186:227–235
13. Brophy CM et al (2009) Rat hepatocyte spheroids formed by rocked technique maintain differentiated hepatocyte gene expression and function. Hepatology 49:578–586
14. Kelm JM, Timmins NE, Brown CJ, Fussenegger M, Nielsen LK (2003) Method for generation of homogeneous multicellular tumor spheroids applicable to a wide variety of cell types. Biotechnol Bioeng 83:173–180
15. Inamori M, Mizumoto H, Kajiwara T (2009) An approach for formation of vascularized liver tissue by endothelial cell-covered hepatocyte spheroid integration. Tissue Eng Part A 15:2029–2037
16. Abu-Absi SF, Hansen LK, Hu WS (2004) Three-dimensional co-culture of hepatocytes and stellate cells. Cytotechnology 45:125–140
17. Shteyer E et al (2014) Reduced liver cell death using an alginate scaffold bandage: a novel approach for liver reconstruction after extended partial hepatectomy. Acta Biomater 10:3209–3216
18. Lin J et al (2015) Use an alginate scaffold-bone marrow stromal cell (BMSC) complex for the treatment of acute liver failure in rats. Int J Clin Exp Med 8:12593–12600
19. Lin N et al (2010) Differentiation of bone marrow-derived mesenchymal stem cells into hepatocyte-like cells in an alginate scaffold. Cell Prolif 43:427–434
20. Dvir-Ginzberg M, Elkayam T, Cohen S (2008) Induced differentiation and maturation of newborn liver cells into functional hepatic tissue in macroporous alginate scaffolds. FASEB J: official publication of the Federation of American Societies for Experimental Biology 22:1440–1449
21. Shang Y et al (2014) Hybrid sponge comprised of galactosylated chitosan and hyaluronic acid mediates the co-culture of hepatocytes and endothelial cells. J Biosci Bioeng 117:99–106

22. Chien HW, Lai JY, Tsai WB (2014) Galactosylated electrospun membranes for hepatocyte sandwich culture. Colloids Surf B Biointerfaces 116:576–581
23. Berthiaume F, Moghe PV, Toner M, Yarmush ML (1996) Effect of extracellular matrix topology on cell structure, function, and physiological responsiveness: hepatocytes cultured in a sandwich configuration. FASEB J: official publication of the Federation of American Societies for Experimental Biology 10:1471–1484
24. Melgar-Lesmes P, Balcells M, Edelman ER (2017) Implantation of healthy matrix-embedded endothelial cells rescues dysfunctional endothelium and ischaemic tissue in liver engraftment. Gut 66:1297–1305
25. Ranucci CS, Kumar A, Batra SP, Moghe PV (2000) Control of hepatocyte function on collagen foams: sizing matrix pores toward selective induction of 2-D and 3-D cellular morphogenesis. Biomaterials 21:783–793
26. Turner WS et al (2007) Human hepatoblast phenotype maintained by hyaluronan hydrogels. J Biom Mat Res Part B Appl Biom 82:156–168
27. Katsuda T, Teratani T, Ochiya T, Sakai Y (2010) Transplantation of a fetal liver cell-loaded hyaluronic acid sponge onto the mesentery recovers a Wilson's disease model rat. J Biochem 148:281–288
28. Kaihara S et al (2000) Survival and function of rat hepatocytes cocultured with nonparenchymal cells or sinusoidal endothelial cells on biodegradable polymers under flow conditions. J Pediatr Surg 35:1287–1290
29. Kim SS et al (2000) Dynamic seeding and in vitro culture of hepatocytes in a flow perfusion system. Tissue Eng 6:39–44
30. Rad AT et al (2014) Conducting scaffolds for liver tissue engineering. J Biomed Mater Res A 102:4169–4181
31. Kanninen LK et al (2016) Hepatic differentiation of human pluripotent stem cells on human liver progenitor HepaRG-derived acellular matrix. Exp Cell Res 341:207–217
32. Tiwari A et al (2016) Expansion of human hematopoietic stem/progenitor cells on decellularized matrix scaffolds. Curr Protoc Stem Cell Biol 36:1C 15 11–11C 15 16
33. Baptista PM et al (2011) The use of whole organ decellularization for the generation of a vascularized liver organoid. Hepatology 53:604–617
34. Sabetkish S et al (2015) Whole-organ tissue engineering: decellularization and recellularization of three-dimensional matrix liver scaffolds. J Biomed Mater Res A 103:1498–1508
35. Wang Y et al (2015) Method for perfusion decellularization of porcine whole liver and kidney for use as a scaffold for clinical-scale bioengineering engrafts. Xenotransplantation 22:48–61
36. Buhler NE, Schulze-Osthoff K, Konigsrainer A, Schenk M (2015) Controlled processing of a full-sized porcine liver to a decellularized matrix in 24 h. J Biosci Bioeng 119:609–613
37. Struecker B et al (2015) Porcine liver decellularization under oscillating pressure conditions: a technical refinement to improve the homogeneity of the decellularization process. Tissue Eng Part C Methods 21:303–313
38. Soto-Gutierrez A et al (2011) A whole-organ regenerative medicine approach for liver replacement. Tissue Eng Part C Methods 17:677–686
39. Nari GA et al (2013) Preparation of a three-dimensional extracellular matrix by decellularization of rabbit livers. Revista espanola de enfermedades digestivas : organo oficial de la Sociedad Espanola de Patologia Digestiva 105:138–143
40. Baptista PM et al (2016) Fluid flow regulation of revascularization and cellular organization in a bioengineered liver platform. Tissue Eng Part C Methods 22:199–207
41. Mazza G et al (2015) Decellularized human liver as a natural 3D-scaffold for liver bioengineering and transplantation. Sci Rep 5:13079
42. Chang R, Emami K, Wu H, Sun W (2010) Biofabrication of a three-dimensional liver micro-organ as an in vitro drug metabolism model. Biofabrication 2:045004
43. Faulkner-Jones A et al (2015) Bioprinting of human pluripotent stem cells and their directed differentiation into hepatocyte-like cells for the generation of mini-livers in 3D. Biofabrication 7:044102

44. Gong H, Agustin J, Wootton D, Zhou JG (2014) Biomimetic design and fabrication of porous chitosan-gelatin liver scaffolds with hierarchical channel network. J Mater Sci Mater Med 25:113–120
45. Dickson I (2016) Liver: bioprinted liver lobules. Nat Rev Gastroenterol Hepatol 13:190
46. Skardal A et al (2015) A hydrogel bioink toolkit for mimicking native tissue biochemical and mechanical properties in bioprinted tissue constructs. Acta Biomater 25:24–34
47. Takebe T et al (2013) Vascularized and functional human liver from an iPSC-derived organ bud transplant. Nature 499:481–484
48. Takebe T et al (2014) Generation of a vascularized and functional human liver from an iPSC-derived organ bud transplant. Nat Protoc 9:396–409
49. Huch M et al (2013) In vitro expansion of single Lgr5+ liver stem cells induced by Wnt-driven regeneration. Nature 494:247–250
50. Nantasanti S et al (2015) Disease modeling and gene therapy of copper storage disease in canine hepatic organoids. Stem Cell Rep 5:895–907
51. Cheng N, Wauthier E, Reid LM (2008) Mature human hepatocytes from ex vivo differentiation of alginate-encapsulated hepatoblasts. Tissue Eng Part A 14:1–7
52. Faulk DM, Wildemann JD, Badylak SF (2015) Decellularization and cell seeding of whole liver biologic scaffolds composed of extracellular matrix. J Clin Exp Hepatol 5:69–80
53. Skardal A, Devarasetty M, Soker S, Hall AR (2015) In situ patterned micro 3D liver constructs for parallel toxicology testing in a fluidic device. Biofabrication 7:031001
54. Rawlins MD (2004) Cutting the cost of drug development? Nat Rev Drug Discov 3:360–364
55. Kola I, Landis J (2004) Can the pharmaceutical industry reduce attrition rates? Nat Rev Drug Discov 3:711–715
56. Kaplowitz N (2005) Idiosyncratic drug hepatotoxicity. Nat Rev Drug Discov 4:489–499
57. Rizzetto M, Ciancio A (2012) Epidemiology of hepatitis D. Semin Liver Dis 32:211–219
58. WHO (2016) World Malaria Report 2015. WHO
59. Smith BW, Adams LA (2011) Nonalcoholic fatty liver disease and diabetes mellitus: pathogenesis and treatment. Nat Rev Endocrinol 7:456–465
60. Cusi K (2009) Nonalcoholic fatty liver disease in type 2 diabetes mellitus. Curr Opin Endocrinol Diabetes Obes 16:141–149
61. Koppe SWP (2014) Obesity and the liver: nonalcoholic fatty liver disease. Transl Res: the journal of laboratory and clinical medicine 164:312–322
62. McGuire S (2016) World cancer report 2014. Geneva, Switzerland: World Health Organization, International Agency for Research on Cancer, WHO Press, 2015. Adv Nutr (Bethesda, MD) 7:418–419
63. LeCluyse EL, Witek RP, Andersen ME, Powers MJ (2012) Organotypic liver culture models: meeting current challenges in toxicity testing. Crit Rev Toxicol 42:501–548
64. Hewitt NJ et al (2007) Primary hepatocytes: current understanding of the regulation of metabolic enzymes and transporter proteins, and pharmaceutical practice for the use of hepatocytes in metabolism, enzyme induction, transporter, clearance, and hepatotoxicity studies. Drug Metab Rev 39:159–234
65. Terry C, Hughes RD, Mitry RR, Lehec SC, Dhawan A (2007) Cryopreservation-induced non-attachment of human hepatocytes: role of adhesion molecules. Cell Transplant 16:639–647
66. Gómez-Lechón MJ, Tolosa L, Conde I, Donato MT (2014) Competency of different cell models to predict human hepatotoxic drugs. Expert Opin Drug Metab Toxicol 10:1553–1568
67. Rowe C et al (2010) Network analysis of primary hepatocyte dedifferentiation using a shotgun proteomics approach. J Proteome Res 9:2658–2668
68. Bale SS et al (2015) Long-term coculture strategies for primary hepatocytes and liver sinusoidal endothelial cells. Tissue Eng Part C Methods 21:413–422
69. Krause P, Saghatolislam F, Koenig S, Unthan-Fechner K, Probst I (2009) Maintaining hepatocyte differentiation in vitro through co-culture with hepatic stellate cells. In Vitro Cell Dev Biol Anim 45:205–212

70. Ohno M, Motojima K, Okano T, Taniguchi A (2008) Up-regulation of drug-metabolizing enzyme genes in layered co-culture of a human liver cell line and endothelial cells. Tissue Eng Part A 14:1861–1869
71. Tukov FF et al (2006) Modeling inflammation-drug interactions in vitro: a rat Kupffer cell-hepatocyte coculture system. ToxicolIn Vitro : an international journal published in association with BIBRA 20:1488–1499
72. Luebke-Wheeler JL, Nedredal G, Yee L, Amiot BP, Nyberg SL (2009) E-cadherin protects primary hepatocyte spheroids from cell death by a caspase-independent mechanism. Cell Transplant 18:1281–1287
73. Sakai Y, Yamagami S, Nakazawa K (2010) Comparative analysis of gene expression in rat liver tissue and monolayer- and spheroid-cultured hepatocytes. Cells Tissues Organs 191:281–288
74. Usta OB et al (2015) Microengineered cell and tissue systems for drug screening and toxicology applications: evolution of in-vitro liver technologies. Technology 3:1–26
75. Chan TS et al (2013) Meeting the challenge of predicting hepatic clearance of compounds slowly metabolized by cytochrome P450 using a novel hepatocyte model. Hepato Pac Drug Metab Dispos: the biological fate of chemicals 41:2024–2032
76. Schütte J et al (2010) A method for patterned in situ biofunctionalization in injection-molded microfluidic devices. Lab Chip 10:2551–2558
77. Baxter GT (2009) Hurel – an in vivo-surrogate assay platform for cell-based studies. Altern Lab Anim: ATLA 37(Suppl 1):11–18
78. Guillouzo A, Guguen-Guillouzo C (2008) Evolving concepts in liver tissue modeling and implications for in vitro toxicology. Expert Opin Drug Metab Toxicol 4:1279–1294
79. Au SH, Chamberlain MD, Mahesh S, Sefton MV, Wheeler AR (2014) Hepatic organoids for microfluidic drug screening. Lab Chip 14:3290–3299
80. Vernetti LA et al (2016) A human liver microphysiology platform for investigating physiology, drug safety, and disease models. Exp Biol Med (Maywood) 241:101–114
81. Schmelzer E et al (2010) Three-dimensional perfusion bioreactor culture supports differentiation of human fetal liver cells. Tissue Eng Part A 16:2007–2016
82. Zeilinger K et al (2011) Scaling down of a clinical three-dimensional perfusion multicompartment hollow fiber liver bioreactor developed for extracorporeal liver support to an analytical scale device useful for hepatic pharmacological in vitro studies. Tissue Eng Part C Methods 17:549–556
83. Uygun BE et al (2010) Organ reengineering through development of a transplantable recellularized liver graft using decellularized liver matrix. Nat Med 16:814–820
84. Skardal A, Devarasetty M, Rodman C, Atala A, Soker S (2015) Liver-tumor hybrid organoids for modeling tumor growth and drug response in vitro. Ann Biomed Eng 43:2361–2373
85. Leite SB et al (2016) Novel human hepatic organoid model enables testing of drug-induced liver fibrosis in vitro. Biomaterials 78:1–10
86. Lee J et al (2016) A 3D alcoholic liver disease model on a chip. Integr Biol: quantitative biosciences from nano to macro 8:302–308
87. Huch M et al (2015) Long-term culture of genome-stable bipotent stem cells from adult human liver. Cell 160:299–312
88. Bruix J, Reig M, Sherman M (2016) Evidence-based diagnosis, staging, and treatment of patients with hepatocellular carcinoma. Gastroenterology 150:835–853
89. Young M, Ordonez L, Clarke AR (2013) What are the best routes to effectively model human colorectal cancer? Mol Oncol 7:178–189
90. Saito M et al (2006) Reconstruction of liver organoid using a bioreactor. World J Gastroenterol 12:1881–1888
91. Dedhia PH, Bertaux-Skeirik N, Zavros Y, Spence JR (2016) Organoid models of human gastrointestinal development and disease. Gastroenterology 150:1098–1112
92. Kosaka T et al (1996) Spheroid cultures of human hepatoblastoma cells (HuH-6 line) and their application for cytotoxicity assay of alcohols. Acta Med Okayama 50:61–66

Mammary Gland Organoids

Rocío Sampayo, Sol Recouvreux, María Inés Diaz Bessone, and Marina Simian

Abstract The study of the mechanisms that regulate development and tumorigenesis is a complex undertaking that requires a variety of model systems to test hypothesis that embrace all levels of organization: from single cells to organs. In the mammary gland field, the use of three-dimensional culture systems has provided a platform to study, in a physiologically relevant setting, cell biology in context. In the late 50's methods to isolate primary mammary organoids were established and since then they have been increasingly used to understand cell behavior. In this chapter we embrace, in a historical perspective, the key findings carried out using primary mammary organoids considering that the broadening of our knowledge will, in the future, rely increasingly on this kind of tridimensional culture setting.

Keywords Mammary gland • Organoids • Cell culture • Morphogenesis • Branching • Hormones • Gene expression • Regulation • Matrigel • Collagen I • 3D cultures • 2D cultures

R. Sampayo, PhD
Instituto de Nanosistemas, Universidad Nacional de San Martín,
San Martín, Buenos Aires, Argentina
e-mail: ro.sampayo@gmail.com

S. Recouvreux, MSc
Instituto de Oncología "Angel H. Roffo",
Avda San Martín, 5481 Ciudad de Buenos Aires, Argentina
e-mail: solrecu@gmail.com

M.I.D. Bessone, PhD • M. Simian, PhD (✉)
Instituto de Nanosistemas, Universidad Nacional de San Martín,
San Martín 1650, Buenos Aires, Argentina
e-mail: mariadiazbessone@hotmail.com; marina.simian@galuzzi.com

© Springer International Publishing AG 2018
S. Soker, A. Skardal (eds.), *Tumor Organoids*, Cancer Drug Discovery and Development, DOI 10.1007/978-3-319-60511-1_3

1   The Mammary Gland

The mammary gland is a particular organ given that most of its development occurs postnatally. The overall pattern of growth and differentiation is similar between rodents and humans, thus much of what we know about mammary gland biology and the mechanisms leading to breast cancer derive from experiments carried out in mice and rats. In all species, mammary glands are composed by an epithelium and a stroma, separated by the basement membrane. The epithelial compartment is composed of two cell types, luminal epithelial cells that conform the ducts and become milk secretory during lactation and myoepithelial cells that surround the luminal cells and enable the expulsion of milk from the alveoli [1, 2].

Even though most of mammary gland development takes place postnatally, six stages can be identified in this process: embryonic, post-natal, pubertal, pregnant, lactating and involuting. Hormones, especially estrogen and progesterone, together with growth factors play key roles in the regulation of these stages. Importantly, when development goes awry, signaling of these pathways is also altered.

The embryonic stage of development is characterized by the formation of rudimentary epithelial structures from the mammary placodes that invades the surrounding adipose tissue. This process begins at embryonic day (E) 10, with the development of milk lines or bilateral stripes of multilayered ectoderm that initiate at the forelimb bud and extend towards the hindlimb on the ventral surface of the embryo. The mammary line resolves into five pairs of placodes by E11.5. Interestingly, the placodes do not arise from proliferation, but from the migration and aggregation of ectodermal cells at the mammary line [3]. Pioneering work by Cunha determined through tissue recombination experiments that the embryonic mesenchyme underlying the mammary line delivers signals that govern the differentiation of mammary epithelial cells [4]. The placodes expand and by E14 form a round mass of cells that stem into the underlying mesenchyme [5]. A thin layer of fibroblasts surrounds the epithelium. By E16 the epithelial cells reach the fat pad, which at this stage is composed of a small number of preadipocytes . This leads to the subsequent development of a rudimentary dichotomous branching system. Interestingly, these branches are generated without the influence of hormones and are only modified with the advent of puberty. Lumen formation takes place between E16 and E18 [6]. Apoptosis, autophagy and remodeling are implicated in this process [7, 8]. Finally, the formation of the nipple takes place by changes in the skin overlying the mammary mesenchyme [9].

At birth the gland is thus a basic ductal system that will accompany body growth but will only suffer further development with the onset of puberty, with the rise in circulating estrogen levels at week three. The terminal end buds, which are club-shaped assemblies consisting of an outer layer of cap cells surrounding a multilayered core of body cells, appear at the end of the ducts and are responsible for the invasion of the fat pad [10]. Cap cells give rise to myoepitelial cells, forming the basal layer of the ductal structures, surrounding the inner luminal cells [11]. The ducts elongate and give rise to secondary branches as a result of a process called bifurcation. This tree like pattern occupies approximately 60% of the mammary fat pad, which will reach its maximum degree of epithelial development under the influence of the hormonal changes that occur with pregnancy. The process of branching morphogenesis is complex and regulated by a broad range of factors both local and systemic: growth factors, extracellular matrix components, proteases, morphogens, and hormones. Estrogen, growth hormone and IGF1 are key regulators of branching morphogenesis in puberty [10, 12]. Growth hormone induces the production of IGF1 by the liver, and together with locally produced IGF1 and circulating estrogens are responsible for the formation of the terminal end buds and ductal branching [13]. Estrogen, together with IGF1, is responsible for the proliferative surge that is required for branching morphogenesis [14]. Interestingly, estrogen receptor is expressed in only a subset of epithelial cells and induces the release of amphiregulin that signals through the stroma inducing the production of additional growth factors such as FGFs that contribute to the branching process [15–17]. Studies in estrogen receptor knockout mice established that signaling through estrogen receptor is critical for terminal end bud maintenance and invasion of the fat pad [18]. During pregnancy, signaling downstream of progesterone and prolactin regulate the increase in side branching and the formation of alveolar structures which will be responsible for milk production [19, 12]. Adipose tissue is reduced as proliferating epithelial cells grow into the interductal spaces. Simultaneously, there is an increase in vascularization [20]. In progesterone receptor knock out mice both proliferation and differentiation associated to pregnancy are hampered [21]. As with estrogen receptor, progesterone receptor in the adult mammary gland is expressed in a subset of epithelial cells. RANKL (receptor activator of NFKB1 ligand) has been shown to be a key mediator of proliferation induced by progesterone receptor [22]. Knock out mice for *Rank* or *Rankl* do not develop alveolar structures during pregnancy, similar to the progesterone receptor knock out mice [23]. RANKL is induced by progesterone in luminal epithelial cells and induces proliferation of PR negative neighboring cells [24]. Prolactin, on the other hand, has both systemic and local actions. At the systemic level prolactin, which is produced by the pituitary, regulates ovarian progesterone production [25]. Locally, in the mammary gland, prolactin has been shown to have a direct role on alveolar development and milk production acting through the prolactin receptor expressed in luminal mammary epithelial cells [26].

After weaning the mammary gland regresses though the process of involution which is characterized by massive cell death and tissue remodeling [27], reaching a state similar to the one it had before pregnancy. Involution consists of two phases: an initial reversible phase that is characterized by apoptosis and detachment of alveolar cells. At 48 h phase two begins with the collapse of alveoli, together with protease activation, extracellular matrix remodeling and massive apoptosis. Most of the secretory epithelium is lost by day six, and the mammary gland returns to a structure similar to that found in the virgin mouse [28]. The mammary gland is thus a very versatile organ which lends itself as an ideal model system for the study of various developmental processes, implicated not only in normal organogenesis, but also associated with alterations in tissue structure and consequently the progression to disease.

2   Model Systems to Study Mammary Gland Development: 2D Vs 3D

Traditionally, and probably due to convenience and reproducibility, tissue culture studies have been mostly carried out in two-dimensional (2D) systems. This approach has led to a deep understanding of cell biology centered on single cell behavior, or to paracrine interactions between identical cells. However, we know that cells make up tissues, and these constitute organs that are three-dimensional (3D) and reside in a complex extracellular matrix, that not only provides physical support, but that additionally contributes key cues that are critical for adequate function. Thus, relevant in vitro studies aiming at understanding developmental and pathological cellular mechanisms should consider this degree of complexity. Mammary epithelial cells, in particular, are unable to express tissue-specific genes, such as casein and WAP (whey acidic protein), when cultured on 2D. It is only in the presence of adequate extracellular matrix components that cells organize into structures similar to those found in vivo and thus express tissue-specific genes [29].

The mammary gland field probably is one of the pioneers in establishing complex 3D cultures. Following the work of Michalopoulos and Pitot (1976) who cultured hepatocyes on floating collagen gels [30], the Bissell laboratory used this scheme and laminin-rich extracellular matrix to culture primary murine luminal mammary epithelial cells [31, 32]. Just as an example of the value of physiologically relevant 3D cultures, this system led to the discovery of the cues that regulate milk production in mammary cells, establishing that laminin-rich extracellular matrix leads to in vivo like structural organization, together with the basolateral exposure of the prolactin receptor, enabling the secretion of milk proteins to the lumen [33]. Laminin-111 was actually shown to induce adequate acinar polarity [34]. Thus, even though the general hormonal regulation of milk production was known at that time, setting up a tridimensional model in culture enabled the discovery of the fine mechanistic details that govern milk production. Adequate culture systems have consequently allowed cell biologists to complement the results obtained in vivo and to answer questions that would be difficult to tackle in whole animal systems.

3   Mammary Gland Organoids

The term "organoid" refers to a section of a mammary duct that contains epithelial and myoepithelial cells together with basement membrane components. Organoids are obtained by mechanically and enzymatically digesting the mammary gland. This leads to a suspension of organoids, erythrocytes, stromal cells and muscle fibers together with cell debris. To further isolate the organoids, differential centrifugations are carried out until a clean pellet of organoids is obtained. Several papers clearly explain the methods that lead to the preparation of viable organoids

[35, 36]. However, we strongly recommend a recent publication by Andy Ewald and collaborators in Methods in Molecular Biology where they clearly illustrate the steps that need to be followed to successfully culture primary mammary gland organoids [37]. Figure 1a schematically shows the steps that lead to a successful 3D culture of mammary gland organoids. Figure 1b–f' explicitly illustrate the procedure that should be followed to access and remove the mouse mammary gland.

Depending on the question to be answered, mammary gland organoids can be either cultured in collagen I, in laminin-rich reconstituted basement membrane, such as Matrigel, or in a combination of both. Figure 2a illustrates the different assays that can be carried out with the primary organoids depending on the composition of the matrix. Figure 2b–e show representative frames of DIC time-lapse movies of organoid behavior in different culture conditions.

Mammary gland organoids were first described in the pioneering papers published by Etienne Lasfargues who found that enzymatic digestion of minced mouse mammary glands with bacterial collagenase generated mammary duct fragments devoid of fibroblasts and adipocytes [38, 39]. In the early '80s Nandi and colleagues embedded mammary epithelial cells from virgin or pregnant mice in collagen I gels and showed that they were able to form three-dimensional structures, retaining the cytological appearance of normal mammary epithelial cells [40–42]. Moreover, the addition of lactogenic hormones led to functional differentiation [40]. In 1991, Kathleen Darcy and Margot Ip established an organoid culture system in serum-free, chemically defined medium using Engelbreth-Holm-Swarm sarcoma-derived reconstituted basement membrane [43]. They showed that in these conditions organoids, derived from unprimed virgin female mice, could develop into either alveolar or ductal three-dimensional structures within the same cultures. Epithelial cells in both cases were able to secrete milk proteins such as casein into the luminal compartment. This culture system set the basis for further experimental work that would aid in the identification and characterization of the regulatory factors controlling not only normal morphogenesis, but oncogenesis as well.

4 Key Finding Using Primary Mammary Organoids as a Model of Development

The use of mammary gland organoids as a tool to investigate the biology of the mammary gland has allowed us to understand many of the mechanisms that regulate normal growth and differentiation, as well as malignant transformation. Following the pioneering experiments mentioned above, a series of papers in the last three decades have contributed to a deeper understanding of multiple mechanisms involved in the biology of mammary gland growth and differentiation using primary organoids.

By the late '80s, researchers working on mammary gland biology knew that differentiation was dependent not only on hormones, but that interactions of the epi-

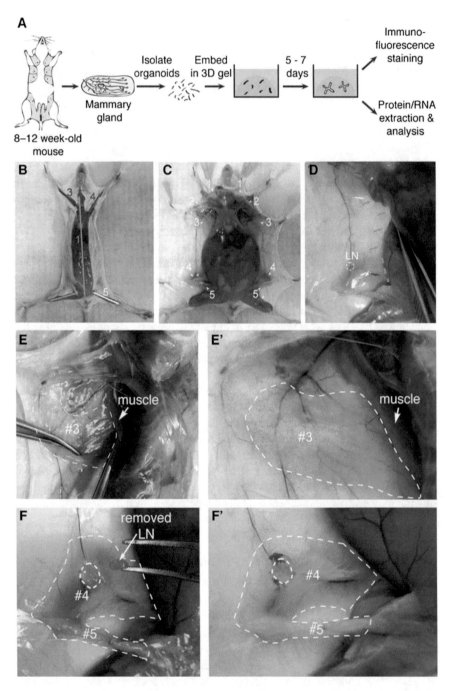

Fig. 1 Collection of mouse mammary glands for organoid isolation and 3D culture. (**a**) Schematic description of isolation and 3D culture of mouse mammary organoids. (**b**) Scheme for surgically accessing the mammary glands. Numbers indicate the order of cuts. (**c**) Locations of the ten mammary glands. (**d**) Expose glands #3,#4, and #5 by pushing back the abdomen (*blue dotted line*) with the back of the Graefe forceps. (**e–e'**) A thin layer of muscle partially covers gland #3 (**e**) and should be pushed back before dissection (**e'**). *Dotted line* in (**e'**) indicates the region of gland #3 to be collected. (**f**) Use the Graefe forceps to pluck out the lymph node in gland #4. *Dotted line* in (**f'**) indicates the approximate region of glands #4 and #5 to be collected (From Nguyen-Ngoc et al. [37], Copyright (2015) Springer)

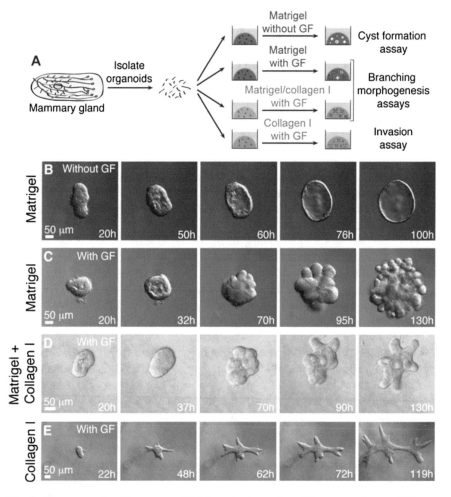

Fig. 2 3D organotypic culture assays. (**a**) Schematic description of four assays that use different extracellular matrix compositions to model specific epithelial behaviors. (**b–e**) Representative frames of DIC time-lapse movies showing cyst formation in Matrigel in basal medium (**b**), branching morphogenesis in Matrigel induced by FGF2 (**c**), branching morphogenesis in a mixture of Matrigel and collagen I induced by FGF2 (**d**), and epithelial cell invasion into pure collagen I induced by FGF2 (**e**) (From Nguyen-Ngoc et al. [37], Copyright (2015) Springer)

thelial cells with the surrounding stromal cells was hypothesized to play a key role as well. However, until then, the study of the regulation of milk protein genes had been hampered by the complexity of the hormonal influences and cell-cell interactions. Organ explant cultures had shown that WAP was controlled by both hydrocortisone and prolactin [44, 45], but cultured epithelial cells, regardless of the substratum, could not be induced to produce the gene [33]. Between November 1989 and January 1990 two papers were published that clearly showed that structural integrity of mammary epithelial cell interactions was critical for WAP transcriptional regulation. Mina Bissel's lab published the first paper in November, showing that when isolated primary mammary cells were cultured on basement membrane-like matrix and allowed to form three-dimensional alveoli-like structures, WAP gene expression was induced and secreted into the lumen of the spheres [29]. Cora-Ann Schoenenberger and collaborators were able to establish a defined culture system where primary mammary organoids derived from mid-pregnant mice were cultured on 3 T3-L1 adipocytes [46]. In this context, they were also able to efficiently induce WAP mRNA by the addition of insulin, hydrocortisone, and prolactin. This paper showed that the structural integrity of the organoid was key for WAP induction and together with the Bissell lab's publication showed why previous attempts to regulate WAP gene transcription in vitro had failed. A subsequent paper using rabbit primary mammary organoids determined that the 6.3 kb rabbit WAP gene upstream fragment carries transcriptional control elements that are sensitive to insulin, prolactin and glucocorticoids [47].

Following the seminal papers on gene regulation, studies on the fine mechanisms that regulate mammary branching morphogenesis was the next subject that was addressed using primary mammary organoids. A series of papers that include publications to this current year led to many interesting findings that would not have been possible using in vivo systems or 2D cultures. In 2001 we used three-dimensional cultures of organoids together with luminal Scp2 cells in collagen I gels to determine that branching morphogenesis is dependent on the interplay of growth factors, morphogens and matrix metalloproteinases (MMP) [35]. Branching stimulated by stromal fibroblasts, epidermal growth factor, fibroblast growth factor 7, fibroblast growth factor 2 and hepatocyte growth factor is strongly hampered by MMP inhibitors. Moreover, we showed that recombinant stromelysin 1/MMP3 alone is sufficient to induce branching in the absence of growth factors in the organoids. However, this is not so in the Scp2 cell clusters, suggesting that MMPs are not enough to drive the branching process, but that additional factors derived from myoepithelial and/or stromal cells are required. We found that plasmin also stimulates branching through an MMP dependent mechanism. To differentiate between signals for proliferation and morphogenesis, we used Scp2 cells, a cloned mammary epithelial cell line that lacks epimorphin, an essential mammary morphogen. Both epimorphin and MMPs are required for morphogenesis, but neither is required for epithelial cell proliferation. These results provided the first direct evidence for a crucial role of MMPs in branching in mammary epithelium and suggested that, in addition to epimorphin, MMP activity is a minimum requirement for branching morphogenesis in the mammary gland.

In 2006, partially based on these results, Celeste Nelson, and Mina Bissell published a seminal paper in Science where they showed that tissue geometry determines the site of branching morphogenesis [48]. Using a micropatterning approach to control the initial three-dimensional structure of mouse mammary epithelial tubules in culture they determined that tubules dictate the position of the branches by defining the local concentration of TGF-β, that acts in this context as an inhibitory morphogen. Figure 3 shows the different stages of the patterning process; the polydimethylsiloxane (PDMS) stamp is used to make a reproducible molded

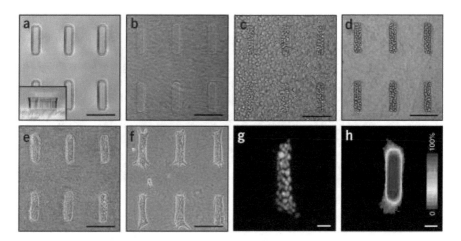

Fig. 3 Images of different stages of the patterning process. (**a**) PDMS stamp (*inset*: vertical section through one post); (**b**) molded collagen gel; (**c**) molded gel during addition of cells (note that cells are both in the wells and on top of the gel); (**d**) molded gel after washing away excess cells; (**e**) tubules; (**f**) branched tissues 24 h after addition of EGF to the sample; (**g**) one branched tissue stained for nuclei with Hoechst 33,258; (**h**) frequency map depicting quantification of 50 branched tissues. Scale bars, 200 μm (**a–f**) and 50 μm (**g**, **h**) (From Nelson et al. 2008, Copyright (2008), Nature Protocols)

collagen gel where the cells are seeded. In this setting, and in the presence of growth factors such as EGF, branching morphogenesis is induced.

Following Nelson's paper, Fata and Bissell described the establishment of a modified 3D culture system for primary mouse mammary organoids: in this case they used a laminin-rich extracellular matrix in 96 well plates to culture the organoids [36]. They showed that the interplay between growth factors, their spatial localization, and the duration of their activation as well as downstream effectors cooperate and choreograph whether mammary branches initiate and/or elongate. To do so they analyzed the relationship between TGFα and FGF7. TGFα induces sustained activation of MAPK^{ERK1,2} for 1 h, and is necessary and sufficient to initiate branching morphogenesis. FGF7, however, leads to a transient 15-minute activation of MAPK^{ERK1,2}, without branching (Fig. 4). Unlike TGFα, FGF7 promotes sustained proliferation as well as ectopic localization of, and increase in, keratin-6 expressing cells. Concurrent stimulation by FGF7 and TGFα indicate that the FGF7 is dominant. Interestingly, FGF7 may prevent branching by suppression of two necessary TGFα-induced morphogenetic effectors: MMP-3 and fibronectin. These findings showed that proliferation, morphogenetic effectors, and cell-type decisions during mammary organoid morphogenesis are closely dependent on the duration of activation of MAPK^{ERK1,2}.

To assess in real time the cellular behavior that leads to branching morphogenesis, Ewald and Werb used the system described above to carry out long-term confocal time-lapse analysis [8, 49]. Mammary primary organoids were obtained from a

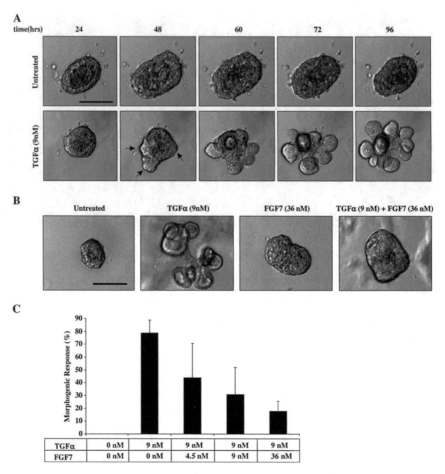

Fig. 4 Organoid response to TGFα and FGF7. (**a**) Untreated organoids fail to undergo major morphological changes, except a slight lumen expansion followed by compression from 48 to 60 h. In contrast, TGFα stimulation initiates bud formation (*arrows*) within 48 h, with the majority of morphogenesis occurring within the 48- to 72-h window. Images represent frames taken from movies (Supplemental Movies 1 and 2). (**b, c**) FGF7 fails to induce branching morphogenesis and suppresses TGFα-induced morphogenesis in a dose-dependent manner. Please see Supplemental Movies 3 and 4. (**c**) Morphometric analysis of branching morphogenesis. Scale bars represent 100 µm. Data are represented as mean morphogenetic response ± standard deviation (SD) and involve counting at least 100 organoids per condition per experiment (From Fata et al. [36], Copyright (2008), Developmental Biology)

reporter mouse in which the keratin-14 promoter drives expression of an actin-EGFP fusion protein [50]. Additionally, all cells were stained with CellTracker Red. Using this system the authors were able to follow the behavior of both the luminal and the myoepithelial cells in real time. They showed that mammary ducts elongate through a distinct type of collective epithelial migration, with no leading cell extensions or leading actin-rich protrusions [8]. This is especially interesting in the context that this is actually so in other models such as border cell migration in *Drosophila* [51] and neuronal precursors in the zebrafish lateral line [52]. Mammary organoids initially reorganize from a quiescent, bilayered epithelium to a preinvasive, highly proliferative, incompletely polarized, multilayered structure. Rac and MLCK are molecular controllers of the transition from this preinvasive state to the launch of new ducts. Moreover, cells within extending ducts dynamically rearrange, but remain adherent and localize E-cadherin and β-catenin to cell-cell contacts [8]. During this process, individual cells within the multilayered region are incompletely polarized. Cells at the elongating tips of ducts have increased staining of pERK1/2 and it is these particular cells that present the highest migration speed [49]. Interestingly, cell proliferation is only required for branch initiation, but elongation is independent of this cellular process [49]. Additionally, cells orient their protrusions in the direction of the branch elongation and Rac signaling is necessary for this process to occur and to sustain the branch elongation process [49].

5 Primary Mammary Organoids as a Platform to Understand Mechanisms Involved in Carcinogenesis

The deep understanding of the mechanisms involved in branching morphogenesis in 3D culture models opens the possibility of developing a platform that could be used to unravel the key determinants of tumorigenesis, in the same way that primary tumor organoids are being used to test in 3D the efficacy of new therapeutic strategies. A clear example to this end was recently published by Zena Werb and Katherine Williams [53]. They used the primary mammary organoid 3D culture model to analyze the direct impact of environmental chemicals on the morphogenetic program of breast cells. The final aim of their venture was to understand how low doses of environmental chemicals such as bisphenol-A, mono-n-butyl phthalate and polychlorinated biphenyl 153 affect mammary gland development. These xenobiotics were selected because they are frequently detected in the serum and/or urine of girls in puberty. The use of this system provides the possibility of testing directly their effects in a physiologically relevant model of mammary development, independently of the effects they may have systemically.

Alternatively, genetic manipulation of primary mammary organoids allows researchers to test the direct contribution certain genes have on cell behaviors that predispose towards cancer development, such as cell migration and invasion. Shamir et al. were successful in using this strategy to determine the contribution of E-cadherin loss and Twist overexpression on the dissemination of mammary epithelial cells out of the epithelium [54]. E-cadherin loss was manipulated by using organoids from mice carrying floxed *E-cad* alleles [55] and a ubiquitously expressed, tamoxifen-inducible Cre recombinase [56]; *Cre-ER;E-cad$^{fl/fl}$* mice. Twist on the other hand, was overexpressed by using organoids from mice carrying a ubiquitously expressed reverse tetracycline transactivator and a Tet-responsive *Twist1* allele

[57]. Using this system the authors determined that E-cadherin is a requisite for normal mammary development but that its loss alone is not sufficient for dissemination. *Twist1* expression, on the other hand, is enough to stimulate normal epithelial cells to propagate out of an epithelium, migrate through the ECM, and establish secondary epithelial sites. Remarkably, the migrating cells display membrane-localized E-cadherin and β-catenin and retained cytokeratin expression.

6 Concluding Remarks

These are examples of the variety of hypothesis that can be tested using primary organoids derived from mammary glands or other organs. In the last years, there has been a surge in the culture of organoids derived from many organs and these are being used to study the mechanisms of development and to understand what pathways are involved when development goes awry [58]. In the case of the mammary gland field few labs so far have systematically used primary mammary organoids in their studies. We look forward to breakthroughs in our understanding of normal development and disease using this system that enables high levels of manipulation in a physiologically relevant setting.

Acknowledgements This book chapter was supported by a grant from the Instituto Nacional del Cáncer, Ministerio de Salud, República Argentina to M.S. M.S. is a career Conicet scientist. S.R. and I.D.B. are supported by Conicet fellowships.

References

1. Nandi S (1958) Endocrine control of mammary gland development and function in C3H/Crgl mouse. J Natl Cancer Inst 21:1039–1063
2. Williams JM, Daniel CW (1983) Mammary ductal elongation: differentiation of myoepithelium and basal lamina during branching morphogenesis. Dev Biol 97(2):274–290
3. Balinsky B (1950) On the prenatal growth of the mammary gland rudiment in the mouse. J Anat 84(Pt 3):227
4. Cunha GR (1994) Role of mesenchymal-epithelial interactions in normal and abnormal development of the mammary gland and prostate. Cancer 74(3 Suppl):1030–1044
5. Cowin P, Wysolmerski J (2010) Molecular mechanisms guiding embryonic mammary gland development. Cold Spring Harb Perspect Biol 2(6):a003251. doi:cshperspect.a003251 [pii] 1101/cshperspect.a003251
6. Hogg NA, Harrison CJ, Tickle C (1983) Lumen formation in the developing mouse mammary gland. J Embryol Exp Morphol 73:39–57
7. Debnath J, Mills KR, Collins NL, Reginato MJ, Muthuswamy SK, Brugge JS (2002) The role of apoptosis in creating and maintaining luminal space within normal and oncogene-expressing mammary acini. Cell 111(1):29–40
8. Ewald AJ, Brenot A, Duong M, Chan BS, Werb Z (2008) Collective epithelial migration and cell rearrangements drive mammary branching morphogenesis. Dev Cell 14(4):570–581. doi:10.1016/j.devcel.2008.03.003

9. Hens JR, Dann P, Zhang JP, Harris S, Robinson GW, Wysolmerski J (2007) BMP4 and PTHrP interact to stimulate ductal outgrowth during embryonic mammary development and to inhibit hair follicle induction. Development 134(6):1221–1230. doi:10.1242/dev.000182

10. Daniel CW, Silberstein GB, Strickland P (1987) Direct action of 17 beta-estradiol on mouse mammary ducts analyzed by sustained release implants and steroid autoradiography. Cancer Res 47(22):6052–6057

11. Ormerod EJ, Rudland PS (1984) Cellular composition and organization of ductal buds in developing rat mammary glands: evidence for morphological intermediates between epithelial and myoepithelial cells. Am J Anat 170(4):631–652. doi:10.1002/aja.1001700408

12. Brisken C, Ataca D (2015) Endocrine hormones and local signals during the development of the mouse mammary gland. Wiley Interdiscip Rev Dev Biol 4(3):181–195. doi:10.1002/wdev.172

13. Ruan W, Kleinberg DL (1999) Insulin-like growth factor I is essential for terminal end bud formation and ductal morphogenesis during mammary development. Endocrinology 140(11):5075–5081. doi:10.1210/endo.140.11.7095

14. Mallepell S, Krust A, Chambon P, Brisken C (2006) Paracrine signaling through the epithelial estrogen receptor alpha is required for proliferation and morphogenesis in the mammary gland. Proc Natl Acad Sci U S A 103(7):2196–2201. doi:10.1073/pnas.0510974103

15. Luetteke NC, Qiu TH, Fenton SE, Troyer KL, Riedel RF, Chang A, Lee DC (1999) Targeted inactivation of the EGF and amphiregulin genes reveals distinct roles for EGF receptor ligands in mouse mammary gland development. Development 126(12):2739–2750

16. Lu P, Ewald AJ, Martin GR, Werb Z (2008) Genetic mosaic analysis reveals FGF receptor 2 function in terminal end buds during mammary gland branching morphogenesis. Dev Biol 321(1):77–87. doi:10.1016/j.ydbio.2008.06.005

17. Coleman-Krnacik S, Rosen JM (1994) Differential temporal and spatial gene expression of fibroblast growth factor family members during mouse mammary gland development. Mol Endocrinol 8(2):218–229

18. Mueller SO, Clark JA, Myers PH, Korach KS (2002) Mammary gland development in adult mice requires epithelial and stromal estrogen receptor alpha. Endocrinology 143(6):2357–2365

19. Shyamala G, Yang X, Cardiff RD, Dale E (2000) Impact of progesterone receptor on cell-fate decisions during mammary gland development. Proc Natl Acad Sci U S A 97(7):3044–3049

20. Djonov V, Andres AC, Ziemiecki A (2001) Vascular remodelling during the normal and malignant life cycle of the mammary gland. Microsc Res Tech 52(2):182–189. doi:10.1002/1097-0029(20010115)52:2<182::AID-JEMT1004>3.0.CO;2-M

21. Lydon JP, DeMayo FJ, Funk CR, Mani SK, Hughes AR, Montgomery CA Jr, Shyamala G, Conneely OM, O'Malley BW (1995) Mice lacking progesterone receptor exhibit pleiotropic reproductive abnormalities. Genes Dev 9(18):2266–2278

22. Gonzalez-Suarez E, Jacob AP, Jones J, Miller R, Roudier-Meyer MP, Erwert R, Pinkas J, Branstetter D, Dougall WC (2010) RANK ligand mediates progestin-induced mammary epithelial proliferation and carcinogenesis. Nature 468(7320):103–107. doi:nature09495 [pii] 1038/nature09495

23. Fata JE, Kong YY, Li J, Sasaki T, Irie-Sasaki J, Moorehead RA, Elliott R, Scully S, Voura EB, Lacey DL, Boyle WJ, Khokha R, Penninger JM (2000) The osteoclast differentiation factor osteoprotegerin-ligand is essential for mammary gland development. Cell 103(1):41–50

24. Fernandez-Valdivia R, Mukherjee A, Creighton CJ, Buser AC, DeMayo FJ, Edwards DP, Lydon JP (2008) Transcriptional response of the murine mammary gland to acute progesterone exposure. Endocrinology 149(12):6236–6250. doi:10.1210/en.2008-0768

25. Brisken C, Kaur S, Chavarria TE, Binart N, Sutherland RL, Weinberg RA, Kelly PA, Ormandy CJ (1999) Prolactin controls mammary gland development via direct and indirect mechanisms. Dev Biol 210(1):96–106. doi:10.1006/dbio.1999.9271

26. Vomachka AJ, Pratt SL, Lockefeer JA, Horseman ND (2000) Prolactin gene-disruption arrests mammary gland development and retards T-antigen-induced tumor growth. Oncogene 19(8):1077–1084. doi:10.1038/sj.onc.1203348

27. Talhouk RS, Bissell MJ, Werb Z (1992) Coordinated expression of extracellular matrix-degrading proteinases and their inhibitors regulates mammary epithelial function during involution. J Cell Biol 118(5):1271–1282

28. Lund LR, Romer J, Thomasset N, Solberg H, Pyke C, Bissell MJ, Dano K, Werb Z (1996) Two distinct phases of apoptosis in mammary gland involution: proteinase-independent and -dependent pathways. Development 122(1):181–193

29. Chen LH, Bissell MJ (1989) A novel regulatory mechanism for whey acidic protein gene expression. Cell Regul 1(1):45–54

30. Michalopoulos G, Sattler CA, Sattler GL, Pitot HC (1976) Cytochrome P-450 induction by phenobarbital and 3-methylcholanthrene in primary cultures of hepatocytes. Science 193(4256):907–909

31. Hall HG, Farson DA, Bissell MJ (1982) Lumen formation by epithelial cell lines in response to collagen overlay: a morphogenetic model in culture. Proc Natl Acad Sci U S A 79(15):4672–4676

32. Li ML, Aggeler J, Farson DA, Hatier C, Hassell J, Bissell MJ (1987) Influence of a reconstituted basement membrane and its components on casein gene expression and secretion in mouse mammary epithelial cells. Proc Natl Acad Sci U S A 84(1):136–140

33. Barcellos-Hoff MH, Aggeler J, Ram TG, Bissell MJ (1989) Functional differentiation and alveolar morphogenesis of primary mammary cultures on reconstituted basement membrane. Development 105(2):223–235

34. Gudjonsson T, Ronnov-Jessen L, Villadsen R, Rank F, Bissell MJ, Petersen OW (2002) Normal and tumor-derived myoepithelial cells differ in their ability to interact with luminal breast epithelial cells for polarity and basement membrane deposition. J Cell Sci 115(Pt 1):39–50

35. Simian M, Hirai Y, Navre M, Werb Z, Lochter A, Bissell MJ (2001) The interplay of matrix metalloproteinases, morphogens and growth factors is necessary for branching of mammary epithelial cells. Development 128(16):3117–3131

36. Fata JE, Mori H, Ewald AJ, Zhang H, Yao E, Werb Z, Bissell MJ (2007) The MAPK(ERK-1,2) pathway integrates distinct and antagonistic signals from TGFalpha and FGF7 in morphogenesis of mouse mammary epithelium. Dev Biol 306(1):193–207. doi:10.1016/j.ydbio.2007.03.013

37. Nguyen-Ngoc KV, Shamir ER, Huebner RJ, Beck JN, Cheung KJ, Ewald AJ (2015) 3D culture assays of murine mammary branching morphogenesis and epithelial invasion. Methods Mol Biol 1189:135–162. doi:10.1007/978-1-4939-1164-6-10

38. Lasfargues EY (1957) Cultivation and behavior in vitro of the normal mammary epithelium of the adult mouse. Anat Rec 127(1):117–129

39. Lasfargues EY (1957) Cultivation and behavior in vitro of the normal mammary epithelium of the adult mouse. II. Observations on the secretory activity. Exp Cell Res 13(3):553–562

40. Flynn D, Yang J, Nandi S (1982) Growth and differentiation of primary cultures of mouse mammary epithelium embedded in collagen gel. Differentiation 22(3):191–194

41. Yang J, Larson L, Flynn D, Elias J, Nandi S (1982) Serum-free primary culture of human normal mammary epithelial cells in collagen gel matrix. Cell Biol Int Rep 6(10):969–975

42. Richards J, Guzman R, Konrad M, Yang J, Nandi S (1982) Growth of mouse mammary gland end buds cultured in a collagen gel matrix. Exp Cell Res 141(2):433–443

43. Darcy KM, Black JD, Hahm HA, Ip MM (1991) Mammary organoids from immature virgin rats undergo ductal and alveolar morphogenesis when grown within a reconstituted basement membrane. Exp Cell Res 196(1):49–65

44. Hobbs AA, Richards DA, Kessler DJ, Rosen JM (1982) Complex hormonal regulation of rat casein gene expression. J Biol Chem 257(7):3598–3605

45. Pittius CW, Sankaran L, Topper YJ, Hennighausen L (1988) Comparison of the regulation of the whey acidic protein gene with that of a hybrid gene containing the whey acidic protein gene promoter in transgenic mice. Mol Endocrinol 2(11):1027–1032

46. Schoenenberger CA, Zuk A, Groner B, Jones W, Andres AC (1990) Induction of the endogenous Whey Acidic Protein (WAP) gene and a Wap-myc hybrid gene in primary murine mammary organoids. Dev Biol 139(2):327–337

47. Devinoy E, Malienou-N'Gassa R, Thepot D, Puissant C, Houdebine LM (1991) Hormone responsive elements within the upstream sequences of the rabbit Whey Acidic Protein (WAP) gene direct Chloramphenicol Acetyl Transferase (CAT) reporter gene expression in transfected rabbit mammary cells. Mol Cell Endocrinol 81(1–3):185–193

48. Nelson CM, Vanduijn MM, Inman JL, Fletcher DA, Bissell MJ (2006) Tissue geometry determines sites of mammary branching morphogenesis in organotypic cultures. Science 314(5797):298–300

49. Huebner RJ, Neumann NM, Ewald AJ (2016) Mammary epithelial tubes elongate through MAPK-dependent coordination of cell migration. Development 143(6):983–993. doi:10.1242/dev.127944

50. Vaezi A, Bauer C, Vasioukhin V, Fuchs E (2002) Actin cable dynamics and Rho/Rock orchestrate a polarized cytoskeletal architecture in the early steps of assembling a stratified epithelium. Dev Cell 3(3):367–381

51. Bianco A, Poukkula M, Cliffe A, Mathieu J, Luque CM, Fulga TA, Rorth P (2007) Two distinct modes of guidance signalling during collective migration of border cells. Nature 448(7151):362–365. doi:10.1038/nature05965

52. Lecaudey V, Gilmour D (2006) Organizing moving groups during morphogenesis. Curr Opin Cell Biol 18(1):102–107. doi:10.1016/j.ceb.2005.12.001

53. Williams KE, Lemieux GA, Hassis ME, Olshen AB, Fisher SJ, Werb Z (2016) Quantitative proteomic analyses of mammary organoids reveals distinct signatures after exposure to environmental chemicals. Proc Natl Acad Sci U S A 113(10):E1343–E1351. doi:10.1073/pnas.1600645113

54. Shamir ER, Pappalardo E, Jorgens DM, Coutinho K, Tsai WT, Aziz K, Auer M, Tran PT, Bader JS, Ewald AJ (2014) Twist1-induced dissemination preserves epithelial identity and requires E-cadherin. J Cell Biol 204(5):839–856. doi:10.1083/jcb.201306088

55. Boussadia O, Kutsch S, Hierholzer A, Delmas V, Kemler R (2002) E-cadherin is a survival factor for the lactating mouse mammary gland. Mech Dev 115(1–2):53–62

56. Badea TC, Wang Y, Nathans J (2003) A noninvasive genetic/pharmacologic strategy for visualizing cell morphology and clonal relationships in the mouse. J Neurosci 23(6):2314–2322

57. Tran PT, Shroff EH, Burns TF, Thiyagarajan S, Das ST, Zabuawala T, Chen J, Cho YJ, Luong R, Tamayo P, Salih T, Aziz K, Adam SJ, Vicent S, Nielsen CH, Withofs N, Sweet-Cordero A, Gambhir SS, Rudin CM, Felsher DW (2012) Twist1 suppresses senescence programs and thereby accelerates and maintains mutant Kras-induced lung tumorigenesis. PLoS Genet 8(5):e1002650. doi:10.1371/journal.pgen.1002650

58. Willyard C (2015) The boom in mini stomachs, brains, breasts, kidneys and more. Nature 523(7562):520–522. doi:10.1038/523520a

Biofabrication Technologies for Developing In Vitro Tumor Models

Andrea Mazzocchi, Shay Soker, and Aleksander Skardal

Abstract Despite having yielded extensive breakthroughs in cancer research, traditional 2D cell cultures have limitations in studying cancer progression and metastasis and screening therapeutic candidates. 3D systems can allow cells to grow, migrate, and interact with each other and the surrounding matrix, resulting in more realistic constructs. Furthermore, interactions between host tissue and developing tumors influence the susceptibility of tumors to drug treatments. The past decade has seen a rapid advancement of the application of 3D cellular systems to cancer research. These 3D tumor models, or tumor organoids, occupy a range of distinct form factors, each with their own strengths and weaknesses, and appropriateness for particular applications. In this chapter we highlight the major categories of tumor organoids and the methods by which they are biofabricated, aiming to provide the reader with an overview of the types of tumor organoids currently employed in cancer research applications.

Keywords Organoids • Biofabrication • Bioprinting • Tissue engineering • Tissue construct • Tumor-on-a-chip

A. Mazzocchi
Wake Forest Institute for Regenerative Medicine, Wake Forest School of Medicine, Medical Center Boulevard, Winston-Salem, NC 27157, USA

Virginia Tech-Wake Forest School of Biomedical Engineering and Sciences, Wake Forest School of Medicine, Medical Center Boulevard, Winston-Salem, NC 27157, USA

S. Soker • A. Skardal (✉)
Wake Forest Institute for Regenerative Medicine, Wake Forest School of Medicine, Medical Center Boulevard, Winston-Salem, NC 27157, USA

Virginia Tech-Wake Forest School of Biomedical Engineering and Sciences, Wake Forest School of Medicine, Medical Center Boulevard, Winston-Salem, NC 27157, USA

Department of Cancer Biology, Wake Forest School of Medicine, Medical Center Boulevard, Winston-Salem, NC 27157, USA

Comprehensive Cancer Center at Wake Forest Baptist, Wake Forest Baptist Health Sciences, Medical Center Boulevard, Winston-Salem, NC 27157, USA
e-mail: askardal@wakehealth.edu

© Springer International Publishing AG 2018   51
S. Soker, A. Skardal (eds.), *Tumor Organoids*, Cancer Drug Discovery
and Development, DOI 10.1007/978-3-319-60511-1_4

1 Introduction

Cancer research has been limited due to the inability to accurately model tumor progression and signaling mechanisms in a controlled environment. Animal models allow limited manipulation and study of these mechanisms, and are not necessarily predictive of results in humans [1]. Traditional in vitro 2D cultures fail to recapitulate the 3D microenvironment of in vivo tissues [2]. Drug diffusion kinetics vary dramatically, drug doses effective in 2D are often ineffective when scaled to patients, and cell-cell/cell-matrix interactions are inaccurate [3, 4]. Tissue culture dishes have three major differences from the tissue where the tumor was isolated: surface topography, surface stiffness, and a 2D rather than 3D architecture. As a consequence, 2D culture places a selective pressure on cells that could substantially alter their molecular and phenotypic properties. We recently demonstrated that on 2D tissue culture dishes, metastatic colorectal cancer (CRC) cells appeared epithelial, but when transitioned into a 3D liver organoid environment they "switched" to a mesenchymal and metastatic phenotype [5]. Such bioengineered platforms better mimic structure and cellular heterogeneity of in vivo tissue, and are therefore more suitable for cancer research. These models can be viable for long periods of time and develop functional properties similar to native tissues. They can also recapitulate the dynamic roles of cell–cell, cell–ECM, and mechanical interactions inside the tumor. Further incorporation of cells representative of the tumor stroma, such as endothelial cells and tumor fibroblasts, and physical matrix components, can mimic the in vivo tumor microenvironment. Thus, bioengineered tumors are an important resource for in vitro study of cancer and development of new and more effective therapies for patients in the clinic. In this chapter, we describe a variety of the technologies researchers employ to create, or biofabricate, 3D in vitro tumor models. These technologies range from the simple – cell aggregates or spheroids – to significantly more complex – bioprinted tumor constructs using extracellular matrix bioinks for example (Fig. 1).

2 Tumor Spheroids

Tumor spheroids represent perhaps some of the earliest forays into creating model systems of tumors with enhanced complexity compared to traditional 2D cell cultures on dishes or well plates. Spheroids are spherical cell aggregates formed by cell-cell adhesions during self-assembly. They are simple and generally quick to produce, thus their widespread appeal [6]. Cell spheroids are generally on the scale of several hundred microns at the maximum, as larger aggregate suffer from poor oxygen and nutrient transport into the center of the spheroid, often resulting in necrotic core regions. However, this feature can mimic necrotic core regions occasionally found in some tumors in vivo. Importantly, the 3D nature of tumor spheroids (and many of the other tumor organoid form factors discussed later) provide a

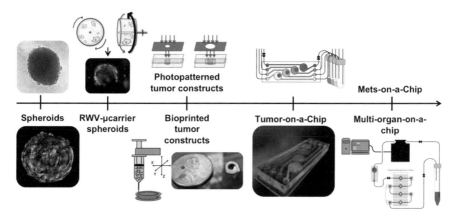

Fig. 1 Tumor organoids vary widely in complexity from simple spheroids to more complicated systems containing multiple organoids in a single platform

variety of characteristics that are superior to traditional 2D cell cultures. Spheroids allow for increased cell-cell interactions as well as interactions between cells and cell-secreted extracellular matrix (ECM) components [7]. Because of the transport limitations described above, spheroids can be used as models for testing drug diffusion kinetics. Likewise, lack of oxygen transport in larger spheroids can create hypoxic regions, which can be an important characteristic of certain types of tumors that drives a variety of end biological behaviors such as proliferation or genetic mutation. Spheroids can be comprised of a single cell population or formed using multiple cell populations, thereby providing opportunities to better model the heterogeneous nature of many tumors. All of these potential features result in model systems that often demonstrate increased chemoresistance to drugs, an outcome observed often in human patient, but less so in 2D cultures [8–10].

Generally, these types of cell-aggregated spheroids are formed using a hanging drop technique. Initially, this could be performed with no specialized equipment. Droplets of a cell suspension would be placed on the underside of a Petri dish or well plate cover and carefully flipped, resulting in drops hanging from the cover. Within these drops, with a lack of a physical substrate, cells aggregate and adhere to one another through cell-cell adhesions such as cadherins and tight junctions (Fig. 2a) [11]. This process has become more streamlined with the development of specific hanging drop plates containing wells with openings at the bottom. Cell suspensions are simply pipetted into each well, and the drop hangs through the bottom of the well. Following cell aggregation, the resulting spheroids can be collected in a 96 or 384 well plate beneath, corresponding to the wells above (Fig. 2b) [12]. More recently, researchers have begun to use ultra-low adhesion round bottom well plates to form spheroids. With the round bottom geometry of the wells, and the inability to adhere to the plastic surfaces in the wells, just as in hanging drop cultures, the cells aggregate with one another into spheroids (Fig. 2c) [13].

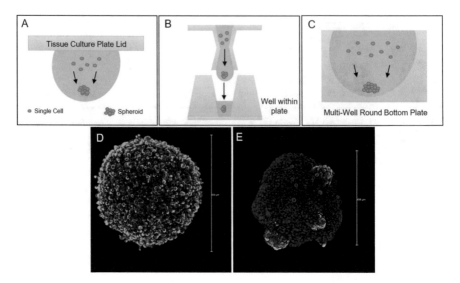

Fig. 2 Tumor spheroids. (**a**) Cells aggregate through cell-cell interactions in the hanging drop. (**b**) Hanging drop commercialized increased throughput well plate format. (**c**) Cell aggregation in round bottom plate. (**d**) Confocal image of a homogeneous mesenchymal stem cell (MSC) organoid and (**e**) a heterogeneous organoid with MSCs in *green* and BxPC3 pancreatic tumor cells in *red*

2.1   Homogeneous Spheroids

Homogeneous spheroids (Fig. 2d) are often used for the study of cancer cell self-assembly and their ability to interact with each other void of other cell types or surfaces. It has been shown that some cell types are unable to aggregate on their own, as they require additional signals or pathways unavailable through only themselves. This in itself has allowed researchers to better understand the requirements of various cancer types and the environmental factors. Surface tension has also been found to play a role in the development of tumor spheroids. This phenomenon was noticed as spheroids appeared to reduce in diameter however metabolic activity was sustained. It has been found that some cell types are more adherent to themselves than others and will form tight junctions reducing the overall size of the spheroid while maintaining a growing population. It has also been shown that over time single cell line tumor spheroids will dissociate and break apart, as they can no longer advantageously attach to each other. This too is specific to cell line and relies on external factors including how long the spheroids are kept in culture.

Drug treatments or external factors can be added to these single cell line tumor spheroids to study direct effects on the cancer aggregation. This allows for direct study of tumor cell behavior in reaction to the drug treatment when stromal cells are not present. Factors that directly influence the spheroid can also be added such as growth factors, conditioned media, or hypoxic conditions, which allow for the tumor spheroid to be better studied.

Currently, outside of academic research, pharmaceutical companies utilize spheroids in high throughput (384 well or greater) screening of compounds before advancing them to Phase I clinical trials. They have found spheroids to be advantageous because of their ability to better replicate an in vivo tumor over 2D culture and offer a platform from which more advance drug screens can be carried out.

2.2 Heterogeneous Spheroids

Heterogeneous spheroids have become of greater interest as cell types related to cancer types, but that are not necessarily tumor cells themselves, are added to improve the robustness of the model (Fig. 2E). Integration of additional cell types allows for natural cell assembly leading to more ideal replication of the tumor architecture. This self-assembly has been studied across many cancer types with numerous stromal cell additions. Tumor behavior is not uniform across all spheroids and can exhibit a variety of behaviors. The cancer cells have been shown to tightly grow together and force the stromal cells to grow as an outer shell around the center tumor spheroid, the cancer cells have also grown together with the stromal cells forming a second grouping grown together next to but attached to the tumor growth, and dispersal of the stromal cells within the tumor spheroid has also been shown. Each of these behaviors can be attributed to multiple factors including cell signaling, cell type adhesion propensity, and surface tension. Interestingly, it has been found that surface tension and cell viscosity play a role in the formation of spheroids, as the collection of cells, or the tissue itself, exhibits fluidic properties over time. This interesting phenomena occurring within the spheroids is that which contributes to cell organization or lack of organization with them. This also can play a role in the interconnection and adhesion of two spheroids grown of different cell lines that are then placed with each other to merge. Dependent on the fluidic properties of each of the cell types, they spheroids will merge in varying ways.

Drug studies are also widely preformed on co-cultured tumor spheroids offering insight into how a more complete tumor environment would react to drug. These studies can show how the tumor cells and stromal cells both behave in the presence of drug and if they play any role in the survival of each other. Heterogeneous spheroids are being further employed in applications such as body- and organ-on-a-chip where they can be placed into devices and studied with other spheroids or with drug via applied flow.

3 Biofabricated Tumor Constructs

Tumor spheroids have become a widely adopted tool for cancer biologists and engineers who wish to model cancer in 3D, using a relatively simple, yet effective methodology. However, this approach can be limited in some applications. For example, many primary tumor cells do not aggregate and self-assembly as easily. Additionally, in the body, tumors do not exist in isolation; they reside in, on, or around other tissues. Therefore, in many studies, one may wish to integrate tumor cells with an extracellular matrix (ECM)-inspired environment or a surrogate for normal tissue. In these cases a wide variety of other technologies can be employed that range in complexity. Often these approaches employ other tools such as bioreactor or microfluidic systems to create supportive environments, or utilize biomaterials such as hydrogels and other scaffolds to serve as ECM analogs.

3.1 Rotating Wall Vessel

While hanging drop cultures employ gravity and a lack of adherent surfaces to form spherical organoids, a similar form factor of organoid can be biofabricated using a lack of gravity, or rather microgravity, and inclusion of adherent surfaces. Rotating wall vessel (RWV) bioreactor culture [14–19] is an established methodology that employs a rotating bioreactor to generate low fluid shear stress rotational forces, which simulates microgravity conditions. Simulated microgravity allows cells to self-aggregate into spheroids or to nucleate around microcarrier beads for adherent suspension cultures (Fig. 3a). To date, a wide variety of tissue types have been modeled as 3D organoids using RWV technology, including lung, colon, intestine, liver, vaginal epithelium, breast, and others [14–16, 18–22].

Our team employed this technology with the help of a custom-developed hydrogel microcarrier technology [19] to create tissue-tumor hybrid organoids. This platform is built on the combination of a modular hydrogel platform [23–25], which has been demonstrated extensively in the application of biofabricating tissue and tumor organoids [5, 19]. Our team recently published a study using this platform to create 3D organoids containing a hepatic cells line, HepG2, and metastatic colorectal cancer cells, HCT116 [5]. The organoids supported HCT116 tumor cell growth over time, induced expression of in *vivo-like* mesenchymal and metastatic markers, including active signaling pathways, and responded to chemotherapeutical drugs (Fig.3b). More recently, we described new 3D liver tumor organoids comprised of more functional primary human hepatocytes, the same HCT116 colorectal cancer cells, and mesenchymal stem cells (MSC) as a surrogate for the stromal component of the liver, the liver stellate cells. We are using this tumor organoid model to observe tumor cell growth and tumor tissue maturation, and perform anti-cancer drug studies. Importantly, the cancer microenvironment is a complex space that contains stromal cells, a multitude of ECM components and proteins, as well as a plethora of signaling, paracrine, and growth factors. Together, these components of the microenvironment push and pull cancer cells between phenotypes and have a significant effect on the long-term progression of a tumor and response to therapy [26, 27]. With this platform, we were able to include a stromal component of the tissue-tumor environment in the form of MSCs. Liver-tumor organoids failed to grow in the absence of MSCs, indicating that the MSCs provide essential support for tumor growth, similar to hepatic stellate cells in liver cancer. By tracking

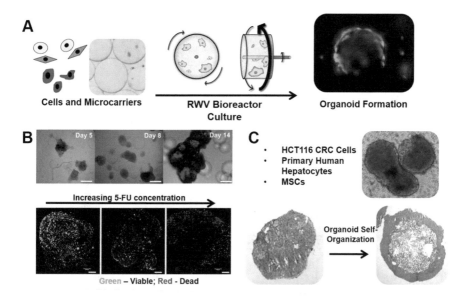

Fig. 3 Generation of tumor organoids in a rotating wall vessel (RWV) bioreactor ssytem. (**a**) AN RWV system with microcarriers supporting cell aggregation. (**b**) Using this technology, organoids can be formed such as liver organoids containing metastatic colorectal cancer cells that allow for screening of chemotherapy drugs. (**c**) Using stromal cell populations, phenomena such as self-organization into distinct stromal and tissue/tumor zones can be observed

fluorescently labeled HCT116 cells we demonstrated the active proliferation of the tumor cells when the MSCs were present. Besides supporting tumor cell growth in the liver organoids, inclusion of MSCs in these organoids resulted in tumor-like tissue organization and maturation. The MSCs migrated to the periphery of the organoid and created an organized shell-like tissue encapsulating the tumor cells and hepatocytes at the core of the organoid (Fig. 3c). Our results demonstrated not only a dose dependent response of the tumor liver organoid to a range of 5-FU drug concentrations but also that more organized organoids were less sensitive to the treatment, similar to results in many studies where the stroma can protect the tumor from therapy [28–30]. These results further demonstrate the capacity of the RWV bioreactor conditions to create a more physiologically relevant tumor models compared with tumor cells in cell culture dishes.

3.2   Three Dimensional Bioprinting

In the last decade and a half, bioprinting, once referred to as "organ printing" [31–34], has emerged as a tool with incredible potential in tissue engineering and regenerative medicine [35]. Bioprinting can be described as additive fabrication using biological building blocks that has the potential to build or pattern living 3D organ-like or tissue

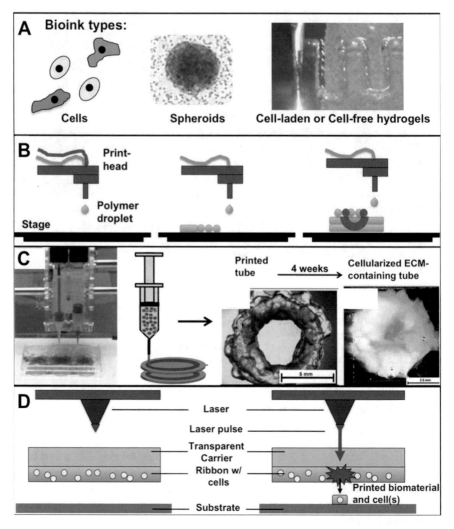

Fig. 4 Bioprinting. (**a**) Types of bioink. (**b**) Inkjet printing. (**c**) Extrusion printing. (**d**) Laser-induced forward transfer (LIFT) printing

structures [36]. In general, bioprinting employs a computer-controlled 3D printing device – the bioprinter – to accurately deposit cells and printable biomaterials into physiologically relevant biological structures. Different bioprinters have different capabilities, but generally are able to print cell aggregates, cells encapsulated in hydrogels or viscous fluids, cell-seeded microcarriers, or cell-free biomaterials – all of which can be referred to as "bioink" (Fig. 4a) [31, 37]. Biologically-derived 3D computer-aid design files, such as .stl or .dwg file formats, can be used to guide the placement of cells and bioinks into geometries that may mimic the macro-architecture of actual tissues and organs. Eventually, the ultimate goal of bioprinting is to print organs, which are subsequently matured into functional tissue constructs or organs [32, 38, 39]. To date, complete fully functional solid organs have not been printed, but this remains the primary long-term goal of bioprinting. However, small-scale tissue and tumor constructs are currently being implemented in a number of applications, including pathology modeling, drug development, and toxicology screening.

A number of bioprinting modalities exist, encompassing use of inkjet-like printers, extrusion devices, and laser-assisted devices. Inkjet printing (Fig. 4b), also refereed to as drop-by-drop bioprinting, is one bioprinting approach that is being explored for creating 3-D biological structures, that is closely related to technologies used for cell patterning. Where basic cell patterning creates a 2-D pattern comprised of cells on a surface, by incorporating a hydrogel or other cell-friendly biomaterial, 3-D cellularized structures can be fabricated drop by drop [40, 41]. Extrusion-based deposition (Fig. 4c), generally from syringe-like equipment, is an additional approach for 3-D bioprinting that relies on the mechanical and temporal properties of the polymer materials being printed. In this modality, the properties of the printed polymer or hydrogel are used to facilitate extrusion through a syringe tip, commonly driven by pneumatic pressure or mechanical pistons controlled by a computer. Laser-induced forward transfer (LIFT)-based bioprinting (Fig.4d) is a recently introduced method that has been adopted from other fields by researchers pursuing bioprinting [42, 43]. LIFT technology was initially developed for high resolution patterning of metals for use in areas such as computer chip fabrication. More recently it has been employed to create micropattern peptides, DNA, and cells. LIFT technology is comprised of a laser beam that is pulsed at desired time lengths and a donor material "ribbon" comprised of the printable material. This is supported on a transport layer such as gold or titanium that absorbs the laser energy and transfers it to the ribbon. When the laser pulses on the ribbon, the focused energy generates an incredibly small, high pressure bubble that propels a droplet of the donor material onto a collecting substrate and stage. By either moving the stage or the laser in relation to the ribbon, material can be patterned on the collecting substrate [44–46]. In the case of LIFT-based bioprinting, the ribbon may be comprised of a biopolymer or protein, and can contain cells within. In this scenario the laser pulse-driven ribbon droplets contain cells, which are then deposited in a pattern on the substrate to create cellular structures and patterns. The ability to print nearly a single cell per droplet [47], has positioned LIFT as a bioprinted modality with much potential in the future. Of these methods each has particular print speeds, resolution, cell densities, and cell viability outcomes that often must be considered when selecting a technology for a given application (Table 1) [35, 48–51].

To date, bioprinting has only for a short time been applied to generating tissue models or organoids. Some notable examples do exist, including using bioprinting to fabricate microfibrous scaffolds to support myocardium and endothelial cells as a cardiac construct in a heart-on-a-chip platform [52]. In addition, our lab has developed a tissue specific hydrogel bioink system for bioprinting that can be used to match both the elastic modulus of a select soft tissue as well as the biochemical growth factor profile of that tissue. We demonstrated this by bioprinting primary human liver organoids [53, 54]. Fewer examples exist still in which bioprinting has

Table 1 Printing parameters for different bioprinting parameters, including resultion, print speed, and cell viability

Printer type	Resolution (μm)	Print speed	Cell viability (%)
Inkjet	>300	5×10^3 drops/s	75–90
Laser – assisted	10–30	9×10^{-8} mL/s	Not available as %
LIFT	30–100	10^2 drops/	95–100
Extrusion	5 μm to millimeters	10–50 μm/s	40–80

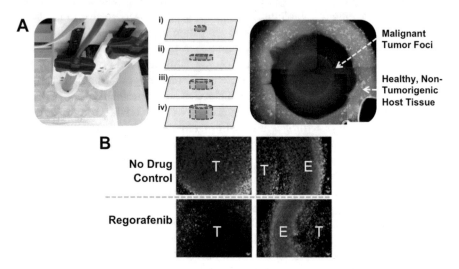

Fig. 5 Bioprinted tumor organoids. (**a**) Multi-zoned tumor organoid printing. (**b**) Biofabrication of multiple zones allows generation of more in vivo-like models, in which the tumor resides inside healthy tissue. This allows drug screens to be performed that demonstrate the capability of targeting the tumor (T), not the healthy tissue (E). In (**b**), green indicates calcein AM-stained viable cells and red indicates ethidium homodimer-stained dead cells

been employed to create tumor organoids, although there is currently work occurring in this area. For instance model systems such as a 3D ovarian cancer coculture model [55] and 3D glioma stem cell-derived brain tumor models have been bioprinted for disease modeling and testing of drug susceptibility [56]. Currently, our team is adapting a long track record of bioprinting experience and bioink development towards printing both cell line-based tumor organoids and primary patient tumor-derived models, incorporating multi-zoned printing to incorporate not only the tumor, but also healthy surrounding tissue in which the tumor resides (Fig. 5a). This is an important feature in these models, as it now allows querying the tumor targeting capabilities of drugs that might be screened. For example, we have shown recently that a broad acting chemotherapeutic agent such as 5-FU can be effective against a tumor population, but also exhibits toxicity in the normal cells surrounding the tumor. Conversely, a drug such as regorafenib that targets a specific mutation of the epidermal growth factor receptor (EGFR) pathway [57] only found in the tumor population, can be effective against the tumor, while being less toxic to the healthy cells (Fig. 5b).

3.3 *Photopatterning*

An alternative strategy for fabricating 3D tissue and tumor constructs is through photopatterning. Specifically, as more and more microfluidic organ-on-a-chip systems evolve [58, 59], strategies that allow integration of 3D constructs inside these devices are becoming more important. The limitation stems from the nature of most microfluidic devices are inherently closed systems, with no direct access to the internal channels and chambers. To address these challenges of integrating 3D cell culture with on-a-chip platforms we have developed a methodology for their in situ fabrication [19] that utilizes widely employed hydrogel biomaterials comprised of photocrosslinkable hyaluronic acid and gelatin [20, 21]. Unlike conventional materials such as collagen, Matrigel, and alginate, these materials are easily integrated with variety of biofabrication techniques, including bioprinting as described above. Furthermore, since HA and gelatin are natural components of native ECM, it provides a truly biomimetic structure in the form of crosslinked HA polysaccharide chains and cell-adherent motifs in the form of hydrolytically degraded collagen gel [23, 53]. In the general approach to fabricating cell culture constructs, HA and gelatin components are mixed with target cells, as well as a crosslinker and photoinitiator to support thiol-acrylate photopolymerization via UV exposure [22, 23]. This mixture is introduced to all microfluidic chambers for a given cell/tissue type and patterning is then performed using a positive-tone photomask to define the shape and location of one or more polymerized construct (Fig. 6a). The cross-linked hydrogel is adherent to the top and bottom surfaces of the chamber, allowing it to be retained following a wash with clean buffer. This photopatterning can be performed simultaneously in an arbitrary number of independent microfluidic chambers. The resulting 3D cell culture constructs can subsequently be kept under circulating flow with long-term viability, and the total system is amenable to analytical investigation, including direct imaging, aliquot sampling, and biochemical administration, such as drug and toxicology screens [19]. Additional patterning (e.g. with additional cell types) can also be used to produce multi-component, concentric structures as well, enabling significant tissue construct complexity to be achieved (Fig. 6b). Notably, the hydrogel platform employed in our work also supports incorporation of components derived directly from tissue ECM, employing heparin pendant changes that can immobilize ECM-derived growth factors, presenting encapsulated cells with additional biomolecular factors *specific to the tissue* [53, 54, 60, 61]. Our studies have shown that such in vitro constructs recapitulate a broad range of physiological activities and reactions observed in vivo [7, 19], highlighting the biomimetic nature of the system. This type of patterning can be used across many types of crosslinkable materials that require activation via UV or visible light and is not restricted to the HA and gelatin gels described above. UV crosslinkable materials are considered those that include thiol groups that can react with free radicals to link with other thiol groups. Versatility is restricted only by materials that are crosslinkable and allows for optimization of each tumor microenvironment being studied. Overall, this fabrication approach is rapid, inexpensive, and modular, with straightforward potential to be expanded to massively parallel investigation.

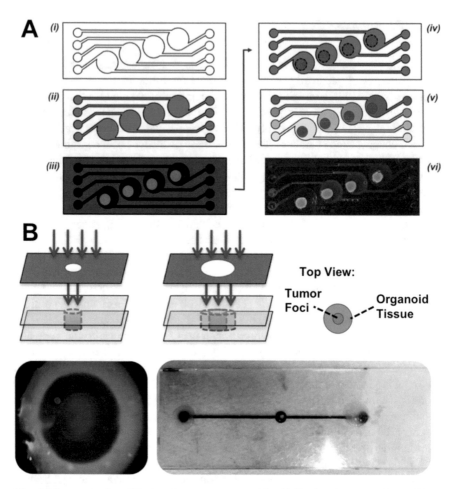

Fig. 6 Photopatterning of hydrogels to create organoids. (**a**) In situ photopatterning within a microfluidic device. A photo-crosslinkable hydrogel precursor solution with cells is injected into the device organoid chambers. A photomask is placed above with apertures allows light exposure to photopolymerize select regions. The uncrosslinked material is washed out leaving 3D organoids within the device chambers. (**b**) Multi-stage photopatterning allows biofabrication of more complex, multi-zoned structures, such as the concentric circle structure shown. These can be fabricated as incredibly small structures, such as the clear circle shown in the middle of the microfluidic device. Blue dye is used to visualize the organoid

3.4 Tumor-on-a-Chip

Further development of bioengineered organ microengineering [62, 63] combined with microfluidic device fabrication has resulted in a growing library of organ-on-a-chip technologies. These kinds of on-a-chip devices and systems can take on a wide variety of forms, from single cell analysis devices to multi-organoid housing systems that can be employed for drug testing, toxicology [64], high throughput screens

[65], and disease modeling (Fig. 7a) [66]. These platforms bring together a variety of important parameters that allow better mimicry of in vivo conditions, including 3D architecture, cell-cell/cell-matrix interactions, circulation, and integration of multiple tissues within one platform. With the biofabrication technologies previously described, tumor-on-a-chip devices can be fabricated in a multitude of ways, which allow for many devices created in parallel for high-throughput screening and research. The tumors organoids are often contained within spheroids or bioinks and placed within the devices and then sealed, resulting in contained systems, which may have open or closed fluidic perfusion. Within these systems, adequate nutrients and oxygen are supplied and external factors can be administered to treat and study the tumor. This technology has been advanced to reduce the overall size of these devices allowing for them to be produced in industry and research on plates as small as 384 wells. With these advances a greater number of studies are able to be conducted in parallel [65].

3.5 *Metastasis-on-a-Chip*

A metastasis-on-a-chip platform, comprised of tumor foci within multiple host tissue constructs, is a concept that to our knowledge has not been widely explored outside our laboratory and our collaborators' laboratories. Metastasis here, is defined as the migration of tumor cells from a primary source to a secondary tissue that is not physically connected to the source, but requires a circulatory system connecting the two sites. This is unlike the study of tumor cells simply in circulation. In the past decade, with the growth of the organ-on-a-chip field, there have also been advances in on-a-chip devices that assess specific scenarios of metastasis. For example, the Kamm group has developed a device that includes endothelium barrier tissue and an adjacent bone construct, facilitating modeling of intravasation of breast cancer cells from circulation into bone [67, 68]. Other platforms of recent years include devices for assessing the effects of interstitial pressure on cell migration [69], multi-channel microfluidic devices that aim to investigate the processes through which aggregated tumor cells migrate through a collagen gels and endothelium [70], and a platforms for increased throughput screening anti-angiogenic drugs [71]. However, there has been an obvious lack of technologies that aim to integrate both primary and metastatic sites, and the features in between (i.e. endothelium and circulatory system) in one device. To address this gap, we employed biofabricated tissue and tumor organoids integrated into a multi-chambered microfluidic device in which the chambers were connected by circulating perfusion (Fig. 7b). By providing circulating flow through the organoid system, we can achieve the dissemination of CRC cells from a colon organoid into circulation, after which metastatic cells can colonize the liver organoid downstream (Fig. 7c) [25]. This model was one the first in vitro models of metastasis recapitulating migration from a 3D primary tissue to a 3D target tissue. This is important and novel because phenotype of cells in the originating malignant tumors and metastases often vary in invasiveness due to genetic

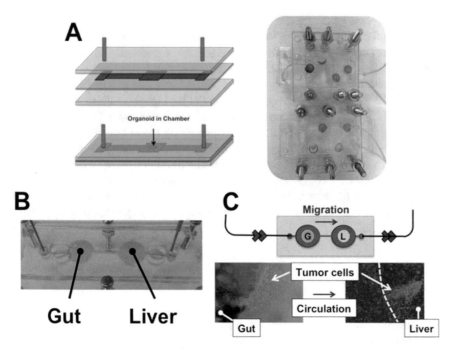

Fig. 7 Cancer-on-a-chip. (**a**) Examples of generic organ-on-a-chip devices. An organoid is housed within a chamber connected to a perfused fluidic system. Linking together of organoid chambers results in a device supporting multiple organoids onboard a single device. (**b**) A metastasis-on-a-chip device, consisting of 2 organoids for modeling colorectal cancer metastasis from the gut to liver

profiles that influence functions such as MMP secretion and stemness [72, 73]. This makes the ability to study both sites and microenvironments extremely important. Notably, we also showed that while metastatic cells metastasized in our system, less malignant non-metastatic tumor cells did not, suggesting that these types of systems can discriminate between different classes of tumors [25]. This opens up potential for new studies that can focus on the mechanistic side of metastasis, or on the other hand, facilitate screening of candidate agents with anti-metastatic properties.

4   Patient-Specific Tumor Models for Personalized Medicine

Precision oncology, whereby tumor DNA is sequenced to identify actionable gene mutations, is poised to become a standard clinical practice for therapeutic decision making of cancer treatment [74–76]. However, in practice, the utility of precision medicine is less clear [77]; even after identification of key mutations, oncologists are often left with several drug options, and for some patients there is no one definitive treatment solution, thus creating a need to further develop a model system to help predict the personalized response to anti-cancer drugs [78, 79]. Novel technologies, capable of extending the diagnostic utility of tissue specimens are critically needed for robust assessment of therapeutic biomarkers and validation of these biomarkers as actionable targets. Moreover, there is a great variability in the biologic behavior of cancer based on histologic type, grade and volume of disease. This variability is currently addressed through precision medicine analysis, by relating genetic mutations to chemotherapy options. However, the efficacy of a given treatment in a specific patient is often unknown. Within research, patient derived xenografts are also used to study patient tumor progression and drug treatment response. These models are lacking in that they require immunodeficient mice to place the biopsies or tumor samples in which causes them to become infiltrated with cells from the mouse. The cells also adapt to their new environment and genetic drift has been shown from the initial samples again making them less ideal. In the clinic, after identification of a mutation through precision medicine, given the unknown impact of the specific mutation on tumor biology and the equally unknown effect of chemotherapy options on the specific cellular phenotype, a modification of a predetermined fixed treatment strategy is a rare event. Bioengineered tumor models derived from patient tumor biospecimens may be more easily attained and less expensive than PDX models, and provide a powerful tool for screening potential therapeutic agents and determining the most efficacious and safest therapy for a particular patient. This is a very new area of tumor organoids, but is one that holds incredible potential for improving cancer patient outcomes.

Such personalized tumor models are currently being developed within our laboratory. With regular access to primary patient samples from biopsies and complete resections, we have been able to dissociate the tumor masses into single cells and use biomaterials and bioinks to biofabricate patient-specific 3D tumor organoids (Fig. 8a) that remain viable in the laboratory (Fig. 8b). Using both bioprinting and photopatterning methods, we have created platforms for testing drugs on these personalized tumor organoids. Figure 8c shows an example of such a drug screening scenario in which tumor organoids created from a gastrointestinal tumor biospecimen responded well to 5-fluorouracil and oxaliplatin (anti-proliferative agents), and regorafenib, an agent targeting a particular EGFR. However, these organoids did not respond to the combination therapy of trametinib and dabrafenib, a therapy often used to treat tumors with a different EGFR mutation profile [57]. These platforms are creating the opportunity for personalized drug treatment optimization in patients that have unclear genetic data that does not respond to standard treatments. We are also able to confirm our models by treating the patient tumor organoids with drugs that the patient responded to in the clinic. Additionally, genetic data can be paired with the patient tumor organoids to study genetic drift and relation to drug response. These tools are still being optimized but show promise for future personalized medicine applications. We anticipate one day having the technology and capabilities to determine the most effective therapy, and just as importantly, the safest therapy, for a given patient prior to any actual treatment administration in the clinic (Fig. 8d). We hope this significantly improves outcomes in patients afflicted with cancer.

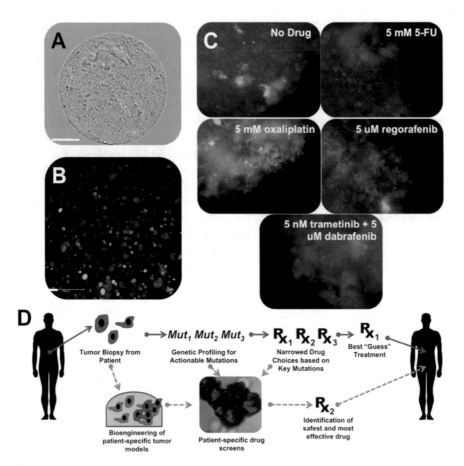

Fig. 8 Patient-derived tumor organoids for personalized medicine. (**a**) Tumor organoids comprised of patient tumor-derived cells encapsulated in 3D extracellular matrix hydrogel constructs (**b**) remain viable in culture (*Green* – viable cells; *Red* – dead cells). (**c**) An example of an in vitro drug screen using these patient-specific tumor organoids. These organoids were more responsive to 5-fluorouracil, oxaliplatin, and regorafenib than a combined treatment of trametinib and dabrafenib (*Green* – viable cells; *Red* – dead cells). (**d**) Typically, precision medicine works by using the patient tumor biospecimen to run genetic analysis with the goal being to identify actionable mutations for which there are drugs available (*red arrows*). However, often multiple mutations and drugs are identified and there is still no clear answer to which will yield the best result for the patient. Patient-specific tumor organoids (*green arrows*) can be used to supplement genetic analyses by allowing drug screens to be performed prior to administration of therapy in the patient, thereby identifying the most effective and safest drug or drug combination

5   Conclusions

Cancer research as a whole, and in particular, development of new, effective therapeutic agents, has been limited due to the inability to accurately model tumor biology, progression, and signaling mechanisms in a controlled environment. Animal models allow limited manipulation and study of these mechanisms, and are not necessarily predictive of results in humans [1]. Traditional in vitro 2D cultures fail to recapitulate the 3D microenvironment of in vivo tissues [2]. Drug diffusion kinetics vary dramatically, drug doses effective in 2D are often ineffective when scaled to patients, and cell-cell/cell-matrix interactions are inaccurate [3, 4]. Furthermore, 2D tissue culture dishes have three major differences from the tissue where the tumor was isolated: surface topography, surface stiffness, and a 2D rather than 3D architecture, which can force alterations of their molecular and phenotypic properties. Bioengineered tumor organoid technologies provide an immense opportunity to change how researchers study cancer and design studies aimed at identifying new treatment options for patients. As described in this chapter, tumor organoids vary greatly in geometry and form factor, cellularity, which combinations of cells are present if more than one population is utilized, inclusion and composition of extracellular matrix components, and how the organoids are formed or biofabricated. Having worked with the range of these organoid types, our philosophy is that no single platform is necessarily the best overarching superior technology. For instance, hanging drop spheroids are simple and inexpensive to fabricate, but often lack in complexity. Conversely, bioprinted tissue-tumor hybrid constructs in a metastasis-on-a-chip system may offer the most complexity in terms of recapitulating cell-matrix interactions, circulation, and multiple tissue sites, but may at this point in time be more difficult to run in a high throughput setting. As such, the different tumor organoid types described here can provide a toolset for researchers, from which a particular organoid form factor can be drawn to address a particular problem or ask a particular question. Nevertheless, tumor organoid technology as a whole provides a significantly improved platform for cancer research compared to traditional approaches, and will in all likelihood continue to advance in a rapid pace in the near future.

References

1. Bhattacharya S, Zhang Q, Carmichael PL, Boekelheide K, Andersen ME (2011) Toxicity testing in the 21 century: defining new risk assessment approaches based on perturbation of intracellular toxicity pathways. PLoS One 6:e20887
2. Kunz-Schughart LA, Freyer JP, Hofstaedter F, Ebner R (2004) The use of 3-D cultures for high-throughput screening: the multicellular spheroid model. J Biomol Screen 9:273–285
3. Ho WJ et al (2010) Incorporation of multicellular spheroids into 3-D polymeric scaffolds provides an improved tumor model for screening anticancer drugs. Cancer Sci 101:2637–2643
4. Drewitz M et al (2011) Towards automated production and drug sensitivity testing using scaffold-free spherical tumor microtissues. Biotechnol J 6:1488–1496
5. Skardal A, Devarasetty M, Rodman C, Atala A, Soker S (2015) Liver-tumor hybrid Organoids for modeling tumor growth and drug response in vitro. Ann Biomed Eng 43:2361–2373
6. Mehta G, Hsiao AY, Ingram M, Luker GD, Takayama S (2012) Opportunities and challenges for use of tumor spheroids as models to test drug delivery and efficacy. J Control Release 164:192–204

7. Hirschhaeuser F et al (2010) Multicellular tumor spheroids: an underestimated tool is catching up again. J Biotechnol 148:3–15
8. Torisawa YS, Takagi A, Shiku H, Yasukawa T, Matsue TA (2005) Multicellular spheroid-based drug sensitivity test by scanning electrochemical microscopy. Oncol Rep 13:1107–1112
9. Kelm JM, Fussenegger M (2004) Microscale tissue engineering using gravity-enforced cell assembly. Trends Biotechnol 22:195–202
10. Lin RZ, Chang HY (2008) Recent advances in three-dimensional multicellular spheroid culture for biomedical research. Biotechnol J 3:1172–1184
11. Amann A et al (2014) Development of an innovative 3D cell culture system to study tumour–stroma interactions in non-small cell lung cancer cells. PLoS One 9:e92511
12. Messner S, Agarkova I, Moritz W, Kelm JM (2013) Multi-cell type human liver microtissues for hepatotoxicity testing. Arch Toxicol 87:209–213
13. Ivanov DP et al (2014) Multiplexing spheroid volume, resazurin and acid phosphatase viability assays for high-throughput screening of tumour spheroids and stem cell neurospheres. PLoS One 9:e103817
14. Barrila J et al (2010) Organotypic 3D cell culture models: using the rotating wall vessel to study host-pathogen interactions. Nat Rev Microbiol 8:791–801
15. Carterson AJ et al (2005) A549 lung epithelial cells grown as three-dimensional aggregates: alternative tissue culture model for Pseudomonas Aeruginosa pathogenesis. Infect Immun 73:1129–1140
16. Honer zu Bentrup K et al (2006) Three-dimensional organotypic models of human colonic epithelium to study the early stages of enteric salmonellosis. Microbes Infect 8:1813–1825
17. Nickerson CA, Ott CM (2004) A new dimension in modeling infectious disease. ASM News 70:169–175
18. Nickerson CA, Richter EG, Ott CM (2007) Studying host-pathogen interactions in 3-D: organotypic models for infectious disease and drug development. J Neuroimmune Pharmacol 2:26–31
19. Skardal A, Sarker SF, Crabbe A, Nickerson CA, Prestwich GD (2010) The generation of 3-D tissue models based on hyaluronan hydrogel-coated microcarriers within a rotating wall vessel bioreactor. Biomaterials 31:8426–8435
20. Barrila J et al (2010) 3-D cell culture models: innovative and predictive platforms for studying human disease pathways and drug design. Nat Rev Microbiol 8:791–801
21. Hjelm BE, Berta AN, Nickerson CA, Arntzen CJ, Herbst-Kralovetz MM (2010) Development and characterization of a three-dimensional organotypic human vaginal epithelial cell model. Biol Reprod 82:617–627
22. Nickerson CA et al (2001) Three-dimensional tissue assemblies: novel models for the study of salmonella enterica serovar Typhimurium pathogenesis. Infect Immun 69:7106–7120
23. Skardal A, Zhang J, Prestwich GD (2010) Bioprinting vessel-like constructs using hyaluronan hydrogels crosslinked with tetrahedral polyethylene glycol tetracrylates. Biomaterials 31:6173–6181
24. Serban MA, Prestwich GD (2008) Modular extracellular matrices: solutions for the puzzle. Methods 45:93–98
25. Skardal A, Devarasetty M, Forsythe SD, Atala A, Soker S (2016) A reductionist metastasis-on-a-chip platform for in vitro tumor progression modeling and drug screening. Biotechnol Bioeng 113(9):2020–2032
26. Fidler IJ, Kim SJ, Langley RR (2007) The role of the organ microenvironment in the biology and therapy of cancer metastasis. J Cell Biochem 101:927–936
27. Langley RR, Fidler IJ (2007) Tumor cell-organ microenvironment interactions in the pathogenesis of cancer metastasis. Endocr Rev 28:297–321
28. Majidinia M, Yousefi B (2017) Breast tumor stroma: a driving force in the development of resistance to therapies. Chem Biol Drug Des 89(3):309–318
29. Dauer P, Nomura A, Saluja A, Banerjee S (2017) Microenvironment in determining chemoresistance in pancreatic cancer: neighborhood matters. Pancreatology 17:7–12
30. Bar-Natan M et al (2017) Bone marrow stroma protects myeloma cells from cytotoxic damage via induction of the oncoprotein MUC1. Br J Haematol 176(6):929–938

31. Mironov V, Boland T, Trusk T, Forgacs G, Markwald RR (2003) Organ printing: computer-aided jet-based 3D tissue engineering. Trends Biotechnol 21:157–161
32. Mironov V, Kasyanov V, Drake C, Markwald RR (2008) Organ printing: promises and challenges. Regen Med 3:93–103
33. Mironov V et al (2009) Organ printing: tissue spheroids as building blocks. Biomaterials 30:2164–2174
34. Prestwich GD (2007) Organ printing. Chem Biol 2:B33–B40
35. Murphy SV, Atala A (2014) 3D bioprinting of tissues and organs. Nat Biotechnol 32:773–785
36. Visconti RP et al (2010) Towards organ printing: engineering an intra-organ branched vascular tree. Expert Opin Biol Ther 10:409–420
37. Fedorovich NE et al (2007) Hydrogels as extracellular matrices for skeletal tissue engineering: state-of-the-art and novel application in organ printing. Tissue Eng 13:1905–1925
38. Boland T, Mironov V, Gutowska A, Roth EA, Markwald RR (2003) Cell and organ printing 2: fusion of cell aggregates in three-dimensional gels. Anat Rec A Discov Mol Cell Evol Biol 272:497–502
39. Derby B (2012) Printing and prototyping of tissues and scaffolds. Science 338:921–926
40. Catros S et al (2011) Laser-assisted bioprinting for creating on-demand patterns of human osteoprogenitor cells and nano-hydroxyapatite. Biofabrication 3:025001
41. Guillotin B, Guillemot F (2011) Cell patterning technologies for organotypic tissue fabrication. Trends Biotechnol 29:183–190
42. Bohandy J, Kim B, Adrian F (1986) Metal deposition from a supported metal film using an excimer laser. J Appl Phys 60:1538
43. Barron JA, Ringeisen BR, Kim H, Spargo BJ, Chrisey DB (2004) Application of laser printing to mammalian cells. Thin Solid Films 453:383–387
44. Chrisey DB (2000) MATERIALS PROCESSING: the power of direct writing. Science 289:879–881
45. Colina M, Serra P, Fernandez-Pradas JM, Sevilla L, Morenza JL (2005) DNA deposition through laser induced forward transfer. Biosens Bioelectron 20:1638–1642
46. Dinca V et al (2008) Directed three-dimensional patterning of self-assembled peptide fibrils. Nano Lett 8:538–543
47. Guillotin B et al (2010) Laser assisted bioprinting of engineered tissue with high cell density and microscale organization. Biomaterials 31:7250–7256
48. Holzl K et al (2016) Bioink properties before, during and after 3D bioprinting. Biofabrication 8:032002
49. Skardal A, Atala A (2015) Biomaterials for integration with 3-d bioprinting. Ann Biomed Eng 43:730–746
50. Li J, Chen M, Fan X, Zhou H (2016) Recent advances in bioprinting techniques: approaches, applications and future prospects. J Transl Med 14:271
51. Malda J et al (2013) 25th anniversary article: engineering hydrogels for biofabrication. Adv Mater 25:5011–5028
52. Zhang YS et al (2016) Bioprinting 3D microfibrous scaffolds for engineering endothelialized myocardium and heart-on-a-chip. Biomaterials 110:45–59
53. Skardal A et al (2015) A hydrogel bioink toolkit for mimicking native tissue biochemical and mechanical properties in bioprinted tissue constructs. Acta Biomater 25:24–34
54. Skardal A et al (2016) Bioprinting Cellularized constructs using a tissue-specific hydrogel Bioink. J Vis Exp (110):e53606
55. Xu F et al (2011) A three-dimensional in vitro ovarian cancer coculture model using a high-throughput cell patterning platform. Biotechnol J 6:204–212
56. Dai X, Ma C, Lan Q, Xu T (2016) 3D bioprinted glioma stem cells for brain tumor model and applications of drug susceptibility. Biofabrication 8:045005
57. Tran NH et al (2015) Precision medicine in colorectal cancer: the molecular profile alters treatment strategies. Ther Adv Med Oncol 7:252–262
58. Bhise NS et al (2014) Organ-on-a-chip platforms for studying drug delivery systems. J Control Release 190:82–93
59. Esch EW, Bahinski A, Huh D (2015) Organs-on-chips at the frontiers of drug discovery. Nat Rev Drug Discov 14:248–260

60. Skardal A et al (2016) A tunable hydrogel system for long-term release of cell-secreted cytokines and bioprinted in situ wound cell delivery. J Biomed Mater Res B Appl Biomater

61. Skardal A et al (2012) Tissue specific synthetic ECM hydrogels for 3-D in vitro maintenance of hepatocyte function. Biomaterials 33:4565–4575

62. Huh D, Hamilton GA, Ingber DE (2011) From 3D cell culture to organs-on-chips. Trends Cell Biol 21:745–754

63. Ghaemmaghami AM, Hancock MJ, Harrington H, Kaji H, Khademhosseini A (2012) Biomimetic tissues on a chip for drug discovery. Drug Discov Today 7(3–4):173–181

64. Skardal A, Devarasetty M, Soker S, Hall AR (2015) In situ patterned micro 3D liver constructs for parallel toxicology testing in a fluidic device. Biofabrication 7:031001

65. Phan DT et al (2017) A vascularized and perfused organ-on-a-chip platform for large-scale drug screening applications. Lab Chip 17:511–520

66. Skardal A, Shupe T, Atala A (2016) Organoid-on-a-chip and body-on-a-chip systems for drug screening and disease modeling. Drug Discov Today 21:1399–1411

67. Bersini S et al (2014) A microfluidic 3D in vitro model for specificity of breast cancer metastasis to bone. Biomaterials 35:2454–2461

68. Bersini S, Jeon JS, Moretti M, Kamm RD (2014) In vitro models of the metastatic cascade: from local invasion to extravasation. Drug Discov Today 19:735–742

69. Polacheck WJ, German AE, Mammoto A, Ingber DE, Kamm RD (2014) Mechanotransduction of fluid stresses governs 3D cell migration. Proc Natl Acad Sci U S A 111:2447–2452

70. Niu Y, Bai J, Kamm RD, Wang Y, Wang C (2014) Validating antimetastatic effects of natural products in an engineered microfluidic platform mimicking tumor microenvironment. Mol Pharm 11:2022–2029

71. Kim C, Kasuya J, Jeon J, Chung S, Kamm RD (2015) A quantitative microfluidic angiogenesis screen for studying anti-angiogenic therapeutic drugs. Lab Chip 15:301–310

72. Karakiulakis G et al (1997) Increased type IV collagen-degrading activity in metastases originating from primary tumors of the human colon. Invasion Metastasis 17:158–168

73. Franci C et al (2013) Biomarkers of residual disease, disseminated tumor cells, and metastases in the MMTV-PyMT breast cancer model. PLoS One 8:e58183

74. Glade Bender J, Verma A, Schiffman JD (2015) Translating genomic discoveries to the clinic in pediatric oncology. Curr Opin Pediatr 27:34–43

75. Andre F et al (2014) Prioritizing targets for precision cancer medicine. Ann Oncol: official journal of the European Society for Medical Oncology / ESMO 25:2295–2303

76. Roychowdhury S, Chinnaiyan AM (2014) Translating genomics for precision cancer medicine. Annu Rev Genomics Hum Genet 15:395–415

77. Hayes DF, Schott AF (2015) Personalized medicine: genomics trials in oncology. Trans Am Clin Climatol Assoc 126:133–143

78. Cantrell MA, Kuo CJ (2015) Organoid modeling for cancer precision medicine. Genome Med 7:32

79. Gao D et al (2014) Organoid cultures derived from patients with advanced prostate cancer. Cell 159:176–187

Three Dimensional In Vitro *Tumor* Platforms for Cancer Discovery

Manasa Gadde, Dan Marrinan, Rhys J. Michna, and Marissa Nichole Rylander

Abstract Traditional experimental platforms to study cancer biology consist of two-dimensional (2D) cell culture systems and animal models. Although 2D cell cultures have yielded fundamental insights into cancer biology, they do not provide a physiologically representative three-dimensional (3D) volume for cell attachment and infiltration. These systems also cannot recapitulate critical features of the tumor microenvironment including hemodynamics, matrix mechanics, cellular crosstalk, and matrix interactions in a dynamic manner, or impose chemical and mechanical gradients. While animal models provide physiologic fidelity, they can be highly variable and cost prohibitive for extensive biological investigation and therapeutic optimization. Furthermore, the interplay of many different microenvironmental variables, such as growth factors, immune reaction, and stromal interactions, make it difficult to isolate the effect of a specific stimulus on cell response using animal models. Due to these limitations, 3D in vitro tumor models have recently emerged as valuable tools for the study of cancer progression as these systems have the ability to overcome many of the limitations of static 2D monolayers and mammalian systems. Initial 3D in vitro models have consisted of static 3D co-culture platforms and have been successful in providing a deeper insight compared to animal and static 2D systems. However, the majority of these existing systems lack the presence of physiological flow, a pivotal stimuli in tumor growth and metastasis and

M. Gadde
Department of Biomedical Engineering, The University of Texas at Austin,
Austin, TX 78712, USA
e-mail: mgadde@utexas.edu

D. Marrinan • R.J. Michna
Department of Mechanical Engineering, The University of Texas at Austin,
Austin, TX 78712, USA
e-mail: dan.marrinan@gmail.com; michnarhys@utexas.edu

M.N. Rylander (✉)
Department of Biomedical Engineering, The University of Texas at Austin,
Austin, TX 78712, USA

Department of Mechanical Engineering, The University of Texas at Austin,
Austin, TX 78712, USA
e-mail: mnr@austin.utexas.edu

© Springer International Publishing AG 2018
S. Soker, A. Skardal (eds.), *Tumor Organoids*, Cancer Drug Discovery
and Development, DOI 10.1007/978-3-319-60511-1_5

71

important consideration for transport of diagnostic or therapeutic agents. In order to consider the influence of flow on cancer progression microfluidic platforms are being widely used. The integration of microfluidic technology and microfabrication techniques with tumor biology has resulted in complex 3D microfluidic platforms capable of investigating various key stages in cancer evolution including angiogenesis and metastasis. 3D microfluidic platforms are able to provide a physiologically representative tumor environment while allowing for dynamic monitoring and simultaneous control of multiple factors such as cellular and extracellular matrix composition, fluid velocity and wall shear stress, and both biochemical and mechanical gradients.

Keywords Collagen type I • Tumor platform • Tumor microenvironment • 3D model • Microfluidics • Angiogenesis • Sprouting • Endothelial • 3D cell culture • In vitro • Tumor model

1   Collagen Characterization for the Use of Tumor Platform

It is well known that three dimensional (3D) cell culture platforms have numerous advantages over their two dimensional (2D) cell monolayer counterparts, as they more accurately represent the tumor environment in vivo [1–4]. Extracellular matrix (ECM) protein collagen I, sourced from tissue, has been widely used for 3D tissue engineering scaffolds and cell culture materials due to its capacity to promote cell adhesion, growth, and proliferation [5–11]. However, challenges arise when collagen hydrogels are used to mimic specific native tissue and ECM properties. Traditionally, gels fabricated from collagen type I for tissue engineering scaffolds possess highly variable material properties as compared to synthetic ECM materials, with these properties being dependent on a number of fabrication parameters [7, 12–14]. Tight control over a broad range of parameters such as collagen source, method of solubilization, polymerization pH and temperature, ionic strength, and concentration of collagen could result in consistently reproducible hydrogel properties. However, the relationship between each of the key fabrication parameters and the functional properties (e.g. matrix stiffness, pore size, fiber structure) of these platforms have not been thoroughly investigated to sufficiently establish a robust methodology for creating platforms that mimic specific tissue microenvironments. These properties and methods for their characterization have been reviewed by the Rylander group [15]. Figure 1 summarizes the wide variability in the distribution of collagen sourcing, collagen extraction methods, and stock collagen concentrations that result from various isolation techniques. Collagen concentrations in the range of 1–5 mg/mL are most commonly used, however, these concentrations are lower than the collagen content of many native tissues [16, 17]. Many types of disease, particularly cancer, can be described using relationships between tissue elasticity and cell response where increased matrix stiffness, together with greater collagen content, is a common trait of many tumors [31, 18, 19].

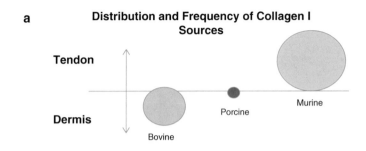

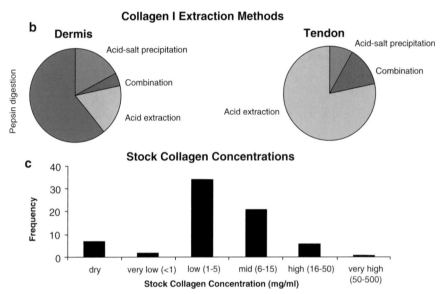

Fig. 1 Synopsis of collagen I sources and solubilization methods. (**a**) Source tissue compared with source animal; (**b**) extraction methods as compared with source tissue; (**c**) collagen concentraton in stock solutions [15]

Other factors that influence hydrogel properties are polymerization temperature and pH at which self-assembly of collagen molecules occurs. Polymerization at high temperatures results in less-ordered structures while low-temperatures create desirable pore sizes for cell proliferation [18, 19]. Elevating pH has been shown to increase collagen gel modulus but there is a decrease in cell viability outside the pH range of 7.4–8.4 [11, 22–26]. Figure 2 shows a summary of established relationships, correlating fabrication parameters and material properties [15]. This figure shows the apparent complexity and breadth of fabrication-property relationships, and it demonstrates the areas where relationships are unknown/unclear/contradictory and need further investigation and characterization. Specifically, the relationships between polymerization temperature and several mechanical properties (compression modulus, tension modulus, shear modulus) and between collagen concentration and fiber diameter require more exploration.

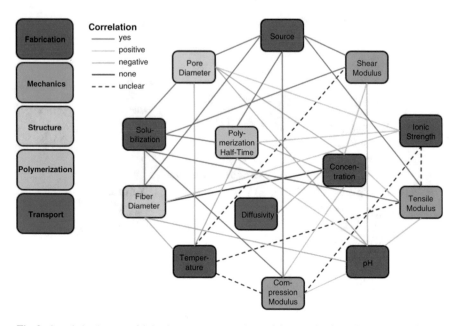

Fig. 2 Correlation between fabrication parameters and material properties for collagen hydrogels [15]

Fiber structure and scaffold stiffness are significant features of engineered cell 3D constructs, as they influence cell membrane stiffness, adhesion, differentiation, morphology, and migration [10, 11, 21, 27–35]. Because of the range of collagen hydrogel fabrication protocols, uniform characterization methods and reproducible material characteristics are needed to create predictable tissue models. In the literature, there is generally poor agreement among quantitative mechanical measurements due to differences in hydrogel fabrication parameters. The Rylander group has extensively characterized collagen type I hydrogels, correlating physiological material and transport properties (stiffness, pore and fiber diameter, diffusivity) and fabrication parameters with the intent of designing hydrogels with matching properties of target tissues. The fabrication parameters that were varied in this study were: (1) collagen concentration, (2) polymerization temperature, and (3) polymerization pH. To study the transport properties of collagen hydrogels, fluorescently tagged dextran of varying hydrodynamic radii comparable to cytokines and other bioactive molecules were used [36].

As one would expect, increased collagen concentration resulted in faster initiation of polymerization but there were no significant relationships between polymerization kinetics and pH. With regard to mechanical properties, experiments showed an increased compression modulus with all three fabrication parameters as shown in Fig. 3a. Hydrogels polymerized at low temperature (Fig. 3b:a, b) exhibited more

Fig. 3 (continued) (**c**) Pore and fiber diameter of collagen hydrogels in relation to fabrication parameters: polymerization pH, polymerization temperature, and absolute collagen concentration. *Blue* markers with dashed lines represent hydrogels polymerized at 23 °C while *red* markers with *solid lines* represent hydrogels polymerized at 37 °C. Data shown are mean + SE with N = 12. Significance was calculated for pH-averaged groups. At each concentration, the difference between means at T-23 °C and T = 37 °C is significant at p < 0.0001 for both fiber diameter and pore diameter [36]

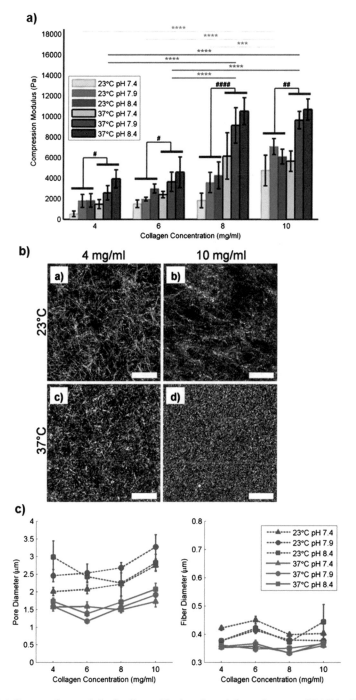

Fig. 3 (**a**) Compression moduli of collagen I hydrogels at deformation rate of 0.1%/s. *Blue bars* with *dashed lines* indicate hydrogels polymerized at 23 °C, and *red bars* with *solid lines* indicate hydrogels polymerized at 37 °C. pH is depicted as color saturation. Data shown are mean + SE with N = 4–16 per bar. Significance was calculated for pH-averaged groups (N = 12–48) as indicated by horizontal black bars. Temperature means comparison is indicated with # while hydrodynamic radius means comparison is indicated with *. (**b**) Fiber structure images obtained using confocal reflectance microscopy. Images shown are for hydrogels polymerized at pH 7.4. Scale bar is 25 μm.

network-like structures while high temperature polymerized hydrogels (Fig. 3b:c, d) resulted in evenly distributed fibers with decreased mesh size. All variations of fabrication parameters and the effects on fiber structure are summarized in Fig. 3c. Diffusivity was largely influenced by hydrodynamic radii of diffusing molecules, with the effects of fabrication parameters made negligible compared to sizes of fluorescent dextran molecules. This study not only illuminated relationships between fabrication parameters and collagen material properties, but these relationships were also used to generate a set of empirical equations that could be applied when designing and optimizing tissue models as shown in Table 1 [36].

2   3D In Vitro Collagen Tumor Models

2D cell monolayers are unable to truly recapitulate the dynamic tumor microenvironment (TME), as they do not incorporate accurate architectural features and critical cell-cell and cell-matrix interactions [37–41]. 3D cell culture models have provided significant insight regarding the role of the TME on tumor growth and development [17, 42–48]. Fischbach, *et al.* have established a number of 3D in vitro tumor models using both native and synthetic polymeric materials for tissue scaffolds [17, 42, 48]. These tumor constructs have shown angiogenic growth factor secretion and drug responsiveness, effects of oxygen tension within tumors and 3D cell-ECM interactions on angiogenic potential, and remodeling of collagen type I ECM by endothelial cells in response to release of angiogenic factors from cancer cells.

A bioengineered collagen type I tumor model developed by the Rylander group is representative of the pre-vascularized stage of solid tumor progression [49]. This stage of tumor growth is characterized by altered TME properties such as uninhibited proliferation, a necrotic core surrounded by hypoxic regions, and activation of genetic factors that lead to the recruitment of local endothelial cells for promoting angiogenesis [50–53]. Hypoxia, an oxygen deficient environment, occurs at a distance of 100 to 200 μm from the nearest vessel. Cells in the core of a growing tumor mass that cannot adapt to hypoxic conditions begin to undergo apoptosis, forming a necrotic core as shown in Fig. 4a. Hypoxia-inducible factor (HIF)-1α is a key marker for hypoxia [50, 53]; HIF-1α is a heterodimeric transcription factor that is protected from degradation when hypoxic levels are reached in the surrounding tissue. Tumors react to the altered hypoxic stress in the TME by progressing from a pre-vascularized to a vascularized state, inducing an angiogenic response. During this progression, tumor cells secrete cytokines and growth factors (e.g. vascular endothelial growth factor A, VEGF-A) that stimulate vascular sprouting and neo-vascularization from proximate endothelial cells [54].

In the bioengineered collagen type I tumor model developed by the Rylander group described in the previous paragraph, MDA-MB-231 breast cancer cells were seeded in collagen type I (8 mg/mL) hydrogel constructs for 7 days as shown in Fig. 4b. By day 3 in culture in the hydrogels, cells developed a stellate, elongated morphology with disorganized nuclei, and by day 7, cells proliferated and aggregated into 3D clusters, exhibiting cell-cell and cell matrix interactions representative

Table 1 Shows the sensitivity of significant hydrogel properties to fabrication parameters

Polymerization half-time ($R^2 = 0.565$)

	C	T	pH
C	−0.78	0.79	–
T	0.79	−1	–
pH	–	–	–

Compression modulus ($R^2 = 0.504$)

	C	T	pH
C	1	–	–
T	–	0.48	–
pH	–	–	0.39

Pore diameter ($R^2 = 0.332$)

	C	T	pH
C	0.40	–	–
T	–	−1	–
pH	–	–	0.27

Diffusivity ($R^2 = 0.867$)

	C	T	pH	r_H^{-1}
C	−0.11	–	–	–
T	–	−0.002	–	–
pH	–	–	−0.03	0.37
r_H^{-1}	–	–	0.37	1

C concentration in mg/mL, *T* temperature in °C, and r_H hydrodynamic radius in nm

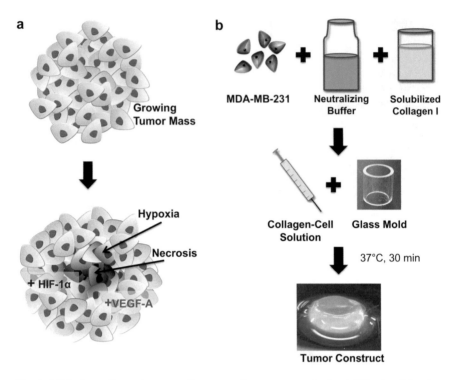

Fig. 4 (**a**) Regions of hypoxia surrounding a necrotic core, as a result of uninhibited proliferation of tumor cells during pre-vascularized stages of in vitro solid tumor development. (**b**) Bioengineered in vitro solid tumor platform consisting of collagen I hydrogels cultured with MBA-MB-231 human breast cancer cells [49]

of in vivo behavior [49]. Cell seeding density (1 or 4 million cells/mL) and scaffold thickness (1.5 or 3 mm) were varied with the intent to promote the development of hypoxia and necrosis via diffusion limitations for oxygen and nutrients. Figure 5 shows the effects of cell seeding density on the nutrient and oxygen availability at depths greater than 150 to 200 μm from the surface of the hydrogels, where cells are in direct contact with oxygenated media. In the hydrogels with 4 million cells/mL density, large amounts of dead cells (stained with propidium iodide) were present at this depth, followed by a space containing no visible cells. The complete absence of cells in this void could be due to cells migrating to the outer boundary to be in closer proximity to oxygen and nutrients. Alternatively, since propidium iodide is a nuclear stain, the void could be indicative of DNA degradation in dead cells nearest the center [55].

To demonstrate that hypoxia is an identifiable precursor to cell death, high-density cell constructs (4 million cell/mL in 3 mm thick hydrogels) were used to induce formation of a necrotic core. Immunofluorescence imaging of HIF-1α was performed to assess intracellular levels of hypoxia. HIF-1α was detected on day 1 with increasing intensity by day 5, attributed to tumor cell proliferation and the subsequent increase in competition for oxygen. It is assumed that cell access to oxygen and nutrients in confined 3D constructs is more difficult than 2D cell monolayers.

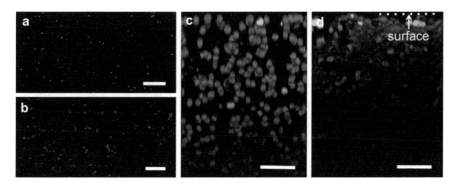

Fig. 5 (**a**) Day 1 of MDA-MB-231 cells that were seeded at 1 million cells/ml in collagen hydrogels. Cells were evenly distributed throughout the hydrogel. (**b**) On day 5, cells show significant proliferation and formation of 3D clusters. (**c**) Cell seeding density was increased to 4 million cells/ml, and on day 1, viable cells (*green*) were evenly distributed throughout the gel with few dead cells (*red*). (**d**) On day 5, the higher-density cell constructs showed viability through 150–200 μm depth below the surface, with limiations in oxygen and nutrients resulting in cell death toward the core of the bioengineered tumor platforms. Scale bars are 250 μm (**a, b**) and 100 μm (**c, d**) ([49])

Therefore, measurable amounts of HIF-1α on day 1 confirm the hypoxic cell reaction to being cultured in 3D. When cells were seeded in 3 mm thick constructs containing 4 million cells/mL, HIF-1α gene expression, analyzed using quantitative RT-PCR, was upregulated on days 3 and 5. By day 7, there was a decrease in HIF-1α expression, attributed to hypoxic cells dying from deficient oxygen and nutrient availability. VEGF-A expression was upregulated on days 3, 5, and 7 compared to day 0, but expression decreased between days 5 and 7. This decrease was likely an effect of down regulation of HIF-1α observed on day 7. When cells were seeded in 3 mm thick constructs at a lower density of 1 million cells/mL, the competition for nutrients and oxygen was alleviated. This led to an initial down regulation of HIF-1α and eventual upregulation of VEGF-A. Expression of HIF-1α was upregulated on days 3 and 5 compared to day 1, and on day 7 compared to day 0. Both HIF-1α and VEGF-A gene expression peaked at day 5 in the high-density (4 million cells/mL) constructs, but in the low-density (1 million cells/mL) constructs, constant upregulation of both markers was observed over the 7-day period [49]. Increased VEGF-A expression is a strong indicator of angiogenic potential in tumors, and a key aspect of tumor maturation is VEGF-A inducement of endothelial cells to promote tumor vascularization [54, 56]. After decreasing scaffold thickness to 1.5 mm while maintaining high-density cell seeding of 4 million cells/mL, no significant upregulation of either HIF-1α or VEGF-A was detected on any day compared to day 0. The reduced thickness diminished diffusion limitations of oxygen and nutrients. This 3D bioengineered tumor model was representative of the pre-vascularized stage of solid tumor progression, and led to the development of multilayered, co-cultured tumor constructs demonstrating the angiogenic and neovascularization processes when cancer cells interacted with endothelial cells [57].

Fig. 6 Bilayer collagen type I hydrogel composed of a collagen type I hydrogel with breast cancer cells on the bottom and an acellular collagen type I hydrogel seeded with TIME cells on top. The bilayer collagen type I hydrogel is housed in a transwell system

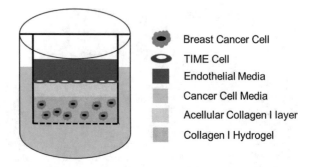

The Rylander group has also developed a 3D bilayer vascular tumor platform to investigate the importance of matrix properties, cell-cell interactions, and growth factors on promoting and supporting angiogenesis [57]. The tumor platform is a bilayer collagen type I hydrogel in which the bottom layer is composed of 8 mg/mL collagen type I seeded with MDA-MB-231 (highly aggressive) or MCF7 (less aggressive) breast cancer cells. The top layer of the platform is an acellular hydrogel composed of collagen type I with telomerase immortalized endothelial (TIME) cells seeded on top as shown in Fig. 6. The acellular region in the bilayer hydrogel was deemed necessary by preliminary studies which showed direct contact between tumor and endothelial cells lead to apoptosis of endothelial cells [58–60]. The bilayer collagen hydrogel was housed in a transwell system allowing for separation of media components for the various cell types and ensures TIME cells from being exposed to the acidic metabolites and wastes generated by the MDA-MB-231 or MCF7 cells. The following parameters in Table 2 were varied by the Rylander group to determine the cellular and matrix properties that influence angiogenesis in a co-culture of TIME and breast cancer cells.

To determine if tumor cells could elicit an angiogenic response from the TIME cells without any exogenous growth factors, TIME cells were grown in 3D bilayer tumor platforms with either MDA-MB-231 or MCF7 cells on either 2, 4, or 8 mg/ mL acellular collagen layers as illustrated in Fig. 6. To remove the influence of exogenous growth factors, TIME cells were cultured in endothelial growth media (EGM) that did not include traditional supplements of vascular endothelial growth factor (VEGF) and basic fibroblast growth factor (bFGF) (promoters of angiogenesis). In both co-culture groups, TIME cells displayed an elongated and aligned morphology and the MDA-MB-231 and TIME co-culture also resulted in an increase in endothelial proliferation with confluence reached by day 7. Conversely, MCF7 co-cultures led to a decrease in endothelial proliferation and confluence of TIME cells was not achieved. This behavior is supported by preliminary studies performed by the Rylander group consisting of MDA-MB-231 and MCF7 mono-cultures grown in collagen type I hydrogels. The results from preliminary studies revealed that from day 1, MDA-MB-231 cells produced VEGF levels much higher than 2 ng/mL present in complete EGM whereas MCF7 cultures required 5 days to produce the amount of VEGF similar to that found in EGM. The increased endothelial proliferation can be attributed to the high levels of VEGF produced by the

Table 2 Details of the various parameters that were investigated for their influence on inducing an angiogenic response

Experimental parameters for testing angiogenic response			
	MDA-Mb-231	MCF7	
Tumor cell density	1×10^6 cells/mL	5×10^6 cells/mL	
TIME cell density	3×10^4	1×10^5	
Acellular collagen type I concentration	2 mg/mL	4 mg/mL	8 mg/mL
Growth factors	EGM with VEGF and bFGF removed	Complete EGM (2 ng/mL VEGF, 4 ng/mL bfGF)	EGM with 10 ng/mL bFGF
Time of TIME cell seeding	1 day into culture	5 days into culture	

MDA-MB-231 cells from the beginning which prompted their proliferation whereas MCF7 cells were unable to produce necessary levels of VEGF at an early time point necessary for the growth of the TIME cells. Additionally, these results were consistent in all three concentrations of acellular collagen layers suggesting that endothelial morphology is influenced by tumor-endothelial interactions but endothelial proliferation is most influenced by the presence of VEGF.

Angiogenic sprouting was studied in bilayer co-cultures of TIME cells with either MDA-MB-231 or MCF7 cells, and in bilayer monoculture of TIME cells with TIME cells grown on a 2, 4, or 8 mg/mL acellular collagen layer. Sprouting of TIME cells was observed on the 2 and 4 mg/mL acellular collagen layers in MDA-MB-231 and TIME co-culture and in the TIME monoculture but not in the MCF7 co-culture with sprouting more prominent on the 2 mg/mL acellular collagen layers. MDA-MB-231 and TIME co-culture produced capillary like tubule networks that penetrated into the acellular collagen, while TIME monoculture showed no signs of tubule formation beneath the surface revealing a connection between matrix concentration (stiffness), presence of tumor cells (aggressive vs non aggressive), and angiogenic sprouting (invasive vs not invasive).

To further elucidate the angiogenic response of tumors, correlation between angiogenic sprouting and growth factors bFGF and VEGF was investigated by altering media composition and initial seeding density of MDA-MB-231 cells. Following the results from the previous experiment, TIME cells were cultured on either 2 or 4 mg/mL acellular collagen as these levels were capable of inducing sprouting. To determine if MDA-MB-231 cells can induce sprouting without exogenous growth factors, TIME cells were cultured in either complete EGM (2 ng/mL VEGF and 4 ng/mL bFGF), complete EGM supplemented with additional bFGF (2 ng/mL VEGF and 10 ng/mL bFGF), or EGM without the addition of VEGF and bFGF supplements. MDA-MB-231 and TIME co-cultures grown in EGM with bFGF and VEGF present showed enhanced angiogenic sprouting compared to media with exogenous growth factors lacking as presented in Fig. 7. Increasing bFGF levels from 4 to 10 ng/mL did not increase sprouting and this behavior persisted regardless of the initial seeding density of MDA-MB-231 cells (1 vs 5 million MDA-MB-231 cells). Even

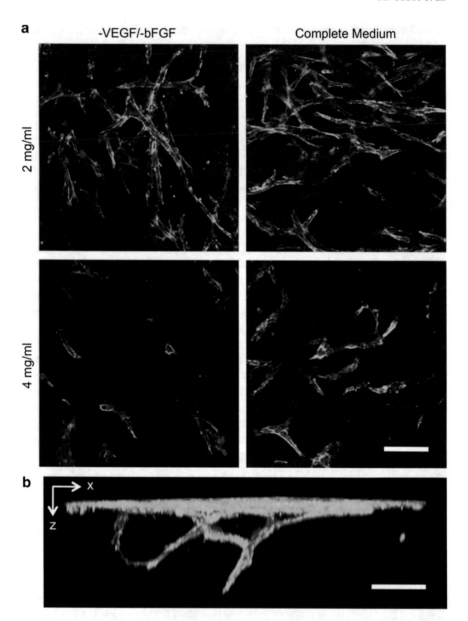

Fig. 7 Influence of matrix concentration and supplemented bFGF on angiogenic sprouting of TIME cells cultured for 7 days on MDA-MB-231 bioengineered tumors. (**a**) Greater degree of angiogenic sprouting was observed within the 2 mg/mL acellular collagen layers as compared with the 4 mg/mL acellular collagen with augmented sprouting in both 2 and 4 mg/mL in the presence of media containing bFGF. (**b**) Three-dimensional image reconstruction shows two separate tubules anastomosing and extending down beneath the surface monolayer (2 mg/mL acellular collagen layer; 10 ng/mL bFGF). *Green*, F-actin; *blue*, nuclei. Scale bars are 50 μm [57]

when exogenous VEGF component was not present in EGM, VEGF wasn't completely absent from the system due to the presence of endogenous VEGF produced by MDA-MB-231 cells. Results revealed that VEGF had an influence on endothelial proliferation and presence of both bFGF and VEGF is necessary for a complete angiogenic response agreeing with previous studies that showed that co-stimulation of bFGF and VEGF augmented angiogenic sprouting in an endothelial monoculture assay [61].

Finally, the Rylander group investigated the influence of TIME cells on angiogenic response by comparing two different seeding densities of TIME cells: low (3×10^4) and high (1×10^5, equivalent to a confluent monolayer). Using the optimal sprouting conditions determined from previous bilayer collage type I hydrogel experiments (MDA-MB-231 co-culture, 2 mg/mL acellular collagen layer, initial MDA-MB-231 seeding density of 1 million cells) they observed that increasing the initial density of TIME cells resulted in an increase in the number of sprouts but the presence of tubule networks occurred at the same time point of 5 days into co-culture regardless of the seeding density. Additionally, the time at which TIME cells were introduced to the co-culture, day 1 vs day 5 (time point at which MDA-MB-231 cells secrete high levels of VEGF), did not increase the rate of tubule formation which once again was observed 5 days into co-culture. These results illustrated that along with necessary levels of VEGF and appropriate matrix concentration, a time dependent tumor-endothelial interaction is necessary for tubule formation. The 3D in vitro vascularized tumor-endothelial co-culture model developed by the Rylander group revealed that the type of tumor cells present, cell-cell interactions, seeding density, matrix concentration, and growth factors are all involved in eliciting an angiogenic response, and it is important to use a system that allows for the presence of all these factors to understand the complexity of tumor developments.

3   Microfluidic Vascularized Tumor Platform

Microfluidic technology was introduced as an analysis tool for biology and chemistry in the early 1990s [62]. It is the manipulation of micro scale volumes of fluids in a microchannel system with dimensions that range from 1 to 1000 μm [63, 64]. The combination of microfluidic technology with cancer biology and drug delivery has enabled development of complex 3D tumor models that provide a more controllable environment while allowing researchers to isolate specific interactions that are absent in 2D models and difficult in animal models [65]. 3D microfluidic platforms are able to recapitulate the complex cell-cell and cell-ECM interactions within dynamic microenvironments characterized by controllable spatial cell distribution and tunable gradients of biochemical and biophysical factors [66].

Microfluidic tumor platforms have a number of advantages over existing tumor models. They use small quantities of cells and reagents and are able to perform experiments with short processing times yielding high resolution and sensitivity [63, 67]. Incorporation of microfabrication techniques has led to development of physiologically relevant TMEs with tissue properties present in vivo such as cross-talk between cells and their microenvironment, vascularization, perfusion, and formation of gradients in nutrients, oxygen, and other soluble factors [68]. Mass transport in microfluidic technology is governed by diffusion due to the small scale resulting in precise spatial and temporal control over gradients of soluble biological factors and cell-cell and cell-ECM interactions. This allows for formation of gradients and the retentions of molecules such as signaling factors and nutrients, in close proximity to cells increasing response sensitivity. Additionally, controlled fluid flow through microchannels simulates the vascular system and interstitial flow and provides constant culture medium refreshment for prolonged culture [65, 69]. Other advantages of 3D microfluidic platforms are that they can mimic important mechanical and biochemical parameters including hypoxia, increased pressure, and shear stress [67, 68]. Finally, multiple microfluidic devices can be connected to form an integrated multi organ platform that allows for a more comprehensive understanding of tumor behavior [70]. These benefits of 3D in vitro microfluidic platforms have resulted in their emergence as powerful systems for gaining a better understanding of cancer progression and development of new therapies.

Dr. Rylander's group has developed an optically clear collagen-based microfluidic vascularized tumor platform that recreates the cancer microenvironment and cellular crosstalk through the incorporation of an endothelialized microchannel within a collagen 3D matrix containing human cancer cells. Their previous studies utilized a 3D in vitro vascularized tumor-endothelial co-culture model to study the influence of paracrine signaling on angiogenesis. Results revealed that the type of tumor cells present, cell-cell interactions, seeding density, matrix concentration, and growth factors are all involved in eliciting an angiogenic response, and it is important to use a system that allows for the presence of all these factors to understand the complexity of tumors To gain a further understanding of cancer and its progression, additional parameters such as flow, pressure and soluble factor gradients, need to be investigated. This led to the development of the collagen-based microfluidic vascularized tumor platform. The platform, shown in Fig. 8 allows for high imaging resolution and dynamic monitoring of drug/nanoparticle transport and angiogenic vessel sprouting [71]. The microchannel is composed of collagen type I embedded with green fluorescent protein (GFP) tagged MDA-MB-231 breast cancer cells with an inner lumen of TIME cells and enclosed in fluorinated ethylene propylene (FEP) capped with polydimethylsiloxane (PDMS) sleeves. Complete details for the development of the microfluidic tumor model can be found in previous publications from the Rylander group [1, 71]. Briefly, collagen type I solution containing MDA-MB-231 cells was injected into the FEP housing with a needle placed through the center. After polymerization, the needle was removed and a solution of TIME cells was injected into the hollow lumen left behind by the needle. Next, a 72 h graded flow preconditioning treatment was applied to the microchannels exposing the TIME cells to shear stress from 0.01 to 0.1 dyn/cm^2 in order to develop a confluent endothelium as displayed in Fig. 8b, c. Once the channels are prepped, the FEP enclosure and a water bath enable refractive matching allowing for undistorted imaging of the system. This system was used to study tumor and

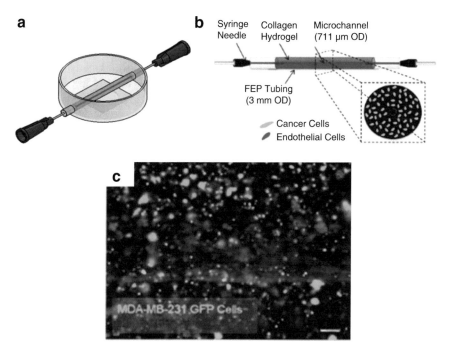

Fig. 8 Tumor-endothelial co-culture in microfluidic collagen hydrogels (**a**) Experimental setup of microfluidic vascularized tumor platform. (**b**) Schematic of a 3D microfluidic tumor vascular model in which cancer cells seeded in the bulk of hydrogel surround endothelial cells lining the lumenal surface of the central microchannel. (**c**) Co-culture maintains growth of MDA-MB-231-GFP breast cancer cells and TIME red fluorescent protein (RFP) cells within physiologically relevant geometries. Image 24 h post-culture. Scale bar is 200 μm [1]

endothelial intercellular signaling and particle transport in response to hemodynamic flow typical of the TME [1, 71, 72].

Using the collagen based microfluidic vascularized tumor model described above, the Rylander group has gained insight into the difference between intracellular signaling in mono vs co-culture and in static vs flow models. They investigated and compared the influence of mono and co-cultures of MDA-MB-231 and TIME cells in 2D tissue culture flasks and in the 3D microfluidic vascularized tumor platform exposed to either static or flow conditions. Perfusion of media through the microchannel was used to impose physical fluid shear stresses on the endothelium as well as simulate tumor-relevant hemodynamic stresses in the system, which are important for regulating reciprocal tumor-endothelial expression of angiogenic growth factors. Studies have shown that fluid shear stresses are linked to endothelial cell transcription, proliferation, barrier transport properties, and modulation of their cytoskeleton [69, 72–77] as well as stimulating and directing the migration of cancer cells [65, 78, 79]. Gene expression measured with reverse transcription polymerase chain reaction (RT-PCR) revealed that MDA-MB-231 cells cultured in static 3D microfluidic platforms compared to 2D culture had a significant increase in expression of matrix metalloproteinase 9 (MMP9), an enzyme that degrades the ECM, as well as proangiogenic factors platelet-derived growth factor B (PDGFB) and angiopoietin 2 (ANG2). In the presence of flow, PDGFB and VEGF-A expressions were higher in comparison to 3D static conditions. Additionally, when co-cultures of MDA-MB-231 and TIME cells were studied, 3D co-culture exposed to flow showed an increased expression of proangiogenic factors of VEGF-A, ANG2, PDGFB, and MMP9 compared to 3D monocultures of MDA-MB-231 cells. In the absence of flow, only VEGFA expression was upregulated [1] These results indicate the importance of multicellular interactions in tumor platforms as well as the presence of hydrodynamic tumor vascular environment.

Subsequent published work by the Rylander group further investigated the effect of shear stress on angiogenic response and barrier function of endothelial cells [71]. They exposed the microfluidic vascularized tumor platform composed of MDA-MB-231 monoculture or co-culture of MDA-MB-231 and TIME cells to three different shear stresses, 4 dyn/cm^2 (normal microvascular wall shear stress), 1 dyn/cm^2 (low microvascular wall shear stress), and 10 dyn/cm^2 (high microvascular wall shear stress). Angiogenic response was quantified by performing PCR and ELISA for the presence of angiogenic markers such as VEGF, bFGF, and angiopoietins 1 and 2 (ANG1, ANG2). Vessel permeability was determined by perfusing the channel with fluorescent nanoparticles ranging from 20 to 1000 nm and fluorescently labeled dextran. The study revealed that the wall shear stress caused by the fluid flow down regulated angiogenic factors released by MDA-MB-231 cells in the presence of an endothelium but had no effect in the MDA-MB-231 mono-cultures as shown in Fig. 9a, suggesting that wall shear stress influences the behavior of the endothelial cells which then in turn regulate the behavior of surrounding tumor cells. Barrier function of the endothelial cells was also shown to be influenced by both the wall shear stress and the presence of tumor cells as revealed in Fig. 9b. Dextran permeability studies revealed that exposure of the endothelium in both mono and co-culture conditions to the three wall shear stresses resulted in decreasing permeability with increasing wall shear stress. Endothelial cells have been shown to elongate and align in the direction of flow and a higher shear stress can lead to the formation of a tighter and confluent endothelium [69, 74, 77]. Additionally under all three flow conditions, co-cultures of tumor and endothelial cells resulted in a leakier vessel compared to an endothelial monoculture. Previous studies have shown that contact between tumor and endothelial cells results in detachment and apoptosis of the endothelial cells [58–60]. This phenomenon combined with the paracrine signaling release of proangiogenic factors could be responsible for the increased vessel permeability in the tumor-endothelial co-culture microfluidic platform. Further permeability studies performed with fluorescently labeled dextran and 1 μm particles depicted in Fig. 10 reveal a size exclusion function of the endothelial barrier as the small dextran particle were able to easily extravasate in the collagen type I matrix whereas the 1 μm particles were too large to cross the endothelium. While the platform developed by the Rylander group has been used primarily to understand breast cancer, the platform has the ability to be employed for a variety of cancers. By tuning the ECM stiffness, composition, porosity, and using

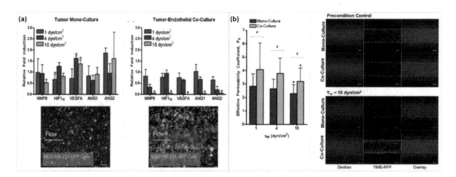

Fig. 9 Effect of wall shear stress on expression of engiogenic factors and endothelial permeability. (**a**) High wall shear stress down-regulates tumor-expressed angiogenic factors in the presence of an endothelium. Tumor mono-cultures or co-cultures with endothelial cells were cultured under the 72 h. preconditioning flow rate, after which the target wall shear stress ($\tau_w = 1, 4,$ or 10 dyn/cm^2) was introduced through the microchannel for a total 6 h. Total tumor mRNA was then isolated for gene expression analysis. Relative mRNA to GAPDH mRNA expressed as a fold induction ± standard deviation (n = 4) *$P < 0.05$. Scale bars are 200 μm [71]. (**b**) Effective permeability coefficient, P_d, decreases as a function of increasing wall shear stress and increases during co-culture with tumor cells. P_d of 70 kDa Oregon Green-conjugated Dextran across the endothelialized microchannel decreases as τ_w increases for both mono-culture and co-culture with tumor cells, with a statistically significant reduction at $\tau_w = 10$ dyn/cm^2 relative to the preconditioned endothelium *$P < 0.05$. P_d during co-culture was significantly increased for all τ_w relative to mono-cultures #$P < 0.05$. Representative images of 70 kDa Oregon Green-conjugated Dextran diffusion across the endothelialized microchannel for the case of $\tau_w = 10$ dyn/cm^2. Scale bar is 200 μm [71]

appropriate cell types, microenvironments of desired properties can be created recapitulating cell-cell and cell-ECM interactions of different cancers by following the same preparation protocol. This model can also be easily adapted to study specific stages of tumor progression such as angiogenesis or metastasis.

In addition to the Rylander group, several other groups have developed microfluidic platforms to investigate tumor mechanisms such as angiogenesis or metastasis. Tien et al. have been developing platforms fabricated from PDMS to house layers of macromolecular hydrogels that can be stacked together to form channels incased by the hydrogel scaffold using additive methods [81]. The Beebe group used a viscous finger patterning method to create endothelialized lumen structures composed of human umbilical vein endothelial cells (HUVECs) within a collagen type I and matrigel hydrogel to study the role of VEGF and 10 T1/2 smooth muscle cells on angiogenesis [81]. They were able to create channels of various geometries with proper endothelial barrier function confirmed through permeability studies of fluorescein isothiocyanate (FITC) labeled bovine serum albumin (BSA). Using their finger patterning method, they created VEGF gradients and showed that HUVEC sprouting occurred in the direction of VEGF source and co-culture of HUVECs with 10 T1/2 cells resulted in a decrease in sprouting regardless of VEGF presence. Other groups have combined additive methods with lithographic techniques to develop in vitro microfluidic vascular networks (μVN) in a three dimensional collagen scaffold for studying angiogenesis and thrombosis [82]. μVNs seeded with

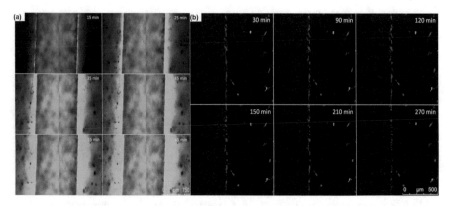

Fig. 10 Extravasation of 70 kDa Oregon Green-conjugated Dextran (**a**) and 1 μm nanoparticles from the microchannel (**b**). (**a**) Each image shows a microfluidic vascularized 3D tumor platform. The two bright *red lines* seen in the first image correspond to TIME-RFP cells that form the border between the microchannel in the *middle* of each image and the collagen surrounding it. Unlabeled MDA-MB-231 breast cancer cells are embedded in the collagen surrounding the microchannel. The *green signal* apparent in each image was produced by 70 kDa Oregon Green-conjugated Dextran. The first image corresponds to 15 min after flow containing the 70 kDa Oregon Green-conjugated Dextran was introduced to the microchannel at a flow rate corresponding to a wall shear stress of $\tau_W = 1$ dyn/ cm^2. Each corresponding image is 10 min after the previous one. As can be seen by the increase in green signal, the 70 kDa Oregon *Green*-conjugated Dextran continuously diffuses out of the microchannel through the endothelium and into the collagen for the duration of the 70 min study. (**b**) Endothelium prevents extravasation of 1 μm nanoparticles from microchannel. Each image shows half of a microfluidic vascularized 3D tumor platform. The *red signal* seen in the left half of the image was produced by 1 μm *red* fluorescent polystyrene nanospheres. The *bright red line* in the *middle* of each image corresponds to TIME-RFP cells which form a barrier between the microchannel and collagen ECM. The *green signal* seen in the right half of each image corresponds to MDA-MB-231-GFP breast cancer cells embedded within the collagen. The first image corresponds to 30 min after flow containing the 1 μm *red* fluorescent plastic nanospheres was introduced to the microchannel at a flow rate corresponding to a wall shear stress of $\tau_W = 1$ dyn/ cm^2. Each corresponding image is 60 min after the previous one. As can be seen, the 1 μm nanospheres are prevented from extravasating out of the microchannel into the collagen by the endothelium for the duration of the 6 hour study

HUVECs demonstrated appropriate endothelial morphology, intracellular junctions, and barrier function. In μVN co-cultures of HUVECs with human brain vascular pericytes (HBVPCs), half of the groups showed sprouting of HUVECs whereas the other half revealed a retracted endothelium from the walls of the microchannels. Additionally, they confirmed that their μVNs could be adapted to study thrombosis.

Another notable group in cancer microfluidics is the Kamm group who has developed multiple cancer microfluidic models to study angiogenesis and metastasis. Examples of their work include using microfluidic platforms to recreate cell-cell signaling present in bone and muscle microenvironments to investigate the metastasis of breast tumor cells to these particular organs [83]. They used 5 mg/ml fibrin gels that were embedded with primary hBM-MSCs, osteo differentiated (OD) hBM-MSCs, and HUVECs to create the bone microenvironment and for the muscle mimic, they replaced the OD hBM MSCs with C2C12 cells. They introduced a MDA-MB-231 cell solution into a neighboring channel and observed the extravasation of the MDAs into the bone microenvironment was much higher than extravasation into the muscle microenvironment. This group has also developed a collagen type I microfluidic model embedded with endothelial cells to study the influence of transendothelial flow as a mechanical regulator of angiogenesis [84]. Endothelial cells were cultured on stiff collagen gels and subjected to no flow (control), apical-to-basal, or basal-to-apical flow for 24 hours. They found basal-to-apical transendo-thelial flow induced sprouting and triggered invadopodia supporting the group's hypothesis that transendothelial pressure gradients produced by basal-to-apical flow promote sprouting angiogenesis.

Other groups developing novel microfluidic platforms for cancer research include Song et al., who have designed a microfluidic vasculature system capable of site specific activation of the endothelium to model the interactions between circu-lating cancer cells and the endothelium during metastasis [85]. They used their microfluidic system to produce site-specific stimulation of endothelium with CXCL12, a chemokine involved in metastasis, on adhesion of circulating breast cancer cells to endothelium. Results from the study demonstrate that circulating breast cancer cells adhere to endothelium when stimulated from the basal side with CXCL12 suggesting the signaling system CXCL12-CXCR4 as a potential target for therapies aimed at blocking metastasis.

In addition to tumor platforms, microfluidic technology has been adapted to cre-ate organ level models such as those for liver and heart tissue with varying degrees of vascularization. These models were primarily developed independently and few attempts have been made to enable the interaction of all these microenvironments to study their collective influence on tumor behavior. Some microfluidic-based organ-on-a-chip systems have multiple cell culture chambers connected with microchannels [70, 86–89]. However, the cell volume in these microsystems is limited and does not allow statistically significant observations. Most of these systems are 2D and cannot truly represent the 3D in vivo cellular microenvironment. In addition, the fabrication and operation of these multi-organ microsystems are costly and cumbersome, and not suited for high-throughput implementation. These limitations need to be addressed because organ level functions and multi-organ interactions are crucial when evaluating drug toxicity or studying metastasis of tumor cells to specific organs. As a result, many groups including the Rylander team, are investigating methods to create multi organ and tumor systems to gain insight into multi-system response.

4   Conclusion

In vitro models have been invaluable tools for gaining improved understanding of cancer biology and progression. Conventional 2D systems and animal models have provided researchers with a framework upon which to elucidate the basic principles of cancer biology but are limited. Attributes such as relative cost and complexity have necessitated the development of 3D models to act as a bridge between conventional 2D cell culture systems and animal models. 3D tumor platforms are able to recapitulate the cell-cell and cell-matrix interactions found in vivo. The introduction of microfluidic technology has resulted in the development of advanced 3D tumor platforms that allow researchers to recreate the dynamic tumor niche. Ongoing cancer research utilizes various 3D models such as transwell assays, polymer hydrogels, spheroids, and microfluidic systems and these models vary from group to group in cell type, ECM protein composition, geometry, and fabrication technique. Currently, no one platform can recreate all the dynamic complexities present in the TME such as stromal cells, various gradients, and the immune response. Advancements in the development of more physiologically relevant platforms will provide a deeper understanding of the complex behavior of tumors and uncover new approaches to diagnosis and treatment.

Acknowledgements We would like to acknowledge funding from the National Institute of Health grant 1R21EB019646 that made this work possible.

References

1. Buchanan C, Voigt E, Szot CS, Freeman JW, Vlachos P, Rylander MN (2013) Three-dimensional microfluidic collagen hydrogels for investigating flow-mediated tumor-endothelial signaling and vascular organization. Tissue Eng Part C Methods 20(1):64–75
2. Ingram M, Techy G, Ward B, Imam S, Atkinson R, Ho H, Taylor C (2010) Tissue engineered tumor models. Biotech Histochem 85:213–229
3. Kumar VA, Brewster LP, Caves JM, Chaikof EL (2011) Tissue engineering of blood vessels: functional requirements, progress, and future challenges. Cardiovasc Eng Technol 2:137–148
4. Sung JH, Shuler ML (2012) Microtechnology for mimicking in vivo tissue environment. Ann Biomed Eng 40:1289–1300
5. Abraham LC, Zuena E, Perez-ramirez B, Kaplan DL (2008) Guide to collagen characterization for biomaterial studies. J Biomed Mater Res B Appl Biomater 87:264–285
6. Charulatha V, Rajaram A (2003) Influence of different crosslinking treatments on the physical properties of collagen membranes. Biomaterials 24:759–767
7. Drury JL, Mooney DJ (2003) Hydrogels for tissue engineering: scaffold design variables and applications. Biomaterials 24:4337–4351
8. Kreger S, Bell B, Bailey J, Stites E, Kuske J, Waisner B, Voytik-harbin S (2010) Polymerization and matrix physical properties as important design considerations for soluble collagen formulations. Biopolymers 93:690–707
9. Parenteau-bareil R, Gauvin R, Berthod F (2010) Collagen-based biomaterials for tissue engineering applications. Materials 3:1863–1887
10. Wolf K, Alexander S, Schacht V, Coussens LM, von Andrian UH, van Rheenen J, Deryugina E, Friedl P (2009. Elsevier) Collagen-based cell migration models in vitro and in vivo. Semin Cell Dev Biol 20(8):931–941
11. Yamamura n, Sudo r, Ikeda M, Tanishita K (2007) Effects of the mechanical properties of collagen gel on the in vitro formation of microvessel networks by endothelial cells. Tissue Eng 13:1443–1453
12. Gribova V, Crouzier T, Picart C (2011) A material's point of view on recent developments of polymeric biomaterials: control of mechanical and biochemical properties. J Mater Chem 21:14354–14366

13. Levy-mishali M, Zoldan J, Levenberg S (2009) Effect of scaffold stiffness on myoblast differentiation. Tissue Eng A 15:935–944
14. Ulrich TA, Jain A, Tanner K, Mackay JL, Kumar S (2010) Probing cellular mechanobiology in three-dimensional culture with collagen–agarose matrices. Biomaterials 31:1875–1884
15. Antoine EE, Vlachos PP, Rylander MN (2014) Review of collagen I hydrogels for bioengineered tissue microenvironments: characterization of mechanics, structure, and transport. Tissue Eng Part B Rev 20:683–696
16. Chrobak KM, Potter DR, Tien J (2006) Formation of perfused, functional microvascular tubes in vitro. Microvasc Res 71:185–196
17. Cross VL, Zheng Y, Choi NW, Verbridge SS, Sutermaster BA, Bonassar LJ, Fischbach C, Stroock AD (2010) Dense type I collagen matrices that support cellular remodeling and microfabrication for studies of tumor angiogenesis and vasculogenesis in vitro. Biomaterials 31:8596–8607
18. Koumoutsakos P, Pivkin I, Milde F (2013) The fluid mechanics of cancer and its therapy. Annual review of fluid mechanics 45:325
19. Polacheck WJ, Zervantonakis IK, Kamm RD (2013) Tumor cell migration in complex microenvironments. Cellular and Molecular Life Sciences 70:1335–1356
20. Raub CB, Suresh V, Krasieva T, Lyubovitsky J, Mih JD, Putnam AJ, Tromberg BJ, George SC (2007) Noninvasive assessment of collagen gel microstructure and mechanics using multiphoton microscopy. Biophys J 92:2212–2222
21. Yang Y-L, Motte S, Kaufman LJ (2010) Pore size variable type I collagen gels and their interaction with glioma cells. Biomaterials 31:5678–5688
22. Achilli M, Mantovani D (2010) Tailoring mechanical properties of collagen-based scaffolds for vascular tissue engineering: the effects of pH, temperature and ionic strength on gelation. Polymers 2:664–680
23. Raub CB, Unruh J, Suresh V, Krasieva T, Lindmo T, Gratton E, Tromberg BJ, George SC (2008) Image correlation spectroscopy of multiphoton images correlates with collagen mechanical properties. Biophys J 94:2361–2373
24. Roeder BA, Kokini K, Voytik-harbin SL (2009) Fibril microstructure affects strain transmission within collagen extracellular matrices. J Biomech Eng 131:031004
25. Naciri M, Kuystermans D, Al-rubeai M (2008) Monitoring pH and dissolved oxygen in mammalian cell culture using optical sensors. Cytotechnology 57:245–250
26. Sung KE, Su G, Pehlke C, Trier SM, Eliceiri KW, Keely PJ, Friedl A, Beebe DJ (2009) Control of 3-dimensional collagen matrix polymerization for reproducible human mammary fibroblast cell culture in microfluidic devices. Biomaterials 30:4833–4841
27. Califano JP, Reinhart-king CA (2010) Exogenous and endogenous force regulation of endothelial cell behavior. J Biomech 43:79–86
28. Carey SP, Kraning-rush CM, Williams RM, Reinhart-king CA (2012) Biophysical control of invasive tumor cell behavior by extracellular matrix microarchitecture. Biomaterials 33:4157–4165
29. Ghousifam N, Mortazavian H, Bhowmick R, Vasquez Y, Blum FD, Gappa-fahlenkamp H (2017) A three-dimensional in vitro model to demonstrate the haptotactic effect of monocyte chemoattractant protein-1 on atherosclerosis-associated monocyte migration. Int J Biol Macromol 97:141–147
30. Gunzer M, Friedl P, Niggemann B, Bröcker E-B, Kämpgen E, Zänker KS (2000) Migration of dendritic cells within 3-D collagen lattices is dependent on tissue origin, state of maturation, and matrix structure and is maintained by proinflammatory cytokines. J Leukoc Biol 67:622–629
31. Haugh MG, Murphy CM, Mckiernan RC, Altenbuchner C, O'brien FJ (2011) Crosslinking and mechanical properties significantly influence cell attachment, proliferation, and migration within collagen glycosaminoglycan scaffolds. Tissue Eng A 17:1201–1208
32. Lo C-M, Wang H-B, Dembo M, Wang Y-L (2000) Cell movement is guided by the rigidity of the substrate. Biophys J 79:144–152

33. Provenzano PP, Inman DR, Eliceiri KW, Knittel JG, Yan L, Rueden CT, White JG, Keely PJ (2008) Collagen density promotes mammary tumor initiation and progression. BMC Med 6:11
34. Sieminski A, Hebbel RP, Gooch KJ (2004) The relative magnitudes of endothelial force generation and matrix stiffness modulate capillary morphogenesis in vitro. Exp Cell Res 297:574–584
35. Wells RG (2008) The role of matrix stiffness in regulating cell behavior. Hepatology 47:1394–1400
36. Antoine EE, Vlachos PP, Rylander MN (2015) Tunable collagen I hydrogels for engineered physiological tissue micro-environments. PLoS One 10:e0122500
37. Griffith LG, Swartz MA (2006) Capturing complex 3D tissue physiology in vitro. Nat Rev Mol Cell Biol 7:211–224
38. Horning JL, Sahoo SK, Vijayaraghavalu S, Dimitrijevic S, Vasir JK, Jain TK, Panda AK, Labhasetwar V (2008) 3-D tumor model for in vitro evaluation of anticancer drugs. Mol Pharm 5:849–862
39. Hutmacher DW, Horch RE, Loessner D, Rizzi S, Sieh S, Reichert JC, Clements JA, Beier JP, Arkudas A, Bleiziffer O (2009) Translating tissue engineering technology platforms into cancer research. J Cell Mol Med 13:1417–1427
40. Kim JB (2005. Elsevier) Three-dimensional tissue culture models in cancer biology. Semin Cancer Biol 15(5):365–377
41. Yamada KM, Cukierman E (2007) Modeling tissue morphogenesis and cancer in 3D. Cell 130:601–610
42. Fischbach C, Chen R, Matsumoto T, Schmelzle T, Brugge JS, Polverini PJ, Mooney DJ (2007) Engineering tumors with 3D scaffolds. Nat Methods 4:855–860
43. Ghajar CM, Bissell MJ (2010) Tumor engineering: the other face of tissue engineering. Tissue Eng A 16:2153–2156
44. Hutmacher DW, Loessner D, Rizzi S, Kaplan DL, Mooney DJ, Clements JA (2010) Can tissue engineering concepts advance tumor biology research? Trends Biotechnol 28:125–133
45. Nelson CM, Bissell MJ (2005. Elsevier) Modeling dynamic reciprocity: engineering three-dimensional culture models of breast architecture, function, and neoplastic transformation. Semin Cancer Biol 15(5):342–352
46. Nelson CM, Inman JL, Bissell MJ (2008) Three-dimensional lithographically defined organo-typic tissue arrays for quantitative analysis of morphogenesis and neoplastic progression. Nat Protoc 3:674–678
47. Raof NA, Raja WK, Castracane J, Xie Y (2011) Bioengineering embryonic stem cell micro-environments for exploring inhibitory effects on metastatic breast cancer cells. Biomaterials 32:4130–4139
48. Verbridge SS, Choi NW, Zheng Y, Brooks DJ, Stroock AD, Fischbach C (2010) Oxygen-controlled three-dimensional cultures to analyze tumor angiogenesis. Tissue Eng A 16:2133–2141
49. Szot CS, Buchanan CF, Freeman JW, Rylander MN (2011) 3D in vitro bioengineered tumors based on collagen I hydrogels. Biomaterials 32:7905–7912
50. Brahimi-Horn MC, Chiche J, Pouysségur J (2007) Hypoxia and cancer. J Mol Med 85:1301–1307
51. Hanahan D, Weinberg RA (2000) The hallmarks of cancer. cell 100:57–70
52. Kilarski W, Bikfalvi A (2007) Recent developments in tumor angiogenesis. Curr Pharm Biotechnol 8:3–9
53. Zhou J, Schmid T, Schnitzer S, Brüne B (2006) Tumor hypoxia and cancer progression. Cancer Lett 237:10–21
54. Hayes A, Huang W, Yu J, Maisonpierre P, Liu A, Kern F, Lippman M, Mcleskey S, Li L (2000) Expression and function of angiopoietin-1 in breast cancer. Br J Cancer 83:1154
55. Nagata S (2000) Apoptotic DNA fragmentation. Exp Cell Res 256:12–18

56. Bos R, van Diest PJ, de Jong JS, van der Groep P, van der Valk P, van der Wall E (2005) Hypoxia-inducible factor-1α is associated with angiogenesis, and expression of bFGF, PDGF-BB, and EGFR in invasive breast cancer. Histopathology 46:31–36
57. Szot CS, Buchanan CF, Freeman JW, Rylander MN (2013) In vitro angiogenesis induced by tumor-endothelial cell co-culture in bilayered, collagen I hydrogel bioengineered tumors. Tissue Eng Part C Methods 19:864–874
58. Kebers F, Lewalle JM, Desreux J, Munaut C, Devy L, Foidart JM, Noel A (1998) Induction of endothelial cell apoptosis by solid tumor cells. Exp Cell Res 240:197–205
59. Lin RZ, Wang TP, Hung RJ, Chuang YJ, Chien CC, Chang HY (2011) Tumor-induced endothelial cell apoptosis: roles of NAD(P)H oxidase-derived reactive oxygen species. J Cell Physiol 226:1750–1762
60. Mcewen A, Emmanuel C, Medbury H, Leick A, Walker DM, Zoellner H (2003) Induction of contact-dependent endothelial apoptosis by osteosarcoma cells suggests a role for endothelial cell apoptosis in blood-borne metastasis. J Pathol 201:395–403
61. Pepper MS, Ferrara N, Orci L, Montesano R (1992) Potent synergism between vascular endothelial growth factor and basic fibroblast growth factor in the induction of angiogenesis in vitro. Biochem Biophys Res Commun 189:824–831
62. Hong JW, Quake SR (2003) Integrated nanoliter systems. Nat Biotechnol 21:1179–1183
63. Whitesides GM (2006) The origins and the future of microfluidics. Nature 442:368–373
64. Zhang Z, Nagrath S (2013) Microfluidics and cancer: are we there yet? Biomed Microdevices 15:595–609
65. Sung KE, Beebe DJ (2014) Microfluidic 3D models of cancer. Adv Drug Deliv Rev 79-80:68–78
66. Bersini S, Moretti M (2015) 3D functional and perfusable microvascular networks for organotypic microfluidic models. J Mater Sci Mater Med 26:180
67. Xu X, Farach-carson MC, Jia X (2014) Three-dimensional in vitro tumor models for cancer research and drug evaluation. Biotechnol Adv 32:1256–1268
68. Stadler M, Walter S, Walzl A, Kramer N, Unger C, Scherzer M, Unterleuthner D, Hengstschlager M, Krupitza G, Dolznig H (2015) Increased complexity in carcinomas: analyzing and modeling the interaction of human cancer cells with their microenvironment. Semin Cancer Biol 35:107–124
69. Buchanan C, Rylander MN (2013) Microfluidic culture models to study the hydrodynamics of tumor progression and therapeutic response. Biotechnol Bioeng 110:2063–2072
70. Park TH, Shuler ML (2003) Integration of cell culture and microfabrication technology. Biotechnol Prog 19:243–253
71. Buchanan CF, Verbridge SS, Vlachos PP, Rylander MN (2014) Flow shear stress regulates endothelial barrier function and expression of angiogenic factors in a 3D microfluidic tumor vascular model. Cell Adhes Migr 8:517–524
72. Antoine E, Buchanan C, Fezzaa K, Lee WK, Rylander MN, Vlachos P (2013) Flow measurements in a blood-perfused collagen vessel using x-ray micro-particle image velocimetry. PLoS One 8:e81198
73. Garcia-cardena G, Comander J, Anderson KR, Blackman BR, Gimbrone MA Jr (2001) Biomechanical activation of vascular endothelium as a determinant of its functional phenotype. Proc Natl Acad Sci U S A 98:4478–4485
74. Levesque MJ, Nerem RM (1985) The elongation and orientation of cultured endothelial cells in response to shear stress. J Biomech Eng 107:341–347
75. Lin K, Hsu PP, Chen BP, Yuan S, Usami S, Shyy JY, LI YS, Chien S (2000) Molecular mechanism of endothelial growth arrest by laminar shear stress. Proc Natl Acad Sci U S A 97:9385–9389
76. Price GM, Wong KH, Truslow JG, Leung AD, Acharya C, Tien J (2010) Effect of mechanical factors on the function of engineered human blood microvessels in microfluidic collagen gels. Biomaterials 31:6182–6189

77. Song JW, Munn LL (2011) Fluid forces control endothelial sprouting. Proc Natl Acad Sci U S A 108:15342–15347
78. Mitchell MJ, King MR (2013) Fluid Shear Stress Sensitizes Cancer Cells to Receptor-Mediated Apoptosis via Trimeric Death Receptors. New J Phys 15:0150r08
79. Shieh AC, Rozansky HA, Hinz B, Swartz MA (2011) Tumor cell invasion is promoted by interstitial flow-induced matrix priming by stromal fibroblasts. Cancer Res 71:790–800
80. Price GM, Chu KK, Truslow JG, Tang-schomer MD, Golden AP, Mertz J, Tien J (2008) Bonding of macromolecular hydrogels using perturbants. J Am Chem Soc 130:6664–6665
81. Bischel LL, Young EW, Mader BR, Beebe DJ (2013) Tubeless microfluidic angiogenesis assay with three-dimensional endothelial-lined microvessels. Biomaterials 34:1471–1477
82. Zheng Y, Chen J, Craven M, Choi NW, Totorica S, Diaz-Santana A, Kermani P, Hempstead B, Fischbach-teschl C, Lopez JA, Stroock AD (2012) In vitro microvessels for the study of angiogenesis and thrombosis. Proc Natl Acad Sci U S A 109:9342–9347
83. Jeon JS, Bersini S, Gilardi M, Dubini G, Charest JL, Moretti M, Kamm RD (2015) Human 3D vascularized organotypic microfluidic assays to study breast cancer cell extravasation. Proc Natl Acad Sci U S A 112:214–219
84. Vickerman V, Kamm RD (2012) Mechanism of a flow-gated angiogenesis switch: early signaling events at cell-matrix and cell-cell junctions. Integr Biol (Camb) 4:863–874
85. Song JW, Cavnar SP, Walker AC, Luker KE, Gupta M, Tung YC, Luker GD, Takayama S (2009) Microfluidic endothelium for studying the intravascular adhesion of metastatic breast cancer cells. PLoS One 4:e5756
86. Heylman C, Sobrino A, Shirure VS, Hughes CC, George SC (2014) A strategy for integrating essential three-dimensional microphysiological systems of human organs for realistic anticancer drug screening. Exp Biol Med (Maywood) 239:1240–1254
87. Imura Y, Sato K, Yoshimura E (2010) Micro total bioassay system for ingested substances: assessment of intestinal absorption, hepatic metabolism, and bioactivity. Anal Chem 82:9983–9988
88. Sung JH, Kam C, Shuler ML (2010) A microfluidic device for a pharmacokinetic–pharmacodynamic (PK–PD) model on a chip. Lab Chip 10:446–455
89. Zhang C, Zhao Z, Abdul RN, van Noort D, Yu H (2009) Towards a human-on-chip: culturing multiple cell types on a chip with compartmentalized microenvironments. Lab Chip 9:3185

Tissue-Engineered Models for Studies of Bone Metastasis

Aaron E. Chiou and Claudia Fischbach

Abstract Patients with advanced cancers are frequently diagnosed with bone metastasis, which is an incurable condition associated with pathological bone remodeling. Despite its widespread impact, understanding of the mechanisms underlying bone metastasis remains relatively limited. While traditional cancer research approaches focus on cancer cells, increasing evidence suggests a role for their surrounding microenvironment in tumorigenesis and metastasis. Therefore, model systems recapitulating physiologically relevant cell-microenvironment interactions are needed in order to study the specific underlying signaling mechanisms. Tissue-engineered, humanized in vitro models may provide an attractive alternative to conventional cell culture and rodent models, as they offer systematic control of microenvironmental aspects relevant to basic and translational studies of bone metastasis. Here, we use breast cancer as an example to review metastasis-associated changes to the bone microenvironment and current approaches to study bone metastasis. In light of their limitations, we discuss tissue-engineered model systems of bone metastasis as a promising alternative, and describe specific design parameters that should be considered when developing such models. Collectively, engineering-inspired culture approaches will be valuable to investigate the functional contribution of the microenvironment to the development, progression, and therapy response of bone metastasis.

Keywords Bone metastasis • Tissue engineering • Tumor microenvironment • Biomaterials • Extracellular Matrix

A.E. Chiou
Nancy E. and Peter C. Meinig School of Biomedical Engineering, Cornell University, Ithaca, NY 14853, USA

C. Fischbach (✉)
Nancy E. and Peter C. Meinig School of Biomedical Engineering, Cornell University, Ithaca, NY 14853, USA

Kavli Institute at Cornell for Nanoscale Science, Cornell University, Ithaca, NY 14853, USA
e-mail: cf99@cornell.edu

© Springer International Publishing AG 2018   95
S. Soker, A. Skardal (eds.), *Tumor Organoids*, Cancer Drug Discovery and Development, DOI 10.1007/978-3-319-60511-1_6

1   Introduction

Metastasis accounts for approximately 90% of cancer-related deaths [1] and very frequently targets the skeleton [2]. In particular, patients with advanced breast and prostate cancer, but also with lung, thyroid, and kidney cancers, are often diagnosed with incurable bone metastasis [3]. The pathological bone remodeling associated with skeletal metastasis increases morbidity and mortality, and can span a wide spectrum of changes that range from excess new bone formation, as in the case of prostate cancer, to complete bone degradation, as often observed with breast cancer [4, 5]. Despite its devastating socioeconomic consequences, our understanding of the molecular, cellular, and tissue-level mechanisms that underlie bone metastasis remains relatively limited.

Traditionally, most cancer research has centered on cancer cells; however, it is now well accepted that the microenvironment in which cancer cells are located is equally important. In fact, an accumulating body of work suggests that tumors can only develop in a permissive context that may, for example, form during the process of aging or inflammation, while a healthy or embryonic microenvironment can prevent tumorigenesis [6]. Although most studies on tumor-microenvironment interactions have been performed in the context of primary tumors, the same concepts apply to secondary tumors that have spread to distant sites including the skeleton. Indeed, the "seed and soil" hypothesis has long argued that metastasis is a non-random process which specifically targets organs that provide fertile ground for tumor cells to seed [7, 8]. Nevertheless, due in part to a lack of relevant model systems, there exists relatively little knowledge about the surrounding "soil", or microenvironment, and what makes it fertile for seeding and progression of metastases.

Historically, bone metastasis has been studied in conventional two-dimensional (2D) cell culture and mouse models. However, both approaches are limited in their ability to recapitulate conditions characteristic of human disease. More specifically, species-specific differences in mice often prevent extrapolation of results to patients, while 2D cultures lack physiologically relevant 3D cell-microenvironment interactions. Nevertheless, these contextual cues are critical regulators of the phenotypic changes that mediate metastasis, including proliferation, differentiation, and gene expression [9]. To address this challenge, cancer biologists increasingly utilize tumor spheroids and organoids. Still, these systems are not easily suited to recapitulate the unique cell-cell and cell-extracellular matrix (ECM) interactions as well as mechanical forces intrinsic to bone metastasis. Tissue-engineered, humanized in vitro models may provide an attractive alternative and advance basic and translational studies of bone metastasis.

In this chapter, we will use breast cancer as an example to introduce biological changes to the bone microenvironment associated with metastasis and review current approaches to study the underlying mechanisms. Subsequently, we will discuss tissue-engineered model systems of bone metastasis as a valuable alternative and define specific design parameters that should be considered when developing such models. Collectively, engineering-inspired culture approaches will be valuable to investigate the functional contribution of the microenvironment to the development, progression, and therapy response of bone metastasis.

2 The Microenvironment in Bone Metastasis

2.1 Bone Structure and Homeostatic Bone Remodeling

The skeleton serves to provide structural support in the body, and is constantly undergoing remodeling (~10% annually [10]) to maintain mechanical strength and integrity. Bone remodeling is a sequential process by which bone is degraded/ resorbed (osteolysis) and then replaced by newly formed bone (osteogenesis). At the cellular level, osteolysis and osteogenesis are carried out by bone-degrading osteoclasts, bone-forming osteoblasts, and mechanosensing osteocytes. Through acid and protease secretion, osteoclasts primarily function to degrade bone matrix, a composite material composed of collagen type I fibrils that are reinforced by hydroxyapatite (HA) nanocrystals [11]. Osteoclasts are hematopoietic in origin and derived from macrophage/monocytes that have differentiated and fused (i.e. osteo-clastogenesis) in the presence of osteoblast-derived cues (e.g. receptor activator of nuclear factor kappa-B ligand [RANKL], macrophage colony-stimulating factor [M-CSF]) [12]. Osteoblasts, on the other hand, are derived from bone marrow mes-enchymal stem cells (BM-MSCs) via transforming growth factor-beta (TGF-β), bone morphogenetic protein (BMP), and WNT signaling [10]. Following behind osteoclasts, osteoblasts deposit new collagen type I matrix for mineralization, then undergo apoptosis or become lining cells or osteocytes. Generally accepted as the primary mechanosensors in bone, osteocytes form an interconnected network embedded within bone matrix, and secrete factors that regulate osteoclastogenesis (e.g. RANKL) and osteoblast differentiation (e.g. TGF-β) in response to physical forces [13]. Critical to the balance of bone resorption and formation is the local strain environment in the bone, which is modulated by external mechanical stimuli. For example, increases in mechanical loading of the bone (e.g. due to physical activity) lead to a net increase in osteogenesis whereas reductions in loading (e.g. due to bed rest) promote osteolysis [14]. In the context of breast cancer, tumor cells deregulate the above-described homeostatic signaling between bone cells and mechanical stimuli to drive their own growth and metastatic potential.

2.2 The Vicious Cycle of Bone Metastasis

Bone metastasis results when cancer cells originating from a primary tumor initiate secondary tumors in the skeleton. The metastatic process is highly selective [8]; primary tumor cells must successfully invade local tissue, intravasate into nearby blood vessels, and circulate systemically while evading the immune system, before localizing and extravasating into bone. Even then, the disseminated cells must survive a period of dormancy before reactivating to establish secondary tumor growth [15]. Survival at each of these steps is rate-limiting and requires crosstalk between a cancer cell and its microenvironment. The bone matrix exemplifies fertile "soil" for cancer cells, as it is packed with morphogens (i.e. growth factors, cytokines, chemokines) that attract tumor cells and feed their growth. For example, the sequestration of osteoblast-secreted stromal-derived factor-1 (SDF-1/CXCL12) in the bone ECM is not only important for homing of CXCR4-expressing immune, hematopoietic, and stem cells, but also plays a role in seeding and proliferation of breast cancer cells in bone [16–19].

Once localized to the bone secondary site, tumor cells modify the microenvironment in their favor by deregulating the signals that govern homeostatic bone remodeling in a feed-forward loop that promotes bone metastatic progression. While osteogenesis appears to be essential for initial seeding of metastasis [20], osteolysis is the primary outcome at later stages of breast cancer bone metastasis. Tumor cells activate the latter process by secreting elevated levels of parathyroid hormone-related peptide (PTHrP), which stimulates the secretion of osteoblast-derived RANKL to increase osteoclast activation and bone resorption [21–23]. Increased bone resorption, in turn, leads to the release of matrix-bound growth factors (e.g. TGF-β, BMPs) that further enhance tumor growth, in a process known as the "vicious cycle" of bone metastasis [4, 11, 24]. This vicious cycle is additionally stimulated by elimination of functional osteoblasts [25]. Furthermore, upregulated RANKL-independent signaling mechanisms may play an important role in bone metastasis, for example, tumor cells expressing elevated levels of interleukin-8 (IL-8) and lysyl oxidase (LOX) also exhibit increased migration [26] and invasiveness [27], and have been correlated with increased osteolysis [28, 29].

More recently, experimental evidence has suggested that tumor cells at the primary site may direct the formation of distant "pre-metastatic niches" primed for metastatic initiation even prior to their own dissemination. Through endocrine-like actions, primary tumor cells release factors that circulate systemically and transform cell behavior from afar in a manner that may ultimately direct organ-specific metastasis [30, 31]. For example, primary breast cancer in rodent models changes bone strength, structure, and mineralization, suggesting that circulating factors may play a role in this process [32]. Indeed, tumor-free mice that were injected with tumor cell-conditioned media similarly present with osteolytic lesions, confirming that systemically circulating tumor-derived factors (e.g. LOX) lead to pre-metastatic conditioning of the bone [33]. However, whether these changes to the bone ECM are critical to bone metastasis remains to be confirmed. Studies with cancer cell-derived extracellular vesicles (e.g. exosomes) strongly suggest this possibility because they have been demonstrated to direct organotropic metastasis via pre-metastatic niche development at sites such as the lungs and the liver [34, 35]. Developing models to specifically investigate the interactions between tumor cells and the bone microenvironment at each stage of the metastatic cascade will further mechanistic understanding of bone metastatic progression (Fig. 1).

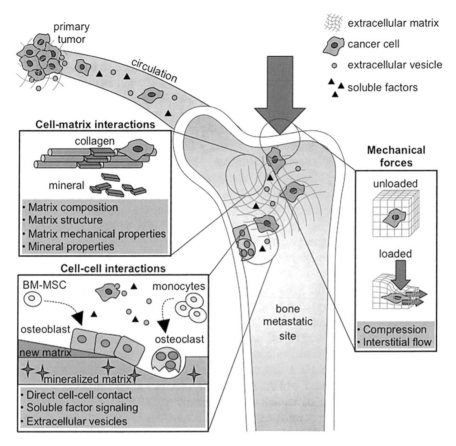

Fig. 1 Design parameters to incorporate into engineered tumor microenvironments for studies of bone metastasis, including cell-matrix interactions, cell-cell interactions, and mechanical forces

3 *In Vivo* Models of Bone Metastasis

Various mouse models of bone metastasis have advanced our knowledge of how tumor cells interact with the bone microenvironment, but not all aspects of human disease may be mimicked with this approach. Transgenic mice reflecting certain genetic mutations found in human breast cancer have facilitated greater under-standing of tumor growth and invasion, and tumor-immune interactions. For example, overexpression of the oncogenes Her2/neu, Ras, and Myc is commonly driven by the Mouse Mammary Tumor Virus (MMTV) promoter [36]. Immune-competent MMTV-driven mice develop spontaneous mammary tumors, but bone metastasis occurs rarely in such models [36]. In fact, most spontaneous breast cancer models in rodents do not metastasize to the bone, and thus other approaches are often utilized.

Inoculation of breast cancer cells through various injection routes has yielded greater rates of bone metastasis compared to transgenic models. Following orthotopic injection into the mammary fat pad, the murine breast cancer line 4T1 has limited ability to spontaneously metastasize to bone after 3–6 weeks, while its clonal subline 4T1.2 exhibits strong bone tropism [37]. The 4T1 model provides the opportunity to study the full bone metastatic cascade in mice, as well as tumor-immune studies in syngeneic BALB/c mice. However, by the time bone metastases become apparent, the tumor burden is typically high at the orthotopic site and in the lungs, leaving a small time window to study bone metastasis [36]. Intracardiac injection through the left ventricle introduces tumor cells directly into the systemic circulation, improving rates of bone metastases [38]. While this model skips key initial steps of the metastatic process, it has enabled study of factors that influence tumor cell seeding and colonization of bones, including the development of bone-tropic sub-lines of the human breast cancer cell line MDA-MB231, as well as the identification of a bone metastasis gene signature [39, 40]. Intraosseous injections, for example by the intratibial route, place tumor cells directly into the bone marrow cavity, allowing study of tumor-bone microenvironmental interactions. This approach is limited to the late stages of the metastatic cascade, but has been especially useful in studying the vicious cycle of bone metastasis [41] and the effectiveness of potential treatments such as bisphosphonates [42], denosumab [43], and even mechanical loading [14]. Collectively, these techniques have shed light on several aspects of breast cancer bone metastasis, however they remain limited by their inability to recapitulate species-specific interactions between human breast cancer cells and human bone in the presence of a functional immune system [44].

Orthotopic injection of human breast cancer cells into mice with implanted human bone tissue may overcome this issue, and confirm a role for human-specific microenvironmental aspects of bone in driving metastasis [45]. The use of patient-derived xenografts (PDX) models, in which tissue from patient primary tumors is transplanted to immunodeficient mice, has been rising because they offer improved predictive value for malignant potential compared to cancer cell lines [46]. Indeed, tumor cells derived from PDX models have displayed spontaneous metastases similar to those of patients, and as such may metastasize to bone in the host mouse [47]. Still, many of these models lack immune interaction, which could be addressed by engrafting human hematopoietic cells within the immunodeficient murine hosts (e.g. nude [48], SCID [49–51], NOD-scid [52]). These humanized models aim to confer partial human immunity to the hosts, however the success of these approaches has been limited by eventual takeover of the hematopoietic compartment by host immune cells and low life spans of mice [53]. Collectively, mouse models of bone metastasis have led to much advancement in our understanding of the disease. Even so, using these models to study the spatiotemporal dynamics of bone metastasis, species-specific differences, and the role of the immune system continues to be a challenge. While certainly limited in their ability to recapitulate full biologic complexity, in vitro culture platforms may address some of these challenges, as they enable the study of human cells under well-defined conditions, in a patient-specific manner, at reduced cost, and with fewer ethical issues relative to animal studies.

4   Tissue-Engineered Models to Study Bone Metastasis

4.1   Dimensionality: 2D Versus 3D

Standard 2D monolayer cultures of human cancer cells have provided valuable insights on cancer biology and informed therapeutic development. However, these 2D culture models are unable to recapitulate most of the heterogeneous interactions within the tumor microenvironment in vivo, including those involving the surrounding extracellular matrix (ECM), as well as other resident cell types, and external physical forces [9, 54]. In fact, cells cultured in 3D compared to 2D exhibit appreciably altered proliferation [55], differentiation [56], metabolism [57], and protein expression [58, 59].

3D cancer cell cultures more appropriately mimic tumors in vivo, as tissue level interactions and dimensionality influence tumor growth [60–62], migration [63], signaling [64, 65], and drug response [66]. For example, multicellular spheroids recapitulating certain aspects of tumor heterogeneity and transport limitations in vivo have led to improved understanding of antitumor drug resistance [67]. Tumor organoids, which are spheroids cultured from primary cells, can retain patient-specific genetic and pathological characteristics, and have helped elucidate genotype-drug interactions and niche contributions to growth, metastasis, and drug response [68–70]. While tumor spheroids and organoids have also been used to study the role of ECM in regulating invasive behavior of tumor cells [71], they typically lack cell-matrix interactions characteristic of bone. Furthermore, they exclude tumor-stromal cell interactions and mechanical stimuli, thus more physiologically relevant 3D models of the bone microenvironment are needed to investigate the mechanisms of bone metastasis [54].

4.2   Cell-Matrix Interactions

4.2.1   Organic Matrix (Collagen, Decellularized Matrices, etc.)

To study tumor-matrix interactions, natural ECM-derived materials such as collagen type I and reconstituted basement membrane (i.e. Matrigel®) are frequently used due to their cytocompatibility, inclusion of cell adhesion sites, remodelability, as well as the ability to control physical matrix properties (e.g. porosity, fiber structure, stiffness) through casting conditions (e.g. temperature, concentration, pH) [72, 73]. Matrigel® and collagen type I hydrogels have also been used to direct stem cell osteogenic differentiation and mineralization [74–78], leading to compositional similarities to organic bone matrix. However, batch-to-batch variability and inability to control specific biological, biochemical, and biophysical characteristics of these matrices [54, 79] limit study reproducibility and thus, mechanistic understanding.

In particular, the ECM composition, structure, and mechanical properties (e.g. stiffness, or elastic modulus) encountered by cells in the bone microenvironment are not reflected or independently controllable in collagen type I or Matrigel®-based hydrogels models. For example, ECMs at common metastatic sites (bone, lung, brain) are complex in their composition and physical properties, yet most naturally-derived hydrogels comprise only one individual component that does not capture the tissue-specific integrin-ECM interactions that critically mediate breast cancer cell adhesion and motility (Fig. 2a) [80]. In addition, the stiffness of bone is orders of magnitude greater than the upper limit possible using natural ECM hydrogels [84]. As substrate mechanics are critical in regulating BM-MSC osteogenic differentiation [85, 86], tumor cell malignancy [87], as well as the progression of bone metastasis (Fig. 2b) [81, 84], the inability to capture bone ECM mechanics inherently limits the physiologic relevance of these models. Furthermore, varying the concentration of collagen gels to control bulk stiffness simultaneously alters fibrillar network structure and adhesive ligand density, which independently modulate cell behavior [88]. Inability to recapitulate biochemical and physical properties of bone matrix restricts the physiologic relevance of cell behavior in hydrogel cultures,

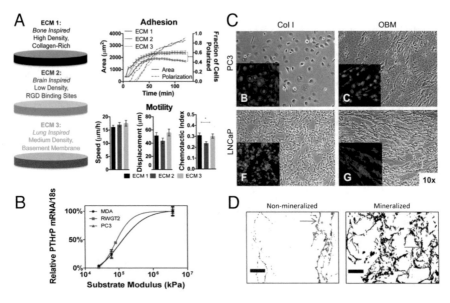

Fig. 2 Cell-matrix interactions. (**a**) Tissue-specific ECM protein density and composition influence breast cancer cell adhesion and motility [80]. (**b**) Osteolytic PTHrP gene expression increases with substrate modulus for bone-metastatic breast (MDA), lung (RWGT2), and prostate (PC3) cancer cell lines [81]. (**c**) Compared to collagen type I matrices (COL I), decellularized osteoblast-derived matrix (OBM) bone tissues induce greater alignment of prostate cancer cell lines (PC3 and LNCaP) [90]. (**d**) Breast cancer cells penetrate deeper into and adhere better onto mineralized, HA-containing scaffolds. Arrows = walls, asterisks = pores, scale bars = 200 μm [83]. (Figures reproduced with permission from Royal Society of Chemistry, Elsevier, and Public Library of Science)

which may be improved by using platforms that allow systematic control of such parameters.

Decellularized matrices, which preserve the natural composition and structure laid down by osteogenic cells, not only direct osteogenic differentiation of BM-MSCs [89], but have also facilitated studies of tumor cell-ECM interactions. Compared to 2D collagen matrices, decellularized matrices derived from primary human osteo-blasts have been shown to enhance alignment, migration, and osteogenic gene expression of prostate cancer cells (Fig. 2c) [90] as well as bone-metastatic breast cancer cells [82]. The feasibility of long-term studies with cell-derived ECMs can be further improved by surface-anchorage, a technique that preserves structural integrity of the ECMs and prevents their detachment in response to cell-mediated traction forces [91]. BM-MSCs in such cultures deposit even more physiologically relevant ECMs under macromolecular crowding conditions [92]. This results in enhanced expansion of hematopoietic progenitor cells, indicating that tumor cells may also respond to such conditions. Still, cell-derived matrices are commonly derived from monolayer cultures. Given that cellular ECM deposition is influenced by the under-lying substrate [93], these ECMs may still not fully recapitulate the in vivo ECM structure and composition that can independently affect availability of ECM binding sites, and subsequent phenotypic changes of secondary cell types [94].

Decellularized bone tissue offers compositional and structural matrix cues inher-ent to native bone that may be explored for studies of bone metastasis. Indeed, decellularized bone tissue alters cellular phenotypes, and can support osteogenic differentiation of progenitor cells (adipose-derived stem cells [95], embryonic stem cells [96], BM-MSCs [97, 98]) as well as studies of tumor cell-bone interactions [99, 100]. However, it is worth noting that bone tissue architecture, marrow mechan-ics, and mineral content can vary greatly within a single bone, let alone across samples and species, limiting reproducibility of these models [101, 102]. These changes are important, for example, as bone mineral materials properties can independently modulate tumor cell behavior [103]. This suggests that bone metas-tasis models of the ECM should not only recapitulate proper organic ECM composi-tion, but also the respective mineral component.

4.2.2 Inorganic Matrix (Mineral)

Along with collagen, HA mineral platelets constitute a fundamental building block of bone matrix, however few bone metastasis models incorporate this inorganic matrix component. Inclusion of HA nanoparticles within 3D scaffolds enhances osteogenic differentiation of stem cells in bone tissue engineering approaches [104–106], but has also been demonstrated to affect breast cancer cell adhesion and secre-tion of pro-osteoclastic IL-8 (Fig. 2d) [83]. Accordingly, biomaterial substrates mineralized by incubation with Simulated Body Fluid (SBF) equally promote adhe-sion and proliferation of breast cancer cells [107]. However, it should be noted that the materials properties of HA itself can vary extensively depending on patient age and disease [108]. In particular, HA particle size, crystallinity, and carbonate substitution are parameters that may vary in the presence of a secondary and/or primary mammary tumor [109, 110]. Hence, synthesis schemes that allow the formation of HA crystals with defined nanoparticle properties have been developed [103, 111]. Indeed, polymeric scaffolds containing HA with differentially controlled particle size and crystallinity impact breast cancer cell adhesion, proliferation, and osteolytic factor secretion as a function of varying HA characteristics [103]. While these in vitro studies strongly suggest a regulatory role of HA materials properties in bone metastasis, the in vivo relevance of these findings will need to be confirmed. Furthermore, HA is associated with collagen type I fibrils in the body. Hence, strategies to mineralize collagen fibrils based on SBF incubation [112, 113] and mineral co-precipitation during fibrillogenesis [114] should be considered to establish platforms that will allow dissection of the individual and combined effects of bone organic and inorganic ECM components during the pathogenesis of bone metastasis.

4.3   Cell-Cell Interactions

4.3.1   Direct: Cell-Cell Contact in Co-cultures of Tumor and Bone Cells

While isolating tumor cell interactions with the bone ECM will be essential for studies of skeletal metastasis, direct interactions of tumor cells with osteoblasts, osteoclasts, and other cells located in the bone are equally important. To design model systems that recapitulate these interactions, a variety of existing co-culture approaches initially developed for regenerative approaches [115–118] or studies of bone biology [119, 120] could be easily adapted. Still, mimicking the bone remodeling process in vitro remains a significant challenge due to the long time frames over which bone cells mature and the need for continuous supplementation of osteogenic precursor cells to carry out bone formation following resorption by osteoclasts. Nevertheless, appropriate combination of culture substrates and cell types can recapitulate conditions observed in vivo and thus, may ultimately reveal novel insights. For example, co-culturing breast cancer cells and osteoclasts within mineralized, collagenous osteoblastic tissue upregulates osteoclast differentiation and downregulates osteoblast differentiation, both of which are features observed in osteolytic bone lesions in vivo [121]. While this specific tri-culture model is very promising and yields physiologically relevant cell behavior, it may not be easily implemented in many conventional biology labs due to the need for custom bioreactors to ensure adequate nutrient and waste transport for the 3D tissue.

   To circumvent the challenge of implementing long-term tri-cultures, a majority of co-culture studies focus solely on the interactions between tumor cells and a single type of bone cell. Several studies have explored the interactions between breast cancer cells and osteoblastic cells in co-culture, demonstrating that their interaction stimulates osteoclast formation [125, 126], exhibits hallmarks of in vivo bone metastatic progression [127, 128], and upregulates expression of the meta-

Fig. 3 Cell-cell interactions. (**a**) Increasing ratios of MSCs co-cultured with breast cancer cells (MDA-MB-231, BrCa) in bone-mimetic scaffolds yield greater metastasis-associated gene expression of metadherin (MTDH) [122]. (**b**) Exosomes derived from prostate cancer cells transform BM-MSCs into pro-migratory, alpha smooth muscle actin (αSMA) expressing myofibroblasts. Scale bars = 100 μm [124]. (Figures reproduced with permission from Elsevier and Impact Journals)

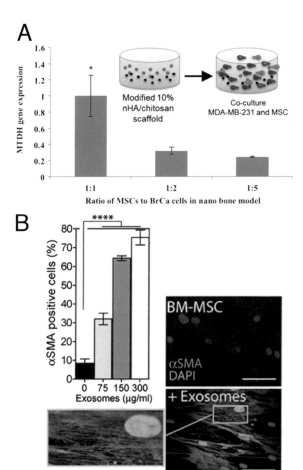

static gene metadherin in breast cancer cells (Fig. 3a) [122]. Biomimetic 3D bone scaffolds have been increasingly used for these co-cultures, as they can help to simulate the behavior of cancer cells in vivo [122, 129]. In addition, co-culture of metastatic breast cancer cells with osteoclast precursor cells supplemented with soluble RANKL can mimic tumor-induced osteolytic activation in culture due to increased osteoclast formation [126]. Together, these studies may further improve understanding of how breast cancer cells alter the signaling between osteoblasts and osteoclasts that is critical to the development of bone metastasis. Nevertheless, current approaches primarily focus on osteoblasts and osteoclasts and typically disregard other bone-resident cells that may play equally important roles. For example, bone marrow progenitor cells such as hematopoietic stem cells are recruited to the bone via similar signaling pathways (e.g. the SDF-1/CXCR4 pathway) as tumor cells and, in fact, directly compete with tumor cells in the bone marrow niche [130–132]. To fully understand the mechanisms of pre-metastatic niche development and the vicious cycle of bone metastasis, culture models that incorporate crosstalk between various different populations of bone-resident cells and tumor cells will be essential. Finally, for effective therapeutic targets to be identified, it will be critical to determine whether phenomena observed in co-cultures are dependent on direct cell-cell contact or on paracrine signaling between cells.

4.3.2   Indirect: Membranes, Cell-Derived Factors, Soluble Cues

Non-contact co-cultures utilizing transwell inserts have enabled study of the effects of bi-directional paracrine signaling between breast cancer cells and osteoclasts [133] as well as between breast cancer cells and BM-MSCs [123] in 2D cultures. To permit more physiologically relevant communication between multiple cell types, non-contact 3D co-cultures have also been established, for example, by placing two scaffolds, each seeded with either breast cancer cells or BM-MSCs, into a single well for culture [123]. Using this method of indirect 3D co-culture, BM-MSC osteogenic differentiation is decreased in the presence of breast cancer cells. While these findings suggest that breast cancer cell-secreted factors reduce osteogenic differentiation of BM-MSCs, the opposite, namely enhanced osteogenic differentiation of BM-MSCs, has also been shown [134]. Hence, it is imperative to consider whether bidirectional paracrine signaling is necessary for the given research question. Indeed, the importance of such feedback is underscored by studies implanting engineered bone microenvironments into tumor-bearing mice, in which BM-MSC migration from implants to mammary tumors in turn affects metastatic growth and frequency [135]. Furthermore, tissue-engineered bone implants have also highlighted that BM-MSCs exposed to BMP-2, a growth factor commonly associated with both osteogenesis [136] and tumorigenesis [137], enhances bone metastatic colonization [138]. Hence, methods to isolate the signaling of specific cell-secreted biomolecules remain relevant.

Historically, the effect of tumor-derived morphogens on cell signaling including BM-MSC migration [139], gene and protein expression [140], and differentiation [134], as well as osteoblast inflammatory response [141] have been frequently isolated with conditioned media. More recently, however, it has become clear that conditioned media not only contains secreted biomolecules, but also tumor cell-shed extracellular vesicles (EVs; e.g. exosomes, microvesicles) and that these EVs may be critical for tumor initiation and progression. More specifically, EVs are membrane-enclosed vesicles that are produced by tumor cells and can be isolated from conditioned media via size-based sorting and filtration techniques [142, 143]. EVs can promote cancer progression via stably transported cargo molecules (e.g. proteins, miRNAs, DNA). Additionally, cancer cell derived-EVs can direct organ-specific metastasis [35], transform the behavior of BM-MSCs and other stromal cells toward cancer-promoting phenotypes (Fig. 3b) [124, 144], and increase the metastatic potential of poorly metastatic cells [145]. However, the exact mechanisms underlying these observations are not well understood. For example, whether tumor cells within bone shed different populations of EVs relative to those located at the primary site, and how these vesicles transmit information to recipient cells remains largely unclear. Studying the biogenesis and signaling mechanisms intrinsic to EVs in physiologically relevant models of bone metastasis promises to shed some light on these phenomena.

4.4 Mechanical Forces

Considering the load-bearing nature of bone and its functional adaptation to mechanical forces, as well as the observation that mechanical cues can affect bone metastatic progression, appropriate mechanical stimuli should be considered when designing bone metastasis models. In the context of bone regeneration, various bioreactor platforms (spinner flasks [146], rotating-wall vessels [147], direct perfusion [148], direct compression [149]) have been developed to impart physical forces that promote bone tissue formation. Similar setups can also be applied to probe the functional impact of such stimuli on the pathogenesis of bone metastasis. In general, tumor growth within bones induces static compression, which can enhance metastatic phenotypes in prostate cancer cells via osteocyte-secreted factors [150]. On the other hand, external cyclic compression of tumor-bearing tibiae to mimic the effect of physical activity has been shown to inhibit secondary tumor growth and osteolysis [14]. Together, these findings indicate that physical forces modulate metastatic progression, but the underlying mechanisms may be diverse. While load-bearing physical activity imparts cyclic compressive loads on bone-resident cells in vivo, it also generates interstitial flow that in and of itself can alter cell behavior due to altered transport of nutrients and waste products as well as small scale mechanical forces (e.g. shear stress, drag forces) [152]. Indeed, introducing interstitial flow into collagen scaffolds using microfluidic approaches influences the direction of breast cancer cell migration (Fig. 4a) [151]. Additionally, flow-derived shear stresses may regulate the drug resistance of tumors as suggested by studies in which tissue-engineered bone tumors were cultured in a flow perfusion bioreactor [153]. Whether these differences were mediated by direct effects on the tumor cells, altered transport of soluble factors, or a combination of the two remains to be investigated. Similarly, direct cyclic compression of HA-containing scaffolds using a custom bioreactor with loading platen upregulates expression of genes associated with bone metastasis by breast cancer cells (Fig. 4b) [14], while the same stimuli promote osteogenic differentiation of BM-MSCs when exposed to breast cancer cell-derived soluble factors [134]. Again, whether these changes are due to direct effects on the tumor cells or altered transport phenomena has yet to be elucidated. Nevertheless, these studies collectively underscore the need to incorporate physiologically relevant mechanical stimuli into bone metastasis models. This approach will be particularly useful in co-culture models involving osteocytes, given the key role of these cells in mechanotransduction [154].

Fig. 4 Mechanical forces. (a) Microfluidic device generating a consistent interstitial flow field via pressure gradient across cell-embedded collagen I gel. Breast cancer cell migration occurs against the flow direction [151]. (b) Direct compression of breast cancer cell-seeded scaffolds in a loading bioreactor reduces expression of osteolysis-associated gene Runx2 [14]. (Figures reproduced with permission from National Academy of Sciences and John Wiley and Sons)

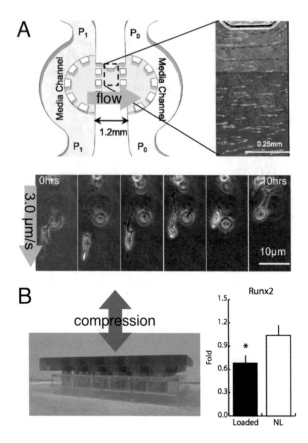

5 Future Perspectives

In conclusion, 3D tissue-engineered models of cancer bone metastasis have the potential to more accurately define the functional interplay between tumor and bone-resident cells that regulates bone metastasis. However, current models remain limited in their ability to fully recapitulate in vivo complexity of microenvironmental factors, including matrix properties (organic and inorganic components, mechanical properties), bone-resident cellular compartments (osteoblasts, osteocytes, osteoclasts, adipocytes, endothelial cells, immune cells), and physical forces (interstitial flow and cyclic compression). Looking forward, thorough characterization of metastasis-associated material changes to the bone microenvironment will be critical to more appropriately model and study their functional consequences. Considering the systemic nature of cancer metastasis, integrating these models with body-on-a-chip systems that also represent other organ sites will enable examination of relative metastatic frequencies as well as mechanistic investigations. The knowledge to be gained from integrative models of bone metastasis will inform therapeutic development, and when using patient-derived cells these models could provide predictive insights for precision medicine.

Acknowledgements We acknowledge financial support through NCI (R01CA173083), the Alexander von Humboldt Foundation (Fellowship for Experienced Researchers to CF), and a fellowship by the Graduate Assistance in Areas of National Need training grant from the Department of Education to AEC (P200A150273).

References

1. Chaffer CL, Weinberg RA (2011) A perspective on cancer cell metastasis. Science 331:1559–1564. doi:10.1126/science.1203543
2. Davila D, Antoniou A, Chaudhry MA (2015) Evaluation of osseous metastasis in bone scintigraphy. Semin Nucl Med 45:3–15. doi:10.1053/j.semnuclmed.2014.07.004
3. Coleman RE (2006) Clinical features of metastatic bone disease and risk of skeletal morbidity. Clin Cancer Res 12:6243s–6249s. doi:10.1158/1078-0432.CCR-06-0931
4. Guise TA (2002) The vicious cycle of bone metastases. J Musculoskelet Neuronal Interact 2:570–572
5. Zheng Y, Zhou H, Dunstan CR et al (2013) The role of the bone microenvironment in skeletal metastasis. J Bone Oncol 2:47–57. doi:10.1016/j.jbo.2012.11.002
6. Brock A, Krause S, Ingber DE (2015) Control of cancer formation by intrinsic genetic noise and microenvironmental cues. Nat Rev Cancer 15:499–509. doi:10.1038/nrc3959
7. Paget S (1889) The distribution of secondary growths in cancer of the breast. Cancer Metastasis Rev 133:571–573. doi:10.1016/S0140-6736(00)49915-0
8. Fidler IJ (2003) The pathogenesis of cancer metastasis: the "seed and soil" hypothesis revisited. Nat Rev Cancer 3:453–458. doi:10.1038/nrc1098
9. Infanger DW, Lynch ME, Fischbach C (2013) Engineered culture models for studies of tumor-microenvironment interactions. Annu Rev Biomed Eng 15:29–53. doi:10.1146/annurev-bioeng-071811-150028
10. Weilbaecher KN, Guise TA, McCauley LK (2011) Cancer to bone: a fatal attraction. Nat Rev Cancer 11:411–425. doi:10.1038/nrc3055
11. Bussard KM, Gay C V, Mastro AM (2008) The bone microenvironment in metastasis; what is special about bone? Cancer Metastasis Rev 27:41–55. doi:10.1007/s10555-007-9109-4
12. Takayanagi H (2007) Osteoclast differentiation and activation. Clin Calcium 17:484–492. doi:10.1038/nature01658
13. Bonewald LF (2011) The amazing osteocyte. J Bone Miner Res 26:229–238. doi:10.1002/jbmr.320
14. Lynch ME, Brooks D, Mohanan S et al (2013) In vivo tibial compression decreases osteolysis and tumor formation in a human metastatic breast cancer model. J Bone Miner Res 28:2357–2367. doi:10.1002/jbmr.1966
15. Lawson MA, McDonald MM, Kovacic N et al (2015) Osteoclasts control re-activation of dormant myeloma cells by remodeling the endosteal niche. Nat Commun 6:1–15. doi:10.1038/ncomms9983
16. Smith MCP (2004) CXCR4 regulates growth of both primary and metastatic breast cancer. Cancer Res 64:8604–8612. doi:10.1158/0008-5472.CAN-04-1844
17. Lapteva N, Yang A-G, Sanders DE et al (2005) CXCR4 knockdown by small interfering RNA abrogates breast tumor growth in vivo. Cancer Gene Ther 12:84–89. doi:10.1038/sj.cgt.7700770
18. Liang Z, Yoon Y, Votaw J et al (2005) Silencing of CXCR4 blocks breast cancer metastasis silencing of CXCR4 blocks breast cancer metastasis. Cancer Res 65:967–971

19. Teicher BA, Fricker SP (2010) CXCL12 (SDF-1)/CXCR4 pathway in cancer. Clin Cancer Res 16:2927–2931. doi:10.1158/1078-0432.CCR-09-2329
20. Wang H, Yu C, Gao X et al (2015) The osteogenic niche promotes early-stage bone colonization of disseminated breast cancer cells. Cancer Cell 27:193–210. doi:10.1016/j.ccell.2014.11.017
21. Guise TA, Yin JJ, Taylor SD et al (1996) Evidence for a causal role of parathyroid hormone-related protein in the pathogenesis of human breast cancer-mediated osteolysis. J Clin Invest 98:1544–1549. doi:10.1172/JCI118947
22. Yin JJ, Selander K, Chirgwin JM et al (1999) TGF-β signaling blockade inhibits PTHrP secretion by breast cancer cells and bone metastases development. J Clin Invest 103:197–206. doi:10.1172/JCI3523
23. Mundy GR (2002) Metastasis to bone: causes, consequences and therapeutic opportunities. Nat Rev Cancer 2:584–593. doi:10.1038/nrc867
24. Kozlow W, Guise TA (2005) Breast cancer metastasis to bone: mechanisms of osteolysis and implications for therapy. J Mammary Gland Biol Neoplasia 10:169–180. doi:10.1007/s10911-005-5399-8
25. Phadke PA, Mercer RR, Harms JF, Jia Y (2006) Kinetics of metastatic breast cancer cell trafficking in bone. Clin Cancer Res 12:1431–1440
26. Youngs SJ, Ali SA, Taub DD, Rees RC (1997) Chemokines induce migrational responses in human breast carcinoma cell lines. Int J Cancer 71:257–266
27. Kirschmann DA, Seftor EA, Fong SFT et al (2002) A molecular role for lysyl oxidase in breast cancer invasion. Cancer Res 1:4478–4483
28. Bendre MS, Montague DC, Peery T et al (2003) Interleukin-8 stimulation of osteoclastogenesis and bone resorption is a mechanism for the increased osteolysis of metastatic bone disease. Bone 33:28–37. doi:10.1016/S8756-3282(03)00086-3
29. Bendre MS, Margulies AG, Walser B et al (2005) Tumor-derived interleukin-8 stimulates osteolysis independent of the receptor activator of nuclear factor-kappaB ligand pathway. Cancer Res 65:11001–11009. doi:10.1158/0008-5472.CAN-05-2630
30. Kaplan RN, Riba RD, Zacharoulis S et al (2005) VEGFR1-positive haematopoietic bone marrow progenitors initiate the pre-metastatic niche. Nature 438:820–827. doi:10.1038/nature04186
31. Kaplan RN, Rafii S, Lyden D (2006) Preparing the "soil": the premetastatic niche. Cancer Res 66:11089–11093. doi:10.1158/0008-5472.CAN-06-2407
32. Thorpe MP, Valentine RJ, Moulton CJ et al (2011) Breast tumors induced by N-methyl-N-nitrosourea are damaging to bone strength, structure, and mineralization in the absence of metastasis in rats. J Bone Miner Res 26:769–776. doi:10.1002/jbmr.277
33. Cox TR, Rumney RMH, Schoof EM et al (2015) The hypoxic cancer secretome induces pre-metastatic bone lesions through lysyl oxidase. Nature 522:106–110. doi:10.1038/nature14492
34. Costa-Silva B, Aiello NM, Ocean AJ et al (2015) Pancreatic cancer exosomes initiate pre-metastatic niche formation in the liver. Nat Cell Biol 17:1–7. doi:10.1038/ncb3169
35. Hoshino A, Costa-Silva B, Shen T-L et al (2015) Tumour exosome integrins determine organotropic metastasis. Nature:1–19. doi:10.1038/nature15756
36. Kretschmann KL, Welm AL (2012) Mouse models of breast cancer metastasis to bone. Cancer Metastasis Rev 31:579–583. doi:10.1007/s10555-012-9378-4
37. Lelekakis M, Moseley JM, Martin TJ et al (1999) A novel orthotopic model of breast cancer metastasis to bone. Clin Exp Metastasis 17:163–170. doi:10.1023/A:1006689719505
38. Campbell JP, Merkel AR, Masood-Campbell SK et al (2012) Models of bone metastasis. J Vis Exp. doi:10.3791/4260
39. Kang Y, Siegel PM, Shu W et al (2003) A multigenic program mediating breast cancer metastasis to bone. Cancer Cell 3:537–549. doi:10.1016/S1535-6108(03)00132-6
40. Garcia T, Jackson A, Bachelier R et al (2008) A convenient clinically relevant model of human breast cancer bone metastasis. Clin Exp Metastasis 25:33–42. doi:10.1007/s10585-007-9099-1

41. Juárez P, Guise TA (2011) TGF-β in cancer and bone: implications for treatment of bone metastases. Bone 48:23–29. doi:10.1016/j.bone.2010.08.004
42. Mundy GR, Yoneda T, Hiraga T (2001) Preclinical studies with zoledronic acid and other bisphosphonates: impact on the bone microenvironment. Semin Oncol 28:35–44. doi:10.1053/sonc.2001.24158
43. Canon JR, Roudier M, Bryant R et al (2008) Inhibition of RANKL blocks skeletal tumor progression and improves survival in a mouse model of breast cancer bone metastasis. Clin Exp Metastasis 25:119–129. doi:10.1007/s10585-007-9127-1
44. Holzapfel BM, Thibaudeau L, Hesami P et al (2013) Humanised xenograft models of bone metastasis revisited: novel insights into species-specific mechanisms of cancer cell osteotropism. Cancer Metastasis Rev 32:129–145. doi:10.1007/s10555-013-9437-5
45. Kuperwasser C, Dessain S, Bierbaum BE et al (2005) A mouse model of human breast cancer metastasis to human bone. Cancer Res 65:6130–6138. doi:10.1158/0008-5472.CAN-04-1408
46. Whittle JR, Lewis MT, Lindeman GJ, Visvader JE (2015) Patient-derived xenograft models of breast cancer and their predictive power. Breast Cancer Res 17:17. doi:10.1186/s13058-015-0523-1
47. DeRose YS, Wang G, Lin Y-C et al (2011) Tumor grafts derived from women with breast cancer authentically reflect tumor pathology, growth, metastasis and disease outcomes. Nat Med 17:1514–1520. doi:10.1038/nm.2454
48. Ganick DJ, Sarnwick RD, Shahidi NT, Manning DD (1980) Inability of intravenously injected monocellular suspensions of human bone marrow to establish in the nude mouse. Int Arch Allergy Immunol 62:330–333
49. Kyoizumi BS, Baum CM, Kaneshima H et al (1992) Implantation and maintenance of functional human bone marrow in SCID – hu Mice. Blood 79:1704–1711
50. Boynton E, Aubin J, Gross A et al (1996) Human osteoblasts survive and deposit new bone when human bone is implanted in SCID mouse. Bone 18:321–326. doi:10.1016/8756-3282(96)00015-4
51. Christianson SW, Greiner DL, Schweitzer IB et al (1996) Role of natural killer cells on engraftment of human lymphoid cells and on metastasis of human T-lymphoblastoid leukemia cells in C57BL/6J-scid mice and in C57BL/6J-scid bg mice. Cell Immunol 171:186–199. doi:10.1006/cimm.1996.0193
52. Shultz LD, Schweitzer PA, Christianson SW et al (2010) Multiple defects in innate and adaptive immunologic function in NOD / LtSz-scid mice. J Immunol 154:180–191
53. Meyerrose TE, Herrbrich P, Hess DA, Nolta JA (2003) Immune-deficient mouse models for analysis of human stem cells. BioTechniques 35:1262–1272
54. Hutmacher DW, Horch RE, Loessner D et al (2009) Translating tissue engineering technology platforms into cancer research. J Cell Mol Med 13:1417–1427. doi:10.1111/j.1582-4934.2009.00853.x
55. Wang F, Weaver VM, Petersen OW et al (1998) Reciprocal interactions between beta1-integrin and epidermal growth factor receptor in three-dimensional basement membrane breast cultures: a different perspective in epithelial biology. Proc Natl Acad Sci U S A 95:14821–14826. doi:10.1073/pnas.95.25.14821
56. Hosseinkhani H, Hosseinkhani M, Tian F et al (2006) Osteogenic differentiation of mesenchymal stem cells in self-assembled peptide-amphiphile nanofibers. Biomaterials 27:4079–4086. doi:10.1016/j.biomaterials.2006.03.030
57. Rhodes NP, Srivastava JK, Smith RF, Longinotti C (2004) Metabolic and histological analysis of mesenchymal stem cells grown in 3-D hyaluronan-based scaffolds. J Mater Sci Mater Med 15:391–395. doi:10.1023/B:JMSM.0000021108.74004.7e
58. Fischbach C, Chen R, Matsumoto T et al (2007) Engineering tumors with 3D scaffolds. Nat Methods 4:855–860. doi:10.1038/nmeth1085
59. Kenny PA, Lee GY, Myers CA et al (2007) The morphologies of breast cancer cell lines in three-dimensional assays correlate with their profiles of gene expression. Mol Oncol 1:84–96. doi:10.1016/j.molonc.2007.02.004

60. Weaver VM, Petersen OW, Wang F et al (1997) Reversion of the malignant phenotype of human breast cells in three-dimensional culture and in vivo by integrin blocking antibodies. J Cell Biol 137:231–245. doi:10.1083/jcb.137.1.231
61. Weaver VM, Lelièvre S, Lakins JN et al (2002) β4 integrin-dependent formation of polarized three-dimensional architecture confers resistance to apoptosis in normal and malignant mammary epithelium. Cancer Cell 2:205–216. doi:10.1016/S1535-6108(02)00125-3
62. Rizki A, Weaver VM, Lee S-Y et al (2008) A human breast cell model of preinvasive to invasive transition. Cancer Res 68:1378–1387. doi:10.1158/0008-5472.CAN-07-2225
63. Fraley SI, Feng Y, Krishnamurthy R et al (2010) A distinctive role for focal adhesion proteins in three-dimensional cell motility. Nat Cell Biol 12:598–604. doi:10.1038/ncb2062
64. Fischbach C, Kong HJ, Hsiong SX et al (2009) Cancer cell angiogenic capability is regulated by 3D culture and integrin engagement. Proc Natl Acad Sci U S A 106:399–404. doi:10.1073/pnas.0808932106
65. DelNero P, Lane M, Verbridge SS et al (2015) 3D culture broadly regulates tumor cell hypoxia response and angiogenesis via pro-inflammatory pathways. Biomaterials 55:110–118. doi:10.1016/j.biomaterials.2015.03.035
66. Pickl M, Ries CH (2009) Comparison of 3D and 2D tumor models reveals enhanced HER2 activation in 3D associated with an increased response to trastuzumab. Oncogene 28:461–468. doi:10.1038/onc.2008.394
67. Sutherland RM, Eddy HA, Bareham B et al (1979) Resistance to adriamycin in multicellular spheroids. Int J Radiat Oncol Biol Phys 5:1225–1230. doi:10.1016/0360-3016(79)90643-6
68. Sato T, Stange DE, Ferrante M et al (2011) Long-term expansion of epithelial organoids from human colon, adenoma, adenocarcinoma, and Barrett's epithelium. Gastroenterology 141:1762–1772. doi:10.1053/j.gastro.2011.07.050
69. Gao D, Vela I, Sboner A et al (2014) Organoid cultures derived from patients with advanced prostate cancer. Cell 159:176–187. doi:10.1016/j.cell.2014.08.016
70. Van De Wetering M, Francies HE, Francis JM et al (2015) Prospective derivation of a living organoid biobank of colorectal cancer patients. Cell 161:933–945. doi:10.1016/j.cell.2015.03.053
71. Cheung KJ, Gabrielson E, Werb Z, Ewald AJ (2013) Collective invasion in breast cancer requires a conserved basal epithelial program. Cell 155:1639–1651. doi:10.1016/j.cell.2013.11.029
72. Elsdale T, Bard J (1972) Collagen substrata for studies on cell behavior. J Cell Biol 54:626–637. doi:10.1083/jcb.54.3.626
73. Benton G, Kleinman HK, George J, Arnaoutova I (2011) Multiple uses of basement membrane-like matrix (BME/Matrigel) in vitro and in vivo with cancer cells. Int J Cancer 128:1751–1757. doi:10.1002/ijc.25781
74. Kang B-J, Ryu H-H, Park S-S et al (2012) Effect of matrigel on the osteogenic potential of canine adipose tissue-derived mesenchymal stem cells. J Vet Med Sci 74:827–836. doi:10.1292/jvms.11-0484
75. Donzelli E, Salvadè A, Mimo P et al (2007) Mesenchymal stem cells cultured on a collagen scaffold: In vitro osteogenic differentiation. Arch Oral Biol 52:64–73. doi:10.1016/j.archoralbio.2006.07.007
76. Salasznyk RM, Williams WA, Boskey A et al (2004) Adhesion to vitronectin and collagen I promotes osteogenic differentiation of human mesenchymal stem cells. J Biomed Biotechnol 2004:24–34. doi:10.1155/S1110724304306017
77. Evans ND, Gentleman E, Chen X et al (2010) Extracellular matrix-mediated osteogenic differentiation of murine embryonic stem cells. Biomaterials 31:3244–3252. doi:10.1016/j.biomaterials.2010.01.039
78. Shih Y-RV, Tseng K-FF, Lai H-YY et al (2011) Matrix stiffness regulation of integrin-mediated mechanotransduction during osteogenic differentiation of human mesenchymal stem cells. J Bone Miner Res 26:730–738. doi:10.1002/jbmr.278
79. Pampaloni F, Reynaud EG, Stelzer EHK (2007) The third dimension bridges the gap between cell culture and live tissue. Nat Rev Mol Cell Biol 8:839–845. doi:10.1038/nrm2236

80. Barney LE, Dandley EC, Jansen LE et al (2015) A cell–ECM screening method to predict breast cancer metastasis. Integr Biol 7:198–212. doi:10.1039/C4IB00218K
81. Page JM, Merkel AR, Ruppender NS et al (2015) Matrix rigidity regulates the transition of tumor cells to a bone-destructive phenotype through integrin β3 and TGF-β receptor type II. Biomaterials 64:33–44. doi:10.1016/j.biomaterials.2015.06.026
82. Taubenberger A V, Quent VM, Thibaudeau L et al (2013) Delineating breast cancer cell interactions with engineered bone microenvironments. J Bone Miner Res 28:1399–1411. doi:10.1002/jbmr.1875
83. Pathi SP, Kowalczewski C, Tadipatri R, Fischbach C (2010) A novel 3-D mineralized tumor model to study breast cancer bone metastasis. PLoS One. doi:10.1371/journal.pone.0008849
84. Guelcher SA, Sterling JA (2011) Contribution of bone tissue modulus to breast cancer metastasis to bone. Cancer Microenviron 4:247–259. doi:10.1007/s12307-011-0078-3
85. Engler AJ, Sen S, Sweeney HL, Discher DE (2006) Matrix elasticity directs stem cell lineage specification. Cell 126:677–689. doi:10.1016/j.cell.2006.06.044
86. Chaudhuri O, Gu L, Klumpers D et al (2015) Hydrogels with tunable stress relaxation regulate stem cell fate and activity. Nat Mater. doi:10.1038/nmat4489
87. Paszek MJ, Zahir N, Johnson KR et al (2005) Tensional homeostasis and the malignant phenotype. Cancer Cell 8:241–254. doi:10.1016/j.ccr.2005.08.010
88. Baker BM, Trappmann B, Wang WY et al (2015) Cell-mediated fibre recruitment drives extracellular matrix mechanosensing in engineered fibrillar microenvironments. Nat Mater 14:1262–1268. doi:10.1038/nmat4444
89. Datta N, Holtorf HL, Sikavitsas VI et al (2005) Effect of bone extracellular matrix synthesized in vitro on the osteoblastic differentiation of marrow stromal cells. Biomaterials 26:971–977. doi:10.1016/j.biomaterials.2004.04.001
90. Reichert JC, Quent VMC, Burke LJ et al (2010) Mineralized human primary osteoblast matrices as a model system to analyse interactions of prostate cancer cells with the bone microenvironment. Biomaterials 31:7928–7936. doi:10.1016/j.biomaterials.2010.06.055
91. Prewitz MC, Seib FP, von Bonin M et al (2013) Tightly anchored tissue-mimetic matrices as instructive stem cell microenvironments. Nat Methods 10:788–794. doi:10.1038/nmeth.2523
92. Prewitz MC, Stißel A, Friedrichs J et al (2015) Extracellular matrix deposition of bone marrow stroma enhanced by macromolecular crowding. Biomaterials 73:60–69. doi:10.1016/j.biomaterials.2015.09.014
93. Antia M, Baneyx G, Kubow KE, Vogel V (2008) Fibronectin in aging extracellular matrix fibrils is progressively unfolded by cells and elicits an enhanced rigidity response. Faraday Discuss 139:229–249; discussion 309–325, 419–420. doi:10.1039/b718714a
94. Herklotz M, Prewitz MC, Bidan CM et al (2015) Availability of extracellular matrix biopolymers and differentiation state of human mesenchymal stem cells determine tissue-like growth in vitro. Biomaterials 60:121–129. doi:10.1016/j.biomaterials.2015.04.061
95. Fröhlich M, Grayson WL, Marolt D et al (2010) Bone grafts engineered from human adipose-derived stem cells in perfusion bioreactor culture. Tissue Eng Part A 16:179–189
96. Marolt D, Marcos Campos I, Bhumiratana S et al (2012) Engineering bone tissue from human embryonic stem cells. Proc Natl Acad Sci 109:8705–8709. doi:10.1073/pnas.1201830109
97. Mauney JR, Sjostorm S, Blumberg J et al (2004) Mechanical stimulation promotes osteogenic differentiation of human bone marrow stromal cells on 3-D partially demineralized bone scaffolds in vitro. Calcif Tissue Int 74:458–468. doi:10.1007/s00223-003-0104-7
98. Grayson WL, Bhumiratana S, Cannizzaro C et al (2008) Effects of initial seeding density and fluid perfusion rate on formation of tissue-engineered bone. Tissue Eng Part A 14:1809–1820. doi:10.1089/ten.tea.2007.0255
99. Villasante A, Marturano-Kruik A, Vunjak-Novakovic G (2014) Bioengineered human tumor within a bone niche. Biomaterials 35:5785–5794. doi:10.1016/j.biomaterials.2014.03.081
100. Holen I, Nutter F, Wilkinson JM et al (2015) Human breast cancer bone metastasis in vitro and in vivo: a novel 3D model system for studies of tumour cell-bone cell interactions. Clin Exp Metastasis 32:1–14. doi:10.1007/s10585-015-9737-y

101. Marcos-Campos I, Marolt D, Petridis P et al (2012) Bone scaffold architecture modulates the development of mineralized bone matrix by human embryonic stem cells. Biomaterials 33:8329–8342. doi:10.1016/j.biomaterials.2012.08.013

102. Jansen LE, Birch NP, Schiffman JD et al (2015) Mechanics of intact bone marrow. J Mech Behav Biomed Mater 50:299–307. doi:10.1016/j.jmbbm.2015.06.023

103. Pathi SP, Lin DDW, Dorvee JR et al (2011) Hydroxyapatite nanoparticle-containing scaffolds for the study of breast cancer bone metastasis. Biomaterials 32(22):5112. doi:10.1016/j.biomaterials.2011.03.055

104. Kim S-S, Sun Park M, Jeon O et al (2006) Poly(lactide-co-glycolide)/hydroxyapatite composite scaffolds for bone tissue engineering. Biomaterials 27:1399–1409. doi:10.1016/j.biomaterials.2005.08.016

105. Shih Y-RV, Hwang Y, Phadke A et al (2014) Calcium phosphate-bearing matrices induce osteogenic differentiation of stem cells through adenosine signaling. Proc Natl Acad Sci U S A 111:990–995. doi:10.1073/pnas.1321717111

106. Mattei G, Ferretti C, Tirella A et al (2015) Decoupling the role of stiffness from other hydroxyapatite signalling cues in periosteal derived stem cell differentiation. Sci Rep 5:10778. doi:10.1038/srep10778

107. Ye M, Mohanty P, Ghosh G (2014) Biomimetic apatite-coated porous PVA scaffolds promote the growth of breast cancer cells. Mater Sci Eng C 44:310–316. doi:10.1016/j.msec.2014.08.044

108. Boskey A (2003) Bone mineral crystal size. Osteoporos Int 14:S16–S21. doi:10.1007/s00198-003-1468-2

109. Haka AS, Shafer-Peltier KE, Fitzmaurice M et al (2002) Identifying microcalcifications in benign and malignant breast lesions by probing differences in their chemical composition using Raman spectroscopy. Cancer Res 62:5375–5380

110. Bi X, Sterling JA, Merkel AR et al (2013) Prostate cancer metastases alter bone mineral and matrix composition independent of effects on bone architecture in mice–a quantitative study using microCT and Raman spectroscopy. Bone 56:454–460. doi:10.1016/j.bone.2013.07.006

111. Choi S, Coonrod S, Estroff L, Fischbach C (2015) Chemical and physical properties of carbonated hydroxyapatite affect breast cancer cell behavior. Acta Biomater 24:333–342. doi:10.1016/j.actbio.2015.06.001

112. Al-Munajjed AA, Plunkett NA, Gleeson JP et al (2009) Development of a biomimetic collagen-hydroxyapatite scaffold for bone tissue engineering using a SBF immersion technique. J Biomed Mater Res - Part B Appl Biomater 90 B:584–591. doi:10.1002/jbm.b.31320

113. Xia Z, Yu X, Jiang X et al (2013) Fabrication and characterization of biomimetic collagen-apatite scaffolds with tunable structures for bone tissue engineering. Acta Biomater 9:7308–7319. doi:10.1016/j.actbio.2013.03.038

114. Zhang W, Liao SS, Cui FZ (2003) Hierarchical self-assembly of nano-fibrils in mineralized collagen. Chem Mater 15:3221–3226. doi:10.1021/cm030080g

115. Nakagawa K, Abukawa H, Shin MY et al (2004) Osteoclastogenesis on tissue-engineered bone. Tissue Eng 10:93–100. doi:10.1089/107632704322791736

116. Jones GL, Motta A, Marshall MJ et al (2009) Osteoblast: osteoclast co-cultures on silk fibroin, chitosan and PLLA films. Biomaterials 30:5376–5384. doi:10.1016/j.biomaterials.2009.07.028

117. Bernhardt A, Thieme S, Domaschke H et al (2010) Crosstalk of osteoblast and osteoclast precursors on mineralized collagen-towards an in vitro model for bone remodeling. J Biomed Mater Res - Part A 95:848–856. doi:10.1002/jbm.a.32856

118. Heinemann S, Heinemann C, Wenisch S et al (2013) Calcium phosphate phases integrated in silica/collagen nanocomposite xerogels enhance the bioactivity and ultimately manipulate the osteoblast/osteoclast ratio in a human co-culture model. Acta Biomater 9:4878–4888. doi:10.1016/j.actbio.2012.10.010

119. Jimi E, Nakamura I, Amano H et al (1996) Osteoclast function is activated by osteoblastic cells through a mechanism involving cell-to-cell contact. Endocrinology 137:2187–2190. doi:10.1210/endo.137.5.8612568

120. Hikita A, Iimura T, Oshima Y et al (2015) Analyses of bone modeling and remodeling using in vitro reconstitution system with two-photon microscopy. Bone 76:5–17. doi:10.1016/j.bone.2015.02.030

121. Krishnan V, Vogler EA, Sosnoski DM, Mastro AM (2014) In vitro mimics of bone remodeling and the vicious cycle of cancer in bone. J Cell Physiol 229:453–462. doi:10.1002/jcp.24464

122. Zhu W, Wang M, Fu Y et al (2015) Engineering a biomimetic three-dimensional nanostructured bone model for breast cancer bone metastasis study. Acta Biomater 14:164–174. doi:10.1016/j.actbio.2014.12.008

123. Dhawan A, von Bonin M, Bray LJ et al (2016) Functional interference in the bone marrow microenvironment by disseminated breast cancer cells. Stem Cells:1–17. doi:10.1002/stem.2384

124. Chowdhury R, Webber JP, Gurney M et al (2015) Cancer exosomes trigger mesenchymal stem cell differentiation into pro-angiogenic and pro-invasive myofibroblasts. Oncotarget 6:715–731. doi:10.18632/oncotarget.2711

125. Thomas RJ, Guise TA, Yin JJ (1999) Breast cancer cells interact with osteoblasts to support osteoclast formation. Endocrinology 140:4451–4458

126. Mancino AT, Klimberg VS, Yamamoto M et al (2001) Breast cancer increases osteoclastogenesis by secreting M-CSF and upregulating RANKL in stromal cells. J Surg Res 100:18–24. doi:10.1006/jsre.2001.6204

127. Dhurjati R, Krishnan V, Shuman LA et al (2008) Metastatic breast cancer cells colonize and degrade three-dimensional osteoblastic tissue in vitro. Clin Exp Metastasis 25:741–752. doi:10.1007/s10585-008-9185-z

128. Krishnan V, L a S, Sosnoski DM et al (2011) Dynamic interaction between breast cancer cells and osteoblastic tissue: comparison of two- and three-dimensional cultures. J Cell Physiol 226:2150–2158. doi:10.1002/jcp.22550

129. Sieh S, Lubik AA, Clements JA et al (2010) Interactions between human osteoblasts and prostate cancer cells in a novel 3D in vitro model. Organogenesis 6:181–188. doi:10.4161/org.6.3.12041

130. Müller A, Homey B, Soto H et al (2001) Involvement of chemokine receptors in breast cancer metastasis. Nature 410:50–56. doi:10.1038/35065016

131. Shiozawa Y, Pedersen EA, Havens AM et al (2011) Human prostate cancer metastases target the hematopoietic stem cell niche to establish footholds in mouse bone marrow. J Clin Invest 121:1298–1312. doi:10.1172/JCI43414DS1

132. Shiozawa Y, Eber MR, Berry JE, Taichman RS (2015) Bone marrow as a metastatic niche for disseminated tumor cells from solid tumors. Bonekey Rep 4:1–7. doi:10.1038/bonekey.2015.57

133. Pederson L, Winding B, Foged NT et al (1999) Identification of breast cancer cell line-derived paracrine factors that stimulate osteoclast activity. Cancer Res 59:5849–5855

134. Lynch ME, Chiou AE, Lee MJ et al (2016) 3D mechanical loading modulates the osteogenic response of mesenchymal stem cells to tumor-derived soluble signals. Tissue Eng Part A 22:1–10. doi:10.1089/ten.tea.2016.0153

135. Goldstein RH, Reagan MR, Anderson K et al (2010) Human bone marrow-derived MSCs can home to orthotopic breast cancer tumors and promote bone metastasis. Cancer Res 70:10044. doi:10.1158/0008-5472.CAN-10-1254

136. Wozney JM, Rosen V, Celeste a J et al (1988) Novel regulators of bone formation: molecular clones and activities. Science 242:1528–1534. doi:10.1126/science.3201241

137. Katsuno Y, Hanyu A, Kanda H et al (2008) Bone morphogenetic protein signaling enhances invasion and bone metastasis of breast cancer cells through Smad pathway. Oncogene 27:6322–6333. doi:10.1038/onc.2008.232

138. Moreau JE, Anderson K, Mauney JR et al (2007) Tissue-engineered bone serves as a target for metastasis of human breast cancer in a mouse model. Cancer Res 67:10304. doi:10.1158/0008-5472.CAN-07-2483

139. Gao H, Priebe W, Glod J, Banerjee D (2009) Activation of signal transducers and activators of transcription 3 and focal adhesion kinase by stromal cell-derived factor 1 is required for migration of human mesenchymal stem cells in response to tumor cell-conditioned medium. Stem Cells 27:857–865. doi:10.1002/stem.23

140. Wobus M, List C, Dittrich T et al (2015) Breast carcinoma cells modulate the chemoattractive activity of human bone marrow-derived mesenchymal stromal cells by interfering with CXCL12. Int J Cancer 136:44–54. doi:10.1002/ijc.28960

141. Kinder M, Chislock E, Bussard KM et al (2008) Metastatic breast cancer induces an osteoblast inflammatory response. Exp Cell Res 314:173–183. doi:10.1016/j.yexcr.2007.09.021

142. Jia S, Zocco D, Samuels ML et al (2014) Emerging technologies in extracellular vesicle-based molecular diagnostics. Expert Rev Mol Diagn 14:307–321. doi:10.1586/14737159.2014.893828

143. Santana SM, Antonyak MA, Cerione RA, Kirby BJ (2014) Microfluidic isolation of cancer-cell-derived microvesicles from hetergeneous extracellular shed vesicle populations. Biomed Microdevices 16:869–877. doi:10.1007/s10544-014-9891-z

144. Antonyak MA, Li B, Lindsey K et al (2011) Cancer cell-derived microvesicles induce transformation by transferring tissue transglutaminase and fibronectin to recipient cells. Proc Natl Acad Sci 108:17569–17569. doi:10.1073/pnas.1114824108

145. Le MTN, Hamar P, Guo C et al (2014) miR-200 – containing extracellular vesicles promote breast cancer cell metastasis. J Clin Invest 124:5109–5128. doi:10.1172/JCI75695DS1

146. Stiehler M, Bünger C, Baatrup A et al (2009) Effect of dynamic 3-D culture on proliferation, distribution, and osteogenic differentiation of human mesenchymal stem cells. J Biomed Mater Res - Part A 89:96–107. doi:10.1002/jbm.a.31967

147. Song K, Liu T, Cui Z et al (2008) Three-dimensional fabrication of engineered bone with human bio-derived bone scaffolds in a rotating wall vessel bioreactor. J Biomed Mater Res A 86:323–332. doi:10.1002/jbm.a.31624

148. Huang C, Ogawa R (2012) Effect of hydrostatic pressure on bone regeneration using human mesenchymal stem cells. Tissue Eng Part A 18:2106–2113. doi:10.1089/ten.tea.2012.0064

149. Matziolis G, Tuischer J, Kasper G et al (2006) Simulation of cell differentiation in fracture healing: mechanically loaded composite scaffolds in a novel bioreactor system. Tissue Eng 12:201–208. doi:10.1089/ten.2006.12.201

150. Sottnik JL, Dai J, Zhang H et al (2015) Tumor-induced pressure in the bone microenvironment causes osteocytes to promote the growth of prostate cancer bone metastases. Cancer Res 75:2151–2158. doi:10.1158/0008-5472.CAN-14-2493

151. Polacheck WJ, Charest JL, Kamm RD (2011) Interstitial flow influences direction of tumor cell migration through competing mechanisms. Proc Natl Acad Sci U S A 108:11115–11120. doi:10.1073/pnas.1103581108

152. Knothe Tate ML, Knothe U, Niederer P (1998) Experimental elucidation of mechanical load-induced fluid flow and its potential role in bone metabolism and functional adaptation. Am J Med Sci 316:189–195. doi:10.1097/00000441-199809000-00007

153. Santoro M, Lamhamedi-Cherradi S-E, Menegaz BA et al (2015) Flow perfusion effects on three-dimensional culture and drug sensitivity of Ewing sarcoma. Proc Natl Acad Sci U S A 112:1506684112. doi:10.1073/pnas.1506684112

154. Xiong J, Piemontese M, Onal M et al (2015) Osteocytes, not osteoblasts or lining cells, are the main source of the RANKL required for osteoclast formation in remodeling bone. PLoS One 10:e0138189. doi:10.1371/journal.pone.0138189

Building Better Tumor Models: Organoid Systems to Investigate Angiogenesis

Venktesh S. Shirure, Mary Kathryn Sewell-Loftin, Sandra F. Lam,
Tyson D. Todd, Priscilla Y. Hwang, and Steven C. George

Abstract Cancer remains a leading cause of death in the United States and other developed countries. In nearly all cases, the cause of death is related to complications associated with tumor metastasis to distant sites such as the brain, lung, liver, and bone. A central feature of tumor progression is the acquisition of a blood supply, which provides nutrients for the growing tumor as well as conduits for transport of cancer cells. Our understanding of how a tumor acquires and manipulates a blood supply has been gleaned largely from animal models, but more recent advances in tissue engineering and microfabrication have led to clever 3D in vitro models of tumors that include blood vessels. This chapter will first briefly review the process of blood vessel growth including our knowledge of blood vessels within the cancer microenvironment, and discuss the most recent advances to mimic blood vessel growth in the tumor microenvironment using 3D in vitro culture methods. Finally, we discuss several important factors that control blood vessel growth including hypoxia, cellular metabolism, and tissue mechanics, which provide rich opportunities for future investigation.

Keywords 3D models • Tissue engineering • Cancer microenvironment • Hypoxia • Mechanics • Metabolism • Metastasis

1 Introduction

Angiogenesis, the process of vessels sprouting from existing blood vessels, is a critical event in numerous pathophysiological processes, including embryogenesis, wound healing, inflammation, diabetes, and cancer. Early growth of a neoplastic tissue engenders a metabolic deficit (e.g., glucose and oxygen) that limits growth. Compensatory mechanisms that permit additional growth include changes in

Venktesh S. Shirure and Mary Kathryn Sewell-Loftin equally contributed to the manuscript

V.S. Shirure • M.K. Sewell-Loftin • S.F. Lam • T.D. Todd • P.Y. Hwang • S.C. George (✉)
Department of Biomedical Engineering, Washington University in St. Louis,
One Brookings Drive, St. Louis, MO 63130-1097, USA
e-mail: vsshirure@gmail.com; mary.k.sewell@gmail.com; sandra.lam107@gmail.com;
tyson.d.todd@wustl.edu; priscillahwang@wustl.edu; scg@wustl.edu

© Springer International Publishing AG 2018   117
S. Soker, A. Skardal (eds.), *Tumor Organoids*, Cancer Drug Discovery
and Development, DOI 10.1007/978-3-319-60511-1_7

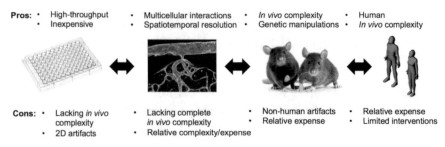

Pros: • High-throughput   • Multicellular interactions   • *In vivo* complexity   • Human
         • Inexpensive   • Spatiotemporal resolution   • Genetic manipulations   • *In vivo* complexity

Cons: • Lacking *in vivo*   • Lacking complete   • Non-human artifacts   • Relative expense
            complexity   *in vivo* complexity   • Relative expense   • Limited interventions
         • 2D artifacts   • Relative complexity/expense

Fig. 1 Advantages and disadvantages of tumor model systems. Experimental model systems of the tumor microenvironment (TME) broadly include four categories: (**a**) traditional 2D monolayer cell culture, (**b**) 3D in vitro multicellular models, (**c**) animal models, and (**d**) human models. While simple and inexpensive, 2D monolayer culture cannot replicate the essential heterotypic cell-cell and cell-matrix interactions that have proven essential in the biology of the TME. Animal models can replicate the integrated response of the whole animal, but many times the immune system is compromised to allow the study of human cells and the temporal and spatial resolution of the TME is severely limited. While humans represent the "perfect" system, studies are limited to more advanced cancers, and most interventions, including genetic manipulation, are not possible. Advanced 3D in vitro multicellular models allow the step-by-step incorporation of key components in the TME, and high spatial and temporal resolution of dynamic events. While it may be difficult to fully recapitulate the TME in vitro, new advances in microfabrication and imaging provide opportunities to tease apart complex cell-cell and cell-matrix dynamics in the TME. The arrows linking the models are purposely two-way as observations made in one system can answer questions, but also generate new hypotheses that can be tested or confirmed in alternate systems. While all four approaches are important, a 3D in vitro model can provide unique opportunities to study angiogenesis in the tumor microenvironment

metabolism and the acquisition of a blood supply. The access to vasculature allows tumors to disseminate cancer cells to distant organ sites, leading to the formation of metastatic lesions. The hypothesis that angiogenesis is required for tumor growth was first proposed by Folkman in 1971 [1]. Thereafter, there has been reaffirmation of this concept by independent groups [2–5]. As a result, anti-angiogenic therapy is part of the treatment regimen for some types of solid cancers including breast, lung, and renal cancers.

The biology of angiogenesis within the tumor microenvironment has been largely studied in either mouse models or simple 2D monolayer culture systems (Fig. 1). Although these classical model systems have provided a wealth of understanding, they have limitations and there remains a need for novel model systems that can further improve our understanding of angiogenesis. Animal models offer a complex tissue environment compared to 2D cell cultures, but the biology of these animal models is simply not human. A more recent model used to study cancer biology is the patient-derived xenograft (PDX) in which a human tumor is implanted either subcutaneously or orthotopically in an immunocompromised mouse. The major limitation in the subcutaneous model is that it lacks important features of the original tumor microenvironment. In contrast, orthotopic tumor xenografts are implanted at the original tumor site and are considered more reliable for studying the biology or predicting drug response in humans. Nonetheless, in both cases the tumor xenografts are surrounded by non-human tissue stroma, developed in the absence of a normal immune response, and take several months to grow [6, 7]. Furthermore, the animal models are expensive to maintain, are not high-throughput, provide barriers to some imaging technologies, and provide inherently limited spatial and temporal resolution. The 2D culture systems, on the other hand, are much easier to develop and utilize. However, these systems lack the fundamental complexity of the multicellular 3D tissue microenvironment. These limitations have led to the development of 3D culture systems, which are positioned between 2D and animal models in terms of advantages and limitations (Fig. 1).

The idea of mimicking 3D tissue function in vitro is not new in cancer research; in fact, tumor spheroids were first presented nearly four decades ago [8]. Since then, the model systems have evolved from 3D tumor spheroids comprised solely of cancerous cells to tumor spheroids composed of a mixture of cancer and stromal cells, vascularized tumors, and more recently perfused vascularized tumors [8–10]. Despite the recent progress that has been made in the field using conventional biological models, we still do not have a complete picture of the impact of microenvironmental factors that dictate the formation and maintenance of cancer-associated blood vessels. Herein we provide a limited discussion of the biological pathways of angiogenesis; unique features of vessels within the cancer microenvironment; the important roles of hypoxia, cellular metabolism, and mechanics on tumor angiogenesis; and tumor metastasis as a backdrop to understand how the creation of in vitro 3D tumor organoids can be used to further augment our understanding of tumor angiogenesis and its role in tumor progression.

2   Cell Signaling Pathways in Tumor Angiogenesis

The growth of blood vessels from existing blood vessels to meet the metabolic needs of a tumor defines tumor angiogenesis (Fig. 2a) [11]. The important proangiogenic factors involved in cancer are vascular endothelial growth factor (VEGF), placental growth factor (PlGF), and angiopoietin-1 (ANG1) [12]. These pro-angiogenic factors activate otherwise quiescent vessels and "turn on" the so-called angiogenic switch. VEGF has been extensively studied for how it activates the angiogenic program [12]. Vessel exposure to proangiogenic factors leads to vasodilation and increased vascular permeability. The endothelial cells lining the vessel degrade the basement membrane by proteolytic activity of matrix metalloproteinases (MMP). The endothelial cells detach and organize into a new branch in which the endothelial cell leading the branch is called a tip cell and the endothelial cells following are called stalk cells (Fig. 2b). The tip cells sense gradients of morphogens and guide the direction of the new sprout. The tip cell restricts the stalk cells from transforming into other tip cells by secreting delta-like ligand 4 and signaling through the NOTCH-mediated pathway. The stalk cells, on the other hand, are responsible for proliferating and forming continuous extension branching from the original vessel. Eventually vessel junctions are reestablished, proteolytic activity is neutralized, the basement membrane is synthesized, and pericytes are recruited

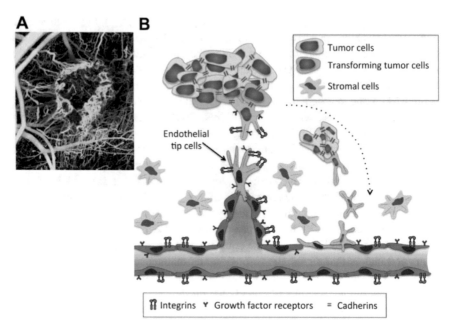

Fig. 2 Angiogenesis in the tumor microenvironment. (**a**) Angiogenesis is required to promote tumor growth. The angiogenesis in tumors of mice was captured using optical frequency domain imaging (OFDI) technique. This high resolution microscopy shows tumor associated vasculature is dense and unorganized compared to surrounding non-tumor tissue. The red and yellow indicate the depth of the tissue and blue indicates lymphatics. Scale bar = 500 mm (reprinted with permission [11]). (**b**) Numerous signaling factors, including soluble growth factors and membrane bound receptors, integrins, and junction proteins, play a role in the development of vasculature during tumor progression. Such signaling is regulated both via tumor cells as well as vascular cells, including the tip cell of blood vessels undergoing angiogenesis

to stabilize the nascent vessels. The processes that stabilize the vessels are conducted by numerous molecular pathways mediated by platelet-derived growth factor B (PDGF-B), ANG-1, transforming growth factor-β (TGF-β), ephrin-B2 and NOTCH. The WNT signaling pathway also plays a role in tumor angiogenesis [13, 14]. Endothelial cells express an array of WNT ligands and their frizzled (FZD) receptors, some of which are essential for stimulating endothelial cell proliferation [14]. One of the regulators of WNT signaling is β-catenin. Activation of WNT/β-catenin signaling can induce numerous tumor growth genes including Myc, Axin2, and Zeb1 in vivo. In contrast, abnormal β-catenin activation and signaling has been associated with solid stress from tumor masses [13, 14].

Another important cell signaling pathway that regulates vessel integrity is the angiopoietin (ANG) and TIE signaling system; this pathway stimulates basement membrane deposition to promote vessel tightness [15, 16]. However, dysregulation of ANG and TIE signaling in sprouting endothelial cells can lead to vascular permeability, inflammation, and defects that allow for tumor metastasis [17]. Finally, p21-activated kinases (PAKs) alter RhoGTPase signaling, causing irregular actomyosin contractility and actin dynamics, and altered cell motility and permeability in endothelial cells [18, 19]. Furthermore, work by Ghosh et al. has shown that endothelial cells in the tumor microenvironment demonstrate aberrant Rho activity and fail to respond to mechanical strain in the same manner as normal endothelial cells [20]. In addition to altering cell motility and permeability, disruption of actin dynamics also changes contractile forces and tension in cells, resulting in changes to the transcriptional regulators YAP and TAZ [21–23]. Studies are beginning to investigate the exact mechanisms that YAP and TAZ have on endothelial cells in cancer-associated blood vessels, but some preliminary work reveals that translocation of YAP/TAZ to the nucleus can upregulate the expression of target genes such as connective tissue growth factor (CTGF) and can lead to an increase in monocyte adhesion to endothelial cells [21].

3 Organoid Systems to Model Angiogenesis

The early 3D systems were mainly devoted to create vessels to study activation of angiogenic programs. In these systems, either a single suspension of endothelial cells or endothelial cell coated microbeads were embedded into extracellular matrix (ECM) gels, such as collagen, fibrin, or Matrigel [24, 25]. These gels were placed in micro-well plates or similar assemblies to generate a 3D culture system. These approaches have successfully yielded capillary microvessels with lumens, but these systems have several limitations. The vasculature was not designed for perfusion of fluid through the vascular lumen, the vasculature formed was not stable over time, and creating controllable temporal and spatial concentration gradients around the vasculature is difficult.

The rapidly emerging "organ-on-a-chip" field utilizes tissue engineering and microfabrication to create in vitro microtissues in platforms that are optically clear, cost-effective, have high spatial and temporal resolution, can capture events in real time, and have the potential to be high-throughput. These systems are proving critical for uncovering novel aspects of angiogenesis. The general method to fabricate the organ-on-a-chip platform begins with the computer-aided design of the device. A mask is printed from these designs, and used to create a master mold. The master mold is fabricated using soft lithography techniques, in which a silicon vapor coated with photoresist, such as SU8, is covered with the mask and exposed to UV. The UV light polymerizes the exposed area of photoresist, which is the area of device design on the mask. The non-polymerized photoresist is etched, and the master mold is used to create numerous replicas of the device design using polymers such as polydimethylsiloxane (PDMS). The devices made of PDMS are ideal for many cell culture applications, including tumor organoids, as they are permeable to oxygen, transparent, and have a similar refractive index to glass to facilitate optical imaging.

We and others have developed several microfluidic platforms that capture features of the human microcirculation (Fig. 3) [26–32]. A critical feature of the

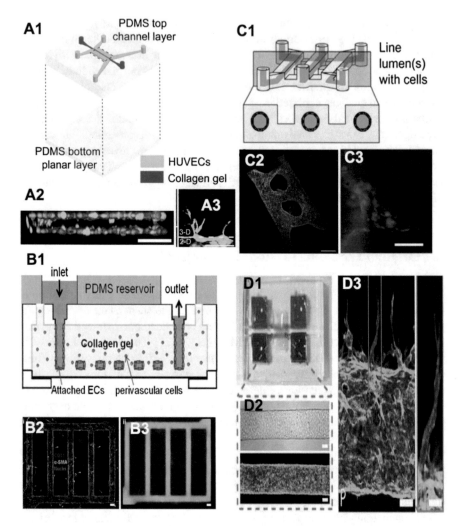

Fig. 3 In vitro blood vessels created by coating microfluidic channels with endothelial cells. (**a1**) Device design for coating endothelial cells on the surfaces of the PDMS and collagen gel. (**a2**) The endothelial cells (*green*) form monolayer in the device, and (**a3**) angiogenesis is observed from 2D coat into 3D collagen gel (reprinted with permission from [30]). (**b1**) Device design to create hollow tubes of circular cross section in collagen gel by using silicon master mold. The surface of the collagen tube are coated with endothelial cells to form a vessel. (**b2**) These vessels stained with endothelial specific CD31 (*red*) sprout and (**b3**) exhibit barrier function as they retain dextran in the lumen (*green*). Scale bar in **b2** and **b3** shows 100 μm (reprinted with permission from [27]). (**c1**) The channels in the hydrogel were developed by using viscous finger patterning and then (**c2**) endothelial cells (*green*) were coated on the hollow structures. (**c3**) These vessels show angiogenic response (*red*) to VEGF concentration gradients. Scale bar in **c2** and **c3** show 500 and 50 μm, respectively (reprinted with permission [32]). (**d1**) PDMS device in which a cylindrical tube is created in collagen gel using needle of 400 μm diameter. (**d2**) The gel cylinder was coated with endothelial cells (*green*). (**d3**) When the vessels exposed to angiogenic factors show angiogenesis. Scale bars in **d2** and **d3** are 100 μm. Scale bar in the insert of **d3** is 50 μm (reprinted with permission from [31])

microcirculation is the hollow capillary structure through which blood or a blood substitute can flow. The studies use mainly two approaches to create these structures. The first approach is lining a conduit with endothelial cells. Some studies first create a perforated rectangular shaped conduit in PDMS, and coat one side or all sides of the conduit with endothelial cells [30]. Others have used a more sophisticated approach of creating a cylindrical conduit in an ECM gel (i.e., collagen or fibrin) and then coat the lumen of the cylinder with endothelial cells [27, 31]. Once the endothelial cells adhere to the wall of the conduit and spread they form tight junctions with physiological permeability coefficients [27]. This method generally creates large diameter (>100 μm) endothelial cell-lined tubes [27, 31, 32]. These endothelial-lined tubes can then be exposed to various levels of concentration gradients, which are created by using additional microfluidic lines. There are several creative designs to establish concentration gradients using microfluidics. These device designs initiate angiogenesis in response to physiological concentration levels of VEGF, bFGF, and several other proangiogenic factors or cocktails of factors [27, 31, 32]. As the endothelial cells are coated, a challenging task is to maintain the density of endothelial cells and shape of the tube to accurately mimic the in vivo vasculature.

The second approach to generate microvessels follows the developmental process of vasculogenesis, in which the endothelial cells are encouraged to self-assemble into capillaries (Fig. 4). In this method, the microvessels are produced from endothelial cells and stromal cells that are initially randomly distributed in an ECM. The stromal cells are a necessary component as they secrete factors necessary to support vessel formation, in particular tube formation and stabilization [33–35]. Our lab has shown that cord blood-derived endothelial cells and human lung fibroblasts in a fibrin gel generate dynamic, interconnected, and perfusable networks of microvessels [29]. When implanted in the mouse, the microvessels anastomose to mouse vasculature and become functional [36, 37].This co-culture system provides a more physiologic alternative, compared to assays using only endothelial cells [27, 31, 32], to mimic in vivo angiogenesis. Moreover the physical dimensions, including diameter, of the microvasculature formed by our assay resembles that of the in vivo microvasculature (<50 μm).

Vasculogenic vessel formation has also been shown to be facilitated by other types of stromal cells, such as bone marrow derived stromal cells [28]. In the context of tumor angiogenesis, such a system could be of interest, as bone marrow is one of the most frequent metastatic sites for multiple types of solid tumors, including breast, and colon cancers. Our lab has been working to develop microfluidic systems to place tumors in the immediate vicinity of perfused microvascular tissue developed by this vasculogenic process [38]. These systems are designed to recapitulate microenvironment of early and advanced tumors and study angiogenesis in response to the microenvironmental perturbations described in the following sections.

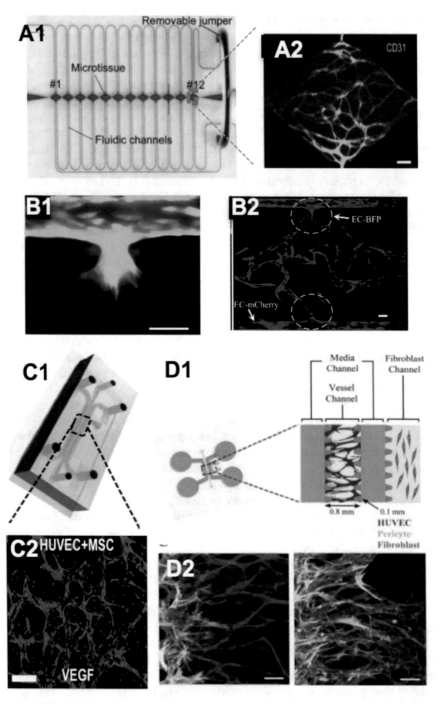

Fig. 4 Microfluidic systems to create in vitro vascular networks by vasculogenesis process. (**a1**) Device design for creating endothelial network from randomly distributed endothelial cells and normal lung fibroblasts in fibrin gel. (**a2**) The endothelial cells (*green*) form interconnected network of vessels (reprinted with permission from [29]). (**b1**) One approach to connect the vessels

4 Hypoxia and Tumor Angiogenesis

4.1 Overview

The deficiency of oxygen, an essential nutrient for cell proliferation and survival, is a critical stimulus for acquiring new blood vessels. Hypoxic tumors activate molecular programs that lead to secretion of proangiogenic factors by the tumor as well as tumor-associated stromal cells. Tumor hypoxia has been associated with poor patient prognosis, with clinical studies showing that advanced breast cancers have a median oxygen tension of 10 mmHg, compared with 65 mmHg in normal breast tissue [39–41]. Hypoxic cores exist in advanced stage tumors [42], and can also exist in tumors as small as 400 μm in diameter [43]. In hypoxic conditions, angiogenesis is primarily regulated by hypoxia inducible factors (HIFs). Of the highly conserved HIF family of transcription factors, HIF-1 has been the best studied [44–46]. It is known to be a heterodimer of α-subunit (HIF-1α) and a β-subunit (HIF-1β), where subunits are members of the basic helix-loop-helix (bHLH)-containing PER-ARNT-SIM (PAS) domain family of transcription factors. In addition to HIF-1α and HIF-1β, there are two additional oxygen regulated α-subunits are (HIF-2α and HIF-3α) and two other constitutively expressed β-subunits (HIF-2β, and HIF-3β). Furthermore, the low oxygen environment stabilizes HIF-1α in endothelial cells as well [47].

The HIF-1 activation follows a series of molecular events. Starting at oxygen concentrations below 6%, HIF-1α stabilizes and translocates from the cytoplasm to the nucleus, where it dimerizes with HIF-1β [48]. HIF-1 then binds to hypoxia responsive elements (HREs) within the promoters of HIF target genes leading to the increased expression of proangiogenic factors such as vascular endothelial growth factor (VEGF), VEGF-R2, angiopoietin 1/2, fibroblast growth factor, platelet-derived growth factor, and the decreased expression of anti-angiogenic factors such as thrombospondin-1 and carbonic anhydrase-9 [49]. In addition to angiogenesis, HIF-1 can activate more than a hundred genes that control important cellular processes such as epithelial-mesenchymal transition, stem-cell maintenance, and metabolism that impact tumor cell invasion, metastasis, metabolic reprograming, and resistance to therapy [4].

Fig. 4 (continued) with the fluidic lines of PDMS device is to coat the fluidic lines with endothelial cells. (**b2**) The endothelial cells in the fluidic line connect with the vessel network in the gel forming a perfused network of vessels (reprinted with permission from [35]). (**c1**) Microfluidic platform design used to create vascular network from bone marrow derived mesenchymal stem cells and endothelial cells in fibrin gel. (**c2**) The micrograph shows endothelial network in this device (*red*). The scale bar is 200 μm (reprinted with permission [28]). (**d1**) Microfluidic platform used for co-culture of endothelial cells and pericytes in fibrin gel. (**d2**) The system supports formation of endothelial network (*red*) formation with pericyte coverage (*green*). The scale bar is 100 μm. The figure is reprinted from [26], and is covered under Creative Commons Attribution (CC BY) license

4.2   Controlling and Measuring Oxygen In Vitro

The traditional method to create hypoxic conditions utilizes cell culture incubators, where blending excess nitrogen with air lowers oxygen concentration. Alternatively, the exchange of oxygen from air can be controlled by an air tight glove box equipment, or hypoxic conditions can simply be generated due to consumption of oxygen by cell culture. Additionally, chemicals that consume oxygen, such as sodium nitrate, can also be used to manipulate oxygen tension [50]. Alternatively, cobalt chloride can stabilize HIF-1α in the presence of normoxia, and allows for more flexible data collection. This "pseudo-hypoxic" condition can simulate the impact of HIF-1α, but cannot fully recapitulate all features that hypoxia has on cell function [51].

Microfluidic devices have become attractive systems to study hypoxia due to their inherently small size, and thus small diffusion distances. A common technique to reduce oxygen in microfluidic devices is to use separate channels containing an oxygen scavenger such as sodium nitrate (Fig. 5). These channels are separated from the tissue chambers by a semipermeable material, such as PDMS, that allows diffusion of oxygen but not water [52–54]. By altering the concentration and flow of the scavenger, the oxygen tension within the device can be controlled with high spatial and temporal resolution. PDMS is ideally suited as a material of construction for these device as it is a highly permeable material with respect to oxygen compared to relatively impermeable materials such as cyclic olefin copolymer, polystyrene, polypropylene, poly(methacrylic acid), polyurethane, and poly(methyl pentene) [55]. By choosing an appropriate coating and/or using an oxygen scavenger, a wide range of oxygen concentrations can be controlled to study tumor hypoxia and its effects.

A major advantage of using in vitro systems is that real time oxygen measurements can be performed in a live tissue culture with minimal disruption of biological processes. The gold standard for the oxygen sensors is Clark-type electrodes which measure oxygen by detecting a current flow caused by the reduction of oxygen [56]. However, the method is operationally complex and less sensitive for oxygen measurement relative to other methods. Recently, more sensitive techniques have been developed that employs an oxygen sensitive luminophore. The luminescence of oxygen sensitive dyes is inversely proportional to the concentration of oxygen. When the dyes are excited by a laser in the presence of oxygen, the excited state energy of the phosphorescent indicator molecule is absorbed by oxygen instead of being emitted as a luminescent photon. In other words, oxygen quenches the phosphorescence, and reduces the lifetime of the phosphorescence decay. Generally, a shorter luminescence lifetime indicates a higher oxygen concentration. The lifetime of the phosphorescence, as opposed to the intensity, is a more robust method as it is insensitive to photobleaching and independent of the concentration of the dye. Detecting the luminescence lifetime generally requires a more complicated experimental setup because a pulsed laser needs to be used [57].

While many research groups have focused on controlling the oxygen environment around tumor spheroids, some groups, including ours, have begun to control

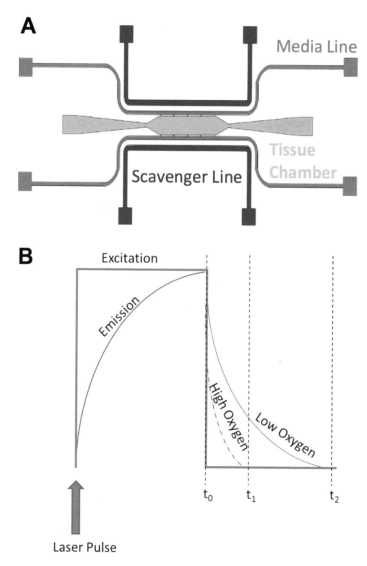

Fig. 5 Manipulating and measuring oxygen concentrations in vitro. (**a**) Oxygen scavenger lines can be designed into microfluidic platforms to generate hypoxic conditions inside tissue chambers. Typically these include materials such as sodium sulfite. (**b**) PhLM is a method used to measure oxygen concentrations in 3D culture systems. Using a pulsed laser to excite the oxygen sensitive dye and measuring the dye's lifetime of decay, a longer phosphorescent lifetimes correspond to lower oxygen concentrations

oxygen tension in vascularized tumors [52, 53, 58]. Due to the role that the vascular network has in oxygen regulation and the interaction between the tumor and the vasculature during hypoxia, the inclusion of these components in the next generation of tumor organoid models is critical for a complete understanding of angiogenesis in the tumor microenvironment.

5 Cellular Metabolism and Angiogenesis in the Tumor Microenvironment

5.1 Overview

Endothelial cells act as a semi-permeable barrier between the circulating blood and various tissues. Being in direct contact with the blood, endothelial cells have the most ready access to the nutrients needed for healthy cell growth, including glucose, glutamine, and oxygen but are also responsible for delivering these nutrients to the surrounding tissue. Endothelial cells are able to balance their own metabolic needs and transport duties by executing a specific metabolic program that shares many similarities with cancer cell metabolism.

Endothelial cells are highly glycolytic and consume glucose at a high rate. Even during quiescence, endothelial cells generate more than 80% of their ATP through glycolysis alone [59, 60]. Glycolysis in endothelial cells tends to favor lactate as its end product, as less than 1% of pyruvate generated by glycolysis is oxidized in the tricarboxylic acid (TCA) cycle. By reducing the utilization of oxidative phosphorylation (OxPhos) and thus reducing the amount of consumed oxygen, they are able to more effectively deliver oxygen to the tissues.

When appropriate signals are received to form tip cells and induce angiogenesis, phosphofructokinase-2/fructose-2,6-bisphosphatase 3 (PFK2 or PFKFB3) expression is upregulated (Fig. 6). PFK2 converts fructose-6-phosphate into fructose-2,6-bisphosphate (F2,6BP), a potent regulator of phosphofructokinase-1 (PFK1) which converts F6P into fructose-1,6-bisphosphate (F1,6BP), considered the first committed step in glycolysis. VEGF and fibroblast growth factor 2 (FGF2) have been shown to increase PFK2 expression and glycolysis. Kruppel-Like Factor 2 (KLF2), a transcription factor which responds to hemodynamic-induced stress on the EC glycocalyx, has been shown to reduce PFK2 expression in quiescent endothelial cells (De Bock et al.; Doddaballapur et al.; De Bock, Georgiadou, and Carmeliet). By upregulating PFK2 and increasing levels of F2,6BP, PFK1 activity and flux through glycolysis are both greatly increased. In many other cells, such as immune cells, this activation would lead to a 20- to 30-fold increase in glycolytic flux but only a twofold increase occurs in endothelial cells. The end products, lactate, can later be used as a mitochondrial fuel by other stromal cells or regenerated through gluconeogenesis after reaching the liver.

Similar to endothelial cells, most tumor cells are highly glycolytic even in the presence of oxygen, known as Warburg Metabolism, and have reduced OxPhos [61]. In contrast to endothelial cells, tumor cells have a high rate of proliferation, and consume large quantities of glucose [61]. The rapid use of glucose and excretion of lactate in the tumor microenvironment stimulates angiogenesis. In low glucose conditions, endothelial cells can utilize Fatty Acid Oxidation (FAO) and amino acid metabolism, especially glutaminolysis, to supplement their energetic and macromolecular needs. FAO catabolizes circulating triglycerides to create acetyl-CoA, which can then be used for energy production in the TCA or for lipid synthesis and

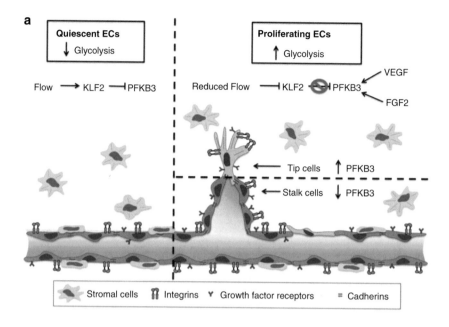

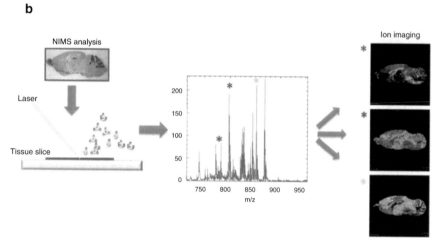

Fig. 6 Endothelial cell metabolism in cancer associated angiogenesis. (**a**) In normal tissues, ECs in blood vessels demonstrate a quiescent phenotype, with limited glycolysis for energy production due to hemodynamic stress-induced stimulation of Kruppel-Like Factor 2 (KLF2). In tip cells, glycolysis is upregulated by several growth factors and downregulation of KLF2 by reduced flow also serves to increase glycolytic flux as ECs become activated to proliferate and develop new vasculature via angiogenesis. (**b**) Nanostructure Imaging Mass Spectrometry of rat brain sections b. to resolve metabolic differences by brain region (reprinted with permission from [62]). An initiator is used, similar in function to the matrix from MALDI techniques, to desorb and ionize metabolites before analysis by mass spectrometry. Each metabolite can be visualized in its own ion image, as shown to the right, which allows for label-free spatial tracking of multiple metabolites in a tissue sample

also yields NADPH as a byproduct. Glutaminolysis catabolizes glutamine, whose concentration in tissues is typically 5 μM, yielding glutamate, which is then converted to α-ketoglutarate and can enter the TCA cycle. Glutamate can also act as a nitrogen source for amino acid or nucleotide synthesis and an NADH source. These alternative energy sources facilitate angiogenesis into the tumor microenvironment, which is typically hypoxic and low in nutrients necessary for proliferation.

5.2   Methods to Characterize Cellular Metabolism In Vitro

There are several techniques that have been utilized to study metabolism in 2D culture and are being adapted to study 3D tissues in vitro. Three promising options include the Seahorse Extracellular Flux (XF) Assay, Fluorescence Lifetime Imaging Microscopy (FLIM), and Mass Spectrometry (MS) based metabolomics analysis. Direct in vitro studies of metabolism in complex tissues, including organoids composed of multiple cell types, create many challenges compared to standard 2D metabolic analyses due to the heterogeneity of the system and the need to analyze multiple focal planes.

The SeaHorse XF assays are useful to characterize a broad metabolic phenotype (i.e., primarily glycolytic or OxPhos) using a microwell plate format. They employ a probe containing an embedded oxygen-sensitive fluorophore and an embedded proton-sensitive fluorophore to monitor minute changes in acidity and oxygen concentration which can then inform the oxygen consumption rate and the extracellular acidification rate. The former is characteristic of OxPhos whereas the latter is indicative of glycolysis with lactate as the terminal end product (Fan et al.). The XF assays were originally developed for 2D cell culture, but have since been adapted to analyze spheroids as well, allowing for the rapid profiling of organoids grown in spheroid plates [62]. This system has the advantage of being label free, high-throughput, customizable for reagent studies, and fully adapted to 3D assays. However, it measures only two of the tens of thousands of possible metabolites, and contains no spatial resolution.

Fluorescence Lifetime Imaging Microscopy (FLIM) utilizes confocal or multi-photon microscopy with rapidly pulsed lasers to detect the lifetime of endogenous fluorophores. FLIM can offer incredible temporal resolution, on the order of nanoseconds, of the chemical state of a system. In vivo and in vitro, NADPH, NADH, and FAD are fluorescent molecules with a myriad of functions tied to the metabolic state of the cell and the ratios of protein bound to unbound forms is indicative of cellular metabolism [63, 64]. FLIM is incredibly sensitive due to the natural sensitivity of the fluorophores to their local chemical environment; bound forms of these molecules show a significant increase in lifetime (for NAD(P)H, 3.2 ns) over their unbound, free solution forms (for NAD(P)H, 0.8 ns) and can thus be used to metabolically profile cells [65, 66]. More recently FLIM has been used in 3D tumor organoids to assess cell proliferation [67]. Because this is a microscopic technique, it also offers high spatial resolution, permitting insight into the subcellular ratios of each of these fluorescent molecules. NADH and NADPH are nearly identical spectrally, but there have been some inroads into differentiating their FLIM signals, which is an important distinction due to the distinct roles of NADH in energy production and NADPH in biomolecule production and redox state maintenance [68, 69]. FLIM, however, is limited to those metabolites which are inherently fluorescent, and requires relatively expensive equipment.

By far the most robust technique for studying metabolism is Liquid Chromatography-Mass Spectrometry (LC-MS). LC-MS allows for the detection and quantification of nearly the entire metabolome of a sample. In 2D cell culture, cells are grown in culture medium, fixed (usually with ice cold methanol), and the metabolites are extracted using a mixture of organic and aqueous solvents before being passed through a chromatography column and analyzed by mass spectrometry. The combination of LC-MS allows for the separation of metabolites based on both the retention time (LC) and mass to charge ratio (MS) that allows for high resolution detection and identification of each metabolite. By comparing the metabolomes or specific metabolites of two nearly identical samples grown in different conditions, known as differential metabolomics, enriched pathways dependent on these differences can be elucidated. In addition, isotope labeling allows for the tracking of metabolites through different pathways through the detection of strong isotope peaks and the use of metabolic flux analysis using isotopically labeled metabolites yields a more complete picture of the metabolic network. The main shortcoming of this technique is that this represents an "average" metabolome for the sample, so extending this technique to 3D tissues results in a total loss of spatial resolution and a lack of cell specificity. To ameliorate the loss of specificity, cell sorting techniques can be used although this also presents its own set of challenges and disadvantages in sample handling.

Mass Spectrometry Imaging (MSI) is a Matrix Assisted Laser Desorption/Ionization (MALDI) variant that uses a laser and specific analyte preparation to desorb and ionize metabolites from finely sectioned tissues before running typical mass spectrometry and analysis. The details of MSI preparation and analysis are active areas of research and have been recently reviewed [70]. However, the result of an MSI experiment recreates the metabolome at each point with sub-micrometer resolution while retaining the spatial organization of the analyzed tissue [62]. By analyzing adjacent tissue sections histologically, metabolic differences between adjacent cells are resolvable as well. Very recently, MSI has been used to investigate tumor organoids in 3D to investigate topics such as drug delivery/penetration and the impact of hypoxia [71–73].

All three techniques outlined here have inherent strengths and weaknesses. Both XF and FLIM techniques can repeat measurements on the same sample and require little preparation, but offer somewhat limited information about the system, while LC-MS and MSI offer more complete information, but require more time, effort, and preparation to execute and analyze and are terminal experiments. As this is still a developing field of research, future advances may offer greater ease or scope for these techniques or new techniques altogether but metabolic studies of complex 3D tissues are finally possible. Being able to analyze cellular metabolism in tumor organoids will create a more complete picture of tumor angiogenesis.

6 Biomechanics in Tumor-Associated Angiogenesis

6.1 Overview

In addition to changes in metabolism and oxygen tension, biomechanical forces can regulate angiogenesis [74, 75]. Physical forces, including extracellular matrix (ECM) stiffness, compressive/contractile forces exerted due to cell proliferation and other cellular activities, and fluid forces exerted by blood and plasma flow have all been shown to be critical regulators of angiogenesis (Fig. 7) [76–82]. The composition, and therefore effective stiffness, as well as the organization of the ECM surrounding the tumor also plays a role in mechanically regulating angiogenesis [83–88]. Increased peritumoral ECM stiffness correlates with increased potential for angiogenesis and metastasis. Furthermore, both tumor cells and endothelial cells

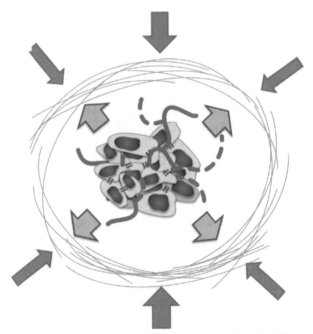

Leaky/Developing Vasculature -> increased interstitial flow
Tumor cell proliferation -> compressive forces
ECM Deposition/Remodeling

Fig. 7 Macromechanical forces in tumor progression. Typically, three different types of forces are considered important in tumor progression. Interstitial flow (*red*) generated by developing vasculature within the tumor promotes vessel growth at the periphery of the mass. Compressive forces and strains (*purple*) increase as tumor cells divide uncontrollably, putting pressure on the surrounding ECM. Finally, ECM surrounding the tumor can apply compressive forces (*green*) as more ECM is deposited by tumor and stromal cells, effectively creating a dense capsule of tissue containing the tumor mass

can actively remodel the ECM to facilitate enhanced angiogenesis as well as promote metastasis. Compressive forces in the tumor microenvironment are a result of the unchecked proliferation of tumor cells that are constrained by surrounding ECM and stromal cells [14, 89]. Finally, at the cellular level, contractile behaviors of cells in the tumor microenvironment can alter angiogenesis and tumor progression [90–93]. Enhanced mechanosignaling from cancer-associated fibroblasts (CAFs) and tumor cells alter ECM alignment and remodeling, promoting both enhanced angiogenesis and tumor cell metastasis [94–99]. Recent work has demonstrated that paracrine regulation to limit the number of tip cells occurs through the Notch pathway, which has been shown to be mechanosensitive [100, 101]. Furthermore, the shift from quiescent vascular endothelial cell to migrating tip cell mimics the phenotypic change seen in epithelial to mesenchymal transformation (EMT). In both cases cell-cell junction proteins are dramatically downregulated and cells become more migratory. Several groups have demonstrated that EMT is regulated through active biomechanical forces including cell-cell tension and contractile forces [92, 102–104].

Endothelial cells are also exquisitely sensitive to fluid flow including intraluminal flow, interstitial flow over and around the basolateral surface, and intercellular (transmural) flow between cell junctions. While interstitial flow of plasma can enhance angiogenic signaling in endothelial cells as well as invasive pathways in tumor cells, luminal flow of blood through vessels limits the angiogenesis [30, 105, 106]. Importantly, the leaky and tortuous nature of blood vessels in the tumor microenvironment impacts the magnitude and variance of all of these flows. Luminal flow exerts shear stress that regulates nitric oxide production by endothelial cells, which in turn limits endothelial cell sprouting and angiogenesis [30]. The interstitial flow of plasma leaks across the capillary wall and is reabsorbed in post capillary venules. Thus, the interstitial flow exerts transmural shear forces on the endothelial junctions, pressure forces from apical to basal, and basal to apical sides of the endothelial tube. The transmural flow has been shown to facilitate angiogenesis in a shear stress dependent manner [107]. Transmural flow is characterized by Starling's Law, in which the driving force is the arithmetic sum of hydrostatic and oncotic pressure differences across the wall of the vessels. The transmural flow exerts shear stress, the magnitude of which not only depends on the flow across the vessels but also on the size of vessel perforations. Interestingly, the vessel perforations in organs throughout the human body vary, indicating differential potential of organs for angiogenesis in response to transmural flow. The basal to apical interstitial flow, like that in post-capillary venules, has been shown to activate and directionally guide angiogenesis [108]. However, apical to basal flow, like that in capillaries, does not activate angiogenesis, indicating the direction of flow is important in activating the angiogenic program (Fig. 8).

Finally, tumor cells themselves can sense shear stress, leading to changes in the production of soluble mediators that directly impact angiogenesis such as VEGF, HIF1, and matrix metalloproteinase 9 [109, 110]. The shear forces are transmitted in cells by several mechanisms, including integrin signaling pathways and surface glycocalyx signaling. Integrins on the surface of endothelial cells attach to the ECM

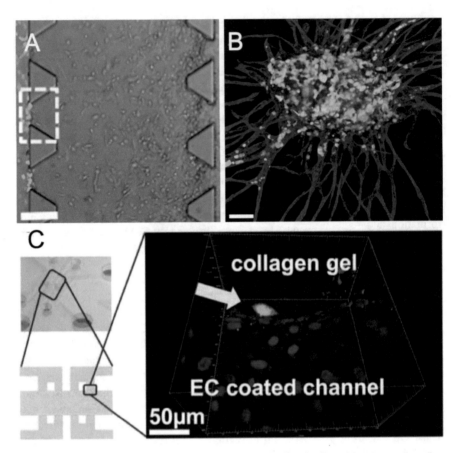

Fig. 8 Angiogenesis models for studying metastasis. (**a**) A microfluidic device that simulates features of intravasation includes a collagen filled central chamber with HT1080 fibrosarcoma cells (*red*) migrating towards an endothelial cell (*green*) lined fluidic line. Scale bar 30 μm (reprinted with permission from [155]). (**b**) An alternate 3D model of intravasation includes a spheroid of cells comprised of both endothelial cells (*red*) and SW620 colon carcinoma cells (*green*) embedded in a collagen gel that contains fibroblasts. Microvessels sprouts from the spheroid and cancer cells intravasate and migrate within the vessel lumen. Scale bar 100 μm (reprinted with permission from [9]). (**c**) A model of tumor cell extravasation using a similar microfluidic device as in (**a**). Here endothelial cells line a fluidic channel (*gray*) and a collagen gel (*green*) is placed adjacent to the abluminal surface at specified regions. Tumor cells (breast cancer, MDA-MB-231) are introduced through the microfluidic channel, and evidence of extravasation is demonstrated (*white arrow*). Red label is VE-cadherin, and *blue* is the DAPI stained nuclei of the endothelial cells (reprinted from [160] and is covered under Creative Commons Attribution (CC BY) license)

surrounding the cells and begin the formation of focal adhesions (FAs) inside the cell. Over 200 proteins have found to be associated with FA formation and many of these or their downstream effectors are either mechanosensors or mechanoregulators. A full review of FA and glycocalyx signaling in tumor-associated angiogenesis is outside the scope of this book chapter but can be found in other excellent reviews [81, 111–116].

6.2 Angiogenesis Models to Elucidate the Impact of Mechanical Forces

Early understanding of biomechanical pathways involved in tumor-associated angiogenesis came exclusively from 2D monolayer cultures, either on uncoated or ECM-protein coated tissue culture plastic or glass. Another level of complexity in 2D monolayers is derived when polyacrylamide (PA) gels are functionalized with collagen or fibronectin before cells are seeded onto the substrate [117–119]. The advantage of this system is that the PA gels can be synthesized over a wide range of stiffness values with great control. ECM proteins, either collagen or fibronectin, can then be covalently bonded to the PA gels permitting cell culture. Numerous groups have used these gels to probe the mechanoregulation of cell behavior including FA formation and regulation of cell contractile behavior. The disadvantage of this widely used system is that it is limited to 2D studies. Recently, work from the Takyama lab has utilized this protocol in conjunction with PDMS-soft lithography and 3D collagen gels to generate hybrid platforms that allow for spatial control over cell seeding with the benefit 3D cell culture in ECM-based gels [120]. The 2D PA system has also been utilized to study the effects of matrix stiffness, specifically crosslinking of collagen by lysyl oxidase, on the upregulation of VEGF in hepatocellular carcinomas [119].

Additionally, there have been several studies that demonstrate remarkable differences in 2D and 3D signaling behavior, especially of endothelial cells [121]. A key demonstration of this occurs in integrin signaling regulation where FAs in 3D are formed and degraded much more quickly than in 2D. FAs are dynamic in 3D and the inhibition of specific integrins can either promote or inhibit faster migration [87, 113, 122, 123]. Results from studies such as these have prompted a new wave of tumor angiogenesis research incorporating the techniques used in tissue engineering to generate 3D organoids to replicate the native tumor microenvironment. These models have gone through several iterations, at first only including tumor cells and then adding more cell lines to recapitulate the complex multicellular environment. This includes stromal or support cells, immunological cells, and endothelial cells in the surrounding blood vessels. While numerous research groups have adopted 3D, multicellular approaches to study specific tumor types, metastatic potential, and cellular pathway regulators, there has been limited investigation of biomechanical regulation of tumor progression, specifically angiogenesis, in this type of model.

Tissue engineering protocols allow for several methods of spatial control over cellular seeding in either synthetic polymer or ECM-derived materials. One of the approaches is a "self-assembled" technique, in which cells are simply mixed together for co-culture before casting of the matrix in a premade mold or dish, and sometimes includes external mechanical stimulation from moving culture platforms including orbital shakers or rotating vessel wall bioreactors [85, 124–127]. Furthermore, many of these studies represent nascent research in developing novel platforms and are limited in their ability to interrogate the role of biomechanics in angiogenesis associated with tumor progression. Bates et al. demonstrated that blocking integrin function in such self-assembled organoid models of colorectal cancer blocked tumor progression [128]. Vascularized liver buds have been generated via these same techniques, with a possible dependence on stromal cell contractile behavior for tissue assembly [129–131]. The advantages of this protocol are that the cells naturally orient themselves in a manner replicating the native in vivo tumor microenvironment. However, there is incomplete spatial control of this process, limiting the type of results that can be gleaned from such studies. However, these models are still important tools to understand tumor angiogenesis, and have demonstrated the importance of CAFs in promotion of tumor associated blood vessel growth through factors including VEGF, HIF-1a, caveolin-1 [31, 97, 132].

Another approach to investigate the role of biomechanics on angiogenesis in 3D tumor organoids involves the use of animal models. A recent study demonstrated the mechanosensitive nature of angiogenesis using the avian choiroallantoic membrane (CAM) model in the developing avian embryo [133]. Rings containing a collagen gel were implanted on top of the membrane, with tension induced in only the outermost layer of tissue. Harvested gels showed invasion of blood vessels due to tensile forces generated by the implant. This same model was utilized by another group to explore how crosslinks affecting biomechanical properties of the collagen gels altered VEGF production in tumor spheroids seeded onto the CAM [134].

Microfluidic model systems, as described above, provide a novel technique to study the effects of luminal and interstitial flow in a 3D tumor microenvironment containing self-assembled vasculature network with the further advantage of high levels over spatiotemporal seeding, flow conditions, and ease of visualization in real time during experiments. By controlling device parameters and fluidic pressures in feeding chambers, the precise direction and magnitude of interstitial flow can be manipulated, allowing for creation and monitoring of soluble signaling factor gradients that alter angiogenesis in the tumor microenvironment. We have developed multiple microfluidic devices that controls interstitial flow and permits tumor growth in the presence of self-assembled vasculature [29, 38, 135–137]. Others have utilized similar techniques to study the effects of ECM composition and stiffness, effects of diffusion of growth factors, alterations in cell phenotypes in co-culture and nascent vasculature biomechanical properties such as permeability [138–142]. The continued advance of model systems will continue to enhance our understanding of the role of mechanical forces on angiogenesis in the tumor microenvironment.

7 Intravasation and Extravasation in Tumor-Associated Angiogenesis

7.1 Overview

Numerous outstanding recent reviews are available that cover the general metastatic process of cancer [143–146], as well as those focusing specifically on the role of the endothelium including intravasation (tumor cells entering the circulation) and extravasation (tumor cells exiting the circulation) [147–150]. In addition, a recent review describes in vitro and in vivo models that have been developed to probe the metastatic process including some of the very recent advances in microfluidic and "organ-on-a-chip" technologies [151]. Thus, this section will succinctly review the metastatic process, features of this process that involve the circulation which have been captured with in vitro models, and then focus on features of the metastatic cascade which specifically involve the circulation that have proven difficult to simulate including possible strategies moving forward.

Tumor metastasis is the process by which a primary tumor is able to successfully move, or metastasize, to another location in the body. While complex, many steps in the metastatic cascade have been described. For an epithelial-based tumor (which comprise approximately 80% of all tumors), the process can be summarized in five steps: (1) dedifferentiation from an epithelial phenotype to a migratory mesenchymal cell phenotype, usually termed epithelial-mesenchymal transition (EMT), (2) intravasation of the mesenchymal phenotype tumor cell, or clusters of tumor cells, from the primary tumor into the circulation, (3) survival within the circulation, (4) attachment to an endothelial cell at a distant site and extravasation from the circulation, and (5) survival and differentiation in a receptive stroma from the mesenchymal tumor cell phenotype back to an epithelial cell phenotype, termed mesenchymal-epithelial transition (MET). Engaging the circulation is a necessary step for successful metastasis. Intravasation, survival in the circulation, and extravasation (steps 2–4) all uniquely require or utilize the vascular network. Although specific features of these events have been demonstrated in vitro, several important features have not, and numerous important questions remain unanswered.

Intravasation occurs in what is generally referred as the metastatic niche, a tumor microenvironment that contains the necessary factors for successful migration and entry into the circulation. The development of the metastatic niche is complex but involves the release of growth factors and trophogens from the endothelium that encourage the clustering of tumor-associated myeloid cells, platelets, and tumor cells towards the vascular supply. For example, endothelial cells in cancer-associated blood vessels have differential expression of adhesion molecules, P- and E- selectin, that recruit attachment of leukocytes to the metastatic niche [74]. Also, increased release of stromal derived factor-1 (SDF1) from endothelial cells leads to recruitment of endothelial progenitor cells to the metastatic niche. The recruitment of additional cell types, along with altered expression on endothelial cells, leads to a cascade of cell secreted factors, such as VEGF, endostatin, and other pro-tumor growth factors that characterize the metastatic niche and contributes to metastasis [74, 152]. Using murine and zebrafish models, and 3D organotypic microvascular niches, Ghajar and co-workers demonstrated that endothelial tip cells of cancer-associated blood vessels have decreased expression of pro-dormancy factor, thrombospondin-1, and enhanced expression of pro-tumor factors, periostin and TGF-β1, that encourages tumor cell migration [153].

7.2   Methods to Investigate Intravasation and Extravasation of Tumor Cells

Intravasation from within the metastatic niche requires the tumor cell(s) to cross the basolateral side of the endothelial cell. This necessitates overcoming the endothelial basement membrane and intercellular functional proteins. There is general consensus that intravasation occurs in vessels that are part of the tumor microenvironment and thus have characteristic features which are different from vessels in noncancerous tissue including increased permeability and less basement membrane. Several relatively sophisticated 3D in vitro models of intravasation have recently been presented. At least two groups have utilized soft lithography to create a microfluidic device to mimic intravasation. In both cases tumor cells could migrate across an ECM hydrogel (collagen or fibrin) and then engage the abluminal surface of an intact layer of endothelial cells [154, 155]. Zervantonakis et al. coated a microfluidic line on the other side of the ECM that was lined with a confluent layer of endothelial cells [155]. The tumor cells could then penetrate the abluminal surface of the endothelial cells, thus mimicking intravasation. Strengths of this approach include the 3D migration of tumor cells in response to controlled gradients, and the controlled migration of tumor cells across an endothelial monolayer. The models are also easily adaptable to include other cells such as macrophages [155], and stromal cells [154]. In either case, the endothelial cell phenotype was not conditioned by the tumor microenvironment and only immortalized cell lines were utilized.

Ehsan et al. presented an alternate strategy to create a 3D in vitro model of intravasation by co-culturing endothelial cells and tumors cells in a spheroid and placing this spheroid in a fibrin gel [9]. A spontaneous vessel network formed within the spheroid and also sprouted from the spheroid. A colon cancer cell line intravasated into the vessel network, and they showed this process was related to EMT and the expression of the transcription factor SNAIL. Strengths of this model include the creation of a vascular network in close proximity to the tumor, and a true 3D vascular network. The surrounding matrix did contain stromal cells, but their work was also limited to immortalized cancer cell linesand there was no flow within the vessel lumens.

Mimicking the step of tumor cell survival in the blood vessel is problematic due to the complexity of blood and its components (e.g., platelets, leukocytes, clotting factors) and the mechanical microenvironment. Most cancer cells in the circulation do not survive; those cancer cells that do survive are able to overcome the shear stress and immune system by aggregating together and/or interacting with platelets [149]. These events have generally been captured using in vivo mice models and post-sacrifice observations of metastasis [156, 157]. This approach has been useful to identify some of the key cells and proteins involved, but lack temporal and spatial resolution. No in vitro model to date has been able to capture these dynamic events.

Extravasation requires the tumor cell(s) to cross from the luminal side of the endothelial cell, and thus crossing the intercellular junctional proteins and basement membrane, in that order. In contrast to intravasation, extravasation occurs at sites distant from the primary tumor and thus the endothelium is generally considered to be normal, but specific to the organ. Many details of how a tumor cell attaches and transmigrates the endothelium have been worked out using Transwell© [158] chambers and 2D laminar flow chambers [159]. Some of the mechanisms parallel the steps of neutrophil adhesion and paracellular transmigration including the expression of PECAM1 and E-Selectin on the endothelial cells and $\alpha_V\beta_3$ integrin and CD44 on the cancer cell. A more advanced 3D microfluidic model was recently reported and demonstrated flow and extravasation of cancer cells through a microfluidic channel lined with endothelial cells [160]. The major weaknesses in the current in vitro models of extravasation are the lack of organ endothelial specificity. Most models have utilized human umbilical vein endothelial cells (HUVECs) [158, 161] cultured on a fibronectin coated membrane of collagen gel, and thus they do not contain organ specific features of the endothelial cell [162] or vascular architecture [163]. Overcoming these challenges in the mimicry of tumor cell extravasation represents a tremendous opportunity to enhance our understanding of tumor progression.

8 Summary and Future Directions

In this chapter, we have discussed the process of angiogenesis in tumor organoids, the development of novel model systems for its study, as well as numerous results garnered from such studies. Increasingly, researchers are trying to recapitulate the complex native in vivo tumor microenvironment to provide an enhanced understanding of tumor progression for the purpose of developing novel therapeutic strategies. Initial research strategies utilized simple co-culture systems, either 2D or 3D, or mouse models, both of which present limited spatial or temporal control in elucidating the cues that regulate angiogenesis and tumor progression. The recent trend is the generation of sophisticated organ-on-a-chip systems where researchers can control spatial and/or temporal patterning of cells in matrices that mimic the native tumor tissue. Furthermore, use of microfluidic systems based on optically transparent materials permits real-time analysis of angiogenesis in the tumor microenvironment. Modular control over factors including hypoxia, shear flow, biomechanical properties, and gradients of growth factors permit interrogation of tumor progression at previously unimaginable resolution and physiological relevance.

As this field develops further, we predict that we will generate models combining the numerous factors discussed in this chapter, to generate in vitro systems that fully recapitulate the complex, native tumor microenvironment. By enhancing our understanding of how these features alter not only tumor cell behavior, but also endothelial cells of tumor-associated vasculature and the processes accompanying tumor development including intravasation/extravasation, we increase the likelihood of a breakthrough scientific discovery that will allow for development of novel anti-cancer treatment strategies, targeting the processes we are only beginning to fully understand due to our refined models of tumor organoid angiogenesis.

References

1. Folkman J (1971) Tumor angiogenesis: therapeutic implications. N Engl J Med 285:1182–1186
2. Carmeliet P, Jain RK (2000) Angiogenesis in cancer and other diseases. Nature 407(6801):249–257. doi:10.1038/35025220
3. Hanahan D, Weinberg RA (2011) Hallmarks of cancer: the next generation. Cell 144(5):646–674. doi:10.1016/j.cell.2011.02.013
4. Semenza GL (2012) Hypoxia-inducible factors: mediators of cancer progression and targets for cancer therapy. Trends Pharmacol Sci 33(4):207–214. doi:10.1016/j.tips.2012.01.005
5. Weidner N, Semple JP, Welch WR, Folkman J (1991) Tumor angiogenesis and metastasis–correlation in invasive breast carcinoma. N Engl J Med 324(1):1–8. doi:10.1056/NEJM199101033240101
6. Morton CL, Houghton PJ (2007) Establishment of human tumor xenografts in immunodeficient mice. Nat Protoc 2(2):247–250. doi:10.1038/nprot.2007.25
7. Richmond A, Su Y (2008) Mouse xenograft models vs GEM models for human cancer therapeutics. Dis Model Mech 1(2–3):78–82. doi:10.1242/dmm.000976
8. Dalen H, Burki HJ (1971) Some observations on the three-dimensional growth of L5178Y cell colonies in soft agar culture. Exp Cell Res 65(2):433–438
9. Ehsan SM, Welch-Reardon KM, Waterman ML, Hughes CCW, George SC (2014) A three-dimensional in vitro model of tumor cell intravasation. Integr Biol (UK) 6(6):603–610. doi:10.1039/c3ib40170g
10. Carver K, Ming X, Juliano RL (2014) Multicellular tumor spheroids as a model for assessing delivery of oligonucleotides in three dimensions. Mol Ther Nucl Acids 3. doi:ARTN e153 10.1038/mtna.2014.5
11. Vakoc BJ, Lanning RM, Tyrrell JA, Padera TP, Bartlett LA, Stylianopoulos T, Munn LL, Tearney GJ, Fukumura D, Jain RK, Bouma BE (2009) Three-dimensional microscopy of the tumor microenvironment in vivo using optical frequency domain imaging. Nat Med 15(10):1219–U1151. doi:10.1038/nm.1971
12. Bergers G, Benjamin LE (2003) Tumorigenesis and the angiogenic switch. Nat Rev Cancer 3(6):401–410. doi:10.1038/nrc1093
13. Fernandez-Sanchez ME, Barbier S, Whitehead J, Bealle G, Michel A, Latorre-Ossa H, Rey C, Fouassier L, Claperon A, Brulle L, Girard E, Servant N, Rio-Frio T, Marie H, Lesieur S, Housset C, Gennisson JL, Tanter M, Menager C, Fre S, Robine S, Farge E (2015) Mechanical induction of the tumorigenic beta-catenin pathway by tumour growth pressure. Nature 523(7558):92–95. doi:10.1038/nature14329
14. Ou G, Weaver VM (2015) Tumor-induced solid stress activates beta-catenin signaling to drive malignant behavior in normal, tumor-adjacent cells. BioEssays 37(12):1293–1297. doi:10.1002/bies.201500090
15. Augustin HG, Koh GY, Thurston G, Alitalo K (2009) Control of vascular morphogenesis and homeostasis through the angiopoietin-Tie system. Nat Rev Mol Cell Biol 10(3):165–177. doi:10.1038/nrm2639
16. Saharinen P, Eklund L, Miettinen J, Wirkkala R, Anisimov A, Winderlich M, Nottebaum A, Vestweber D, Deutsch U, Koh GY, Olsen BR, Alitalo K (2008) Angiopoietins assemble distinct Tie2 signalling complexes in endothelial cell-cell and cell-matrix contacts. Nat Cell Biol 10(5):527–537. doi:10.1038/ncb1715
17. Cascone T, Heymach JV (2012) Targeting the angiopoietin/Tie2 pathway: cutting tumor vessels with a double-edged sword? J Clin Oncol (Official Journal of the American Society of Clinical Oncology) 30(4):441–444. doi:10.1200/jco.2011.38.7621
18. Radu M, Semenova G, Kosoff R, Chernoff J (2014) PAK signalling during the development and progression of cancer. Nat Rev Cancer 14(1):13–25
19. Fryer BH, Field J (2005) Rho, Rac, Pak and angiogenesis: old roles and newly identified responsibilities in endothelial cells. Cancer Lett 229(1):13–23. doi:http://dx.doi.org/10.1016/j.canlet.2004.12.009

20. Ghosh K, Thodeti CK, Dudley AC, Mammoto A, Klagsbrun M, Ingber DE (2008) Tumor-derived endothelial cells exhibit aberrant Rho-mediated mechanosensing and abnormal angiogenesis in vitro. Proc Natl Acad Sci U S A 105(32):11305–11310. doi:10.1073/pnas.0800835105

21. Halder G, Dupont S, Piccolo S (2012) Transduction of mechanical and cytoskeletal cues by YAP and TAZ. Nat Rev Mol Cell Biol 13(9):591–600

22. Dupont S (2016) Role of YAP/TAZ in cell-matrix adhesion-mediated signalling and mechanotransduction. Exp Cell Res. doi:http://dx.doi.org/10.1016/j.yexcr.2015.10.034

23. Piccolo S, Cordenonsi M, Dupont S (2013) Molecular pathways: YAP and TAZ take center stage in organ growth and tumorigenesis. Clin Cancer Res (An Official Journal of the American Association for Cancer Research) 19(18):4925–4930. doi:10.1158/1078-0432.ccr-12-3172

24. Nakatsu MN, Hughes CCW (2008) An optimized three-dimensional in vitro model for the analysis of angiogenesis. Angiogenesis: in vitro systems. Methods Enzymol 443:65. doi:10.1016/S0076-6879(08)02004-1

25. Welch-Reardon KM, Ehsan SM, Wang KH, Wu N, Newman AC, Romero-Lopez M, Fong AH, George SC, Edwards RA, Hughes CCW (2014) Angiogenic sprouting is regulated by endothelial cell expression of Slug. J Cell Sci 127(9):2017–2028. doi:10.1242/jcs.143420

26. Kim J, Chung M, Kim S, Jo DH, Kim JH, Jeon NL (2015) Engineering of a biomimetic pericyte-covered 3D microvascular network. PLoS One 10(7):e0133880. doi:10.1371/journal.pone.0133880

27. Zheng Y, Chen J, Craven M, Choi NW, Totorica S, Diaz-Santana A, Kermani P, Hempstead B, Fischbach-Teschl C, Lopez JA, Stroock AD (2012) In vitro microvessels for the study of angiogenesis and thrombosis. Proc Natl Acad Sci U S A 109(24):9342–9347. doi:10.1073/pnas.1201240109

28. Jeon JS, Bersini S, Whisler JA, Chen MB, Dubini G, Charest JL, Moretti M, Kamm RD (2014) Generation of 3D functional microvascular networks with human mesenchymal stem cells in microfluidic systems. Integr Biol-Uk 6(5):555–563. doi:10.1039/c3ib40267c

29. Moya ML, Hsu YH, Lee AP, Hughes CC, George SC (2013) In vitro perfused human capillary networks. Tissue Eng Part C Methods 19(9):730–737. doi:10.1089/ten.TEC.2012.0430

30. Song JW, Munn LL (2011) Fluid forces control endothelial sprouting. Proc Natl Acad Sci U S A 108(37):15342–15347. doi:10.1073/pnas.1105316108

31. Nguyen DH, Stapleton SC, Yang MT, Cha SS, Choi CK, Galie PA, Chen CS (2013) Biomimetic model to reconstitute angiogenic sprouting morphogenesis in vitro. Proc Natl Acad Sci U S A 110(17):6712–6717. doi:10.1073/pnas.1221526110

32. Bischel LL, Young EW, Mader BR, Beebe DJ (2013) Tubeless microfluidic angiogenesis assay with three-dimensional endothelial-lined microvessels. Biomaterials 34(5):1471–1477. doi:10.1016/j.biomaterials.2012.11.005

33. Newman AC, Chou W, Welch-Reardon KM, Fong AH, Popson SA, Phan DT, Sandoval DR, Nguyen DP, Gershon PD, Hughes CC (2013) Analysis of stromal cell secretomes reveals a critical role for stromal cell-derived hepatocyte growth factor and fibronectin in angiogenesis. Arterioscler Thromb Vasc Biol 33(3):513–522. doi:10.1161/ATVBAHA.112.300782

34. Newman AC, Nakatsu MN, Chou W, Gershon PD, Hughes CC (2011) The requirement for fibroblasts in angiogenesis: fibroblast-derived matrix proteins are essential for endothelial cell lumen formation. Mol Biol Cell 22(20):3791–3800. doi:10.1091/mbc.E11-05-0393

35. Wang XL, Phan DTT, Sobrino A, George SC, Hughes CC, Lee AP (2016) Engineering anastomosis between living capillary networks and endothelial cell-lined microfluidic channels. Lab Chip 16(2):282–290. doi:10.1039/c5lc01050k

36. Chen X, Aledia AS, Ghajar CM, Griffith CK, Putnam AJ, Hughes CC, George SC (2009) Prevascularization of a fibrin-based tissue construct accelerates the formation of functional anastomosis with host vasculature. Tissue Eng Part A 15(6):1363–1371. doi:10.1089/ten.tea.2008.0314

37. Chen X, Aledia AS, Popson SA, Him L, Hughes CC, George SC (2010) Rapid anastomosis of endothelial progenitor cell-derived vessels with host vasculature is promoted by a high density of cotransplanted fibroblasts. Tissue Eng Part A 16(2):585–594. doi:10.1089/ten. TEA.2009.0491

38. Alonzo LF, Moya ML, Shirure VS, George SC (2015) Microfluidic device to control interstitial flow-mediated homotypic and heterotypic cellular communication. Lab Chip 15(17):3521–3529. doi:10.1039/c5lc00507h

39. Gilkes DM, Semenza GL, Wirtz D (2014) Hypoxia and the extracellular matrix: drivers of tumour metastasis. Nat Rev Cancer 14(6):430–439. doi:10.1038/nrc3726

40. Harris AL (2002) Hypoxia–a key regulatory factor in tumour growth. Nat Rev Cancer 2(1):38–47. doi:10.1038/nrc704

41. Vaupel P, Mayer A, Hockel M (2004) Tumor hypoxia and malignant progression. Methods Enzymol 381:335–354. doi:10.1016/S0076-6879(04)81023-1

42. Baudino TA, McKay C, Pendeville-Samain H, Nilsson JA, Maclean KH, White EL, Davis AC, Ihle JN, Cleveland JL (2002) c-Myc is essential for vasculogenesis and angiogenesis during development and tumor progression. Genes Dev 16(19):2530–2543. doi:10.1101/gad.1024602

43. Grimes DR, Kelly C, Bloch K, Partridge M (2014) A method for estimating the oxygen consumption rate in multicellular tumour spheroids. J R Soc Interface 11(92):20131124. doi:10.1098/rsif.2013.1124

44. Adams JM, Difazio LT, Rolandelli RH, Lujan JJ, Hasko G, Csoka B, Selmeczy Z, Nemeth ZH (2009) HIF-1: a key mediator in hypoxia. Acta Physiol Hung 96(1):19–28. doi:10.1556/APhysiol.96.2009.1.2

45. Semenza GL (2007) Hypoxia-inducible factor 1 (HIF-1) pathway. Science's STKE: signal transduction knowledge environment 2007 (407):cm8. doi:10.1126/stke.4072007cm8

46. Ke Q, Costa M (2006) Hypoxia-inducible factor-1 (HIF-1). Mol Pharmacol 70(5):1469–1480. doi:10.1124/mol.106.027029

47. Carmeliet P (2003) Angiogenesis in health and disease. Nat Med 9(6):653–660. doi:10.1038/nm0603-653

48. Zhou W, Dosey TL, Biechele T, Moon RT, Horwitz MS, Ruohola-Baker H (2011) Assessment of hypoxia inducible factor levels in cancer cell lines upon hypoxic induction using a novel reporter construct. PLoS One 6(11):e27460. doi:10.1371/journal.pone.0027460

49. Krock BL, Skuli N, Simon MC (2011) Hypoxia-induced angiogenesis: good and evil. Genes Cancer 2(12):1117–1133. doi:10.1177/1947601911423654

50. Byrne MB, Leslie MT, Gaskins HR, Kenis PJ (2014) Methods to study the tumor microenvironment under controlled oxygen conditions. Trends Biotechnol 32(11):556–563. doi:10.1016/j.tibtech.2014.09.006

51. Piret JP, Mottet D, Raes M, Michiels C (2002) CoCl2, a chemical inducer of hypoxia-inducible factor-1, and hypoxia reduce apoptotic cell death in hepatoma cell line HepG2. Ann N Y Acad Sci 973:443–447

52. Brennan MD, Rexius-Hall ML, Elgass LJ, Eddington DT (2014) Oxygen control with microfluidics. Lab Chip 14(22):4305–4318. doi:10.1039/c4lc00853g

53. Funamoto K, Zervantonakis IK, Liu Y, Ochs CJ, Kim C, Kamm RD (2012) A novel microfluidic platform for high-resolution imaging of a three-dimensional cell culture under a controlled hypoxic environment. Lab Chip 12(22):4855–4863. doi:10.1039/c2lc40306d

54. Wang L, Liu W, Wang Y, Wang JC, Tu Q, Liu R, Wang J (2013) Construction of oxygen and chemical concentration gradients in a single microfluidic device for studying tumor cell-drug interactions in a dynamic hypoxia microenvironment. Lab Chip 13(4):695–705. doi:10.1039/c2lc40661f

55. Ochs CJ, Kasuya J, Pavesi A, Kamm RD (2014) Oxygen levels in thermoplastic microfluidic devices during cell culture. Lab Chip 14(3):459–462. doi:10.1039/c3lc51160j

56. Clark LC Jr, Lyons C (1962) Electrode systems for continuous monitoring in cardiovascular surgery. Ann N Y Acad Sci 102:29–45

57. Esipova TV, Karagodov A, Miller J, Wilson DF, Busch TM, Vinogradov SA (2011) Two new "protected" oxyphors for biological oximetry: properties and application in tumor imaging. Anal Chem 83(22):8756–8765. doi:10.1021/ac2022234
58. Griffith CK, Miller C, Sainson RC, Calvert JW, Jeon NL, Hughes CC, George SC (2005) Diffusion limits of an in vitro thick prevascularized tissue. Tissue Eng 11(1–2):257–266. doi:10.1089/ten.2005.11.257
59. De Bock K, Georgiadou M, Carmeliet P (2013) Role of endothelial cell metabolism in vessel sprouting. Cell Metab 18(5):634–647. doi:10.1016/j.cmet.2013.08.001
60. De Bock K, Georgiadou M, Schoors S, Kuchnio A, Wong BW, Cantelmo AR, Quaegebeur A, Ghesquiere B, Cauwenberghs S, Eelen G, Phng LK, Betz I, Tembuyser B, Brepoels K, Welti J, Geudens I, Segura I, Cruys B, Bifari F, Decimo I, Blanco R, Wyns S, Vangindertael J, Rocha S, Collins RT, Munck S, Daelemans D, Imamura H, Devlieger R, Rider M, Van Veldhoven PP, Schuit F, Bartrons R, Hofkens J, Fraisl P, Telang S, Deberardinis RJ, Schoonjans L, Vinckier S, Chesney J, Gerhardt H, Dewerchin M, Carmeliet P (2013) Role of PFKFB3-driven glycolysis in vessel sprouting. Cell 154(3):651–663. doi:10.1016/j.cell.2013.06.037
61. Verdegem D, Moens S, Stapor P, Carmeliet P (2014) Endothelial cell metabolism: parallels and divergences with cancer cell metabolism. Cancer Metab 2:19. doi:10.1186/2049-3002-2-19
62. Wenzel C, Riefke B, Grundemann S, Krebs A, Christian S, Prinz F, Osterland M, Golfier S, Rase S, Ansari N, Esner M, Bickle M, Pampaloni F, Mattheyer C, Stelzer EH, Parczyk K, Prechtl S, Steigemann P (2014) 3D high-content screening for the identification of compounds that target cells in dormant tumor spheroid regions. Exp Cell Res 323(1):131–143. doi:10.1016/j.yexcr.2014.01.017
63. Wright BK, Andrews LM, Jones MR, Stringari C, Digman MA, Gratton E (2012) Phasor-FLIM analysis of NADH distribution and localization in the nucleus of live progenitor myoblast cells. Microsc Res Tech 75(12):1717–1722. doi:10.1002/jemt.22121
64. Wright BK, Andrews LM, Markham J, Jones MR, Stringari C, Digman MA, Gratton E (2012) NADH distribution in live progenitor stem cells by phasor-fluorescence lifetime image microscopy. Biophys J 103(1):L7–L9. doi:10.1016/j.bpj.2012.05.038
65. Walsh AJ, Cook RS, Sanders ME, Aurisicchio L, Ciliberto G, Arteaga CL, Skala MC (2014) Quantitative optical imaging of primary tumor organoid metabolism predicts drug response in breast cancer. Cancer Res 74(18):5184–5194. doi:10.1158/0008-5472.CAN-14-0663
66. Walsh AJ, Castellanos JA, Nagathihalli NS, Merchant NB, Skala MC (2015) Optical imaging of drug-induced metabolism changes in murine and human pancreatic cancer organoids reveals heterogeneous drug response. Pancreas. doi:10.1097/MPA.0000000000000543
67. Okkelman IA, Dmitriev RI, Foley T, Papkovsky DB (2016) Use of Fluorescence Lifetime Imaging Microscopy (FLIM) as a timer of cell cycle S phase. PLoS One 11(12):e0167385. doi:10.1371/journal.pone.0167385
68. Blacker TS, Mann ZF, Gale JE, Ziegler M, Bain AJ, Szabadkai G, Duchen MR (2014) Separating NADH and NADPH fluorescence in live cells and tissues using FLIM. Nat Commun 5:3936. doi:10.1038/ncomms4936
69. Stringari C, Cinquin A, Cinquin O, Digman MA, Donovan PJ, Gratton E (2011) Phasor approach to fluorescence lifetime microscopy distinguishes different metabolic states of germ cells in a live tissue. Proc Natl Acad Sci U S A 108(33):13582–13587. doi:10.1073/pnas.1108161108
70. Jungmann JH, Heeren RM (2012) Emerging technologies in mass spectrometry imaging. J Proteome 75(16):5077–5092. doi:10.1016/j.jprot.2012.03.022
71. Feist PE, Sidoli S, Liu X, Schroll MM, Rahmy S, Fujiwara R, Garcia BA, Hummon AB (2017) Multicellular tumor spheroids combined with mass spectrometric histone analysis to evaluate epigenetic drugs. Anal Chem 89(5):2773–2781. doi:10.1021/acs.analchem.6b03602
72. Giordano S, Morosi L, Veglianese P, Licandro SA, Frapolli R, Zucchetti M, Cappelletti G, Falciola L, Pifferi V, Visentin S, D'Incalci M, Davoli E (2016) 3D mass spectrometry imaging reveals a very heterogeneous drug distribution in tumors. Sci Rep 6:37027. doi:10.1038/srep37027

73. Jiang L, Chughtai K, Purvine SO, Bhujwalla ZM, Raman V, Pasa-Tolic L, Heeren RM, Glunde K (2015) MALDI-mass spectrometric imaging revealing hypoxia-driven lipids and proteins in a breast tumor model. Anal Chem 87(12):5947–5956. doi:10.1021/ac504503x

74. Psaila B, Lyden D (2009) The metastatic niche: adapting the foreign soil. Nat Rev Cancer 9(4):285–293. doi:10.1038/nrc2621

75. Carmeliet P, Jain RK (2011) Molecular mechanisms and clinical applications of angiogenesis. Nature 473(7347):298–307. doi:10.1038/nature10144

76. Shieh AC, Swartz MA (2011) Regulation of tumor invasion by interstitial fluid flow. Phys Biol 8(1):015012. doi:10.1088/1478-3975/8/1/015012

77. Jean C, Gravelle P, Fournie JJ, Laurent G (2011) Influence of stress on extracellular matrix and integrin biology. Oncogene 30(24):2697–2706. doi:10.1038/onc.2011.27

78. Csikasz-Nagy A, Escudero LM, Guillaud M, Sedwards S, Baum B, Cavaliere M (2013) Cooperation and competition in the dynamics of tissue architecture during homeostasis and tumorigenesis. Semin Cancer Biol 23(4):293–298. doi:10.1016/j.semcancer.2013.05.009

79. Butcher DT, Alliston T, Weaver VM (2009) A tense situation: forcing tumour progression. Nat Rev Cancer 9(2):108–122. doi:10.1038/nrc2544

80. DuFort CC, Paszek MJ, Weaver VM (2011) Balancing forces: architectural control of mechanotransduction. Nat Rev Mol Cell Biol 12(5):308–319. doi:10.1038/nrm3112

81. Fu BM, Tarbell JM (2013) Mechano-sensing and transduction by endothelial surface glycocalyx: composition, structure, and function. Wiley Interdiscip Rev Syst Biol Med 5(3):381–390. doi:10.1002/wsbm.1211

82. Sund M, Xie L, Kalluri R (2004) The contribution of vascular basement membranes and extracellular matrix to the mechanics of tumor angiogenesis. APMIS 112(7–8):450–462. doi:10.1111/j.1600-0463.2004.t01-1-apm11207-0806.x

83. Shen Y, Hou Y, Yao S, Huang P, Yobas L (2015) In vitro epithelial organoid generation induced by substrate nanotopography. Sci Rep 5:9293. doi:10.1038/srep09293

84. Bignon M, Pichol-Thievend C, Hardouin J, Malbouyres M, Brechot N, Nasciutti L, Barret A, Teillon J, Guillon E, Etienne E, Caron M, Joubert-Caron R, Monnot C, Ruggiero F, Muller L, Germain S (2011) Lysyl oxidase-like protein-2 regulates sprouting angiogenesis and type IV collagen assembly in the endothelial basement membrane. Blood 118(14):3979–3989. doi:10.1182/blood-2010-10-313296

85. Yamamura N, Sudo R, Ikeda M, Tanishita K (2007) Effects of the mechanical properties of collagen gel on the in vitro formation of microvessel networks by endothelial cells. Tissue Eng 13(7):1443–1453. doi:10.1089/ten.2006.0333

86. Asparuhova MB, Secondini C, Ruegg C, Chiquet-Ehrismann R (2015) Mechanism of irradiation-induced mammary cancer metastasis: a role for SAP-dependent Mkl1 signaling. Mol Oncol 9(8):1510–1527. doi:10.1016/j.molonc.2015.04.003

87. Levental KR, Yu H, Kass L, Lakins JN, Egeblad M, Erler JT, Fong SF, Csiszar K, Giaccia A, Weninger W, Yamauchi M, Gasser DL, Weaver VM (2009) Matrix crosslinking forces tumor progression by enhancing integrin signaling. Cell 139(5):891–906. doi:10.1016/j.cell.2009.10.027

88. Lu P, Weaver VM, Werb Z (2012) The extracellular matrix: a dynamic niche in cancer progression. J Cell Biol 196(4):395–406. doi:10.1083/jcb.201102147

89. Yu H, Mouw JK, Weaver VM (2011) Forcing form and function: biomechanical regulation of tumor evolution. Trends Cell Biol 21(1):47–56. doi:10.1016/j.tcb.2010.08.015

90. Matsumoto T, Yung YC, Fischbach C, Kong HJ, Nakaoka R, Mooney DJ (2007) Mechanical strain regulates endothelial cell patterning in vitro. Tissue Eng 13(1):207–217. doi:10.1089/ten.2006.0058

91. Hanna M, Liu H, Amir J, Sun Y, Morris SW, Siddiqui MA, Lau LF, Chaqour B (2009) Mechanical regulation of the proangiogenic factor CCN1/CYR61 gene requires the combined activities of MRTF-A and CREB-binding protein histone acetyltransferase. J Biol Chem 284(34):23125–23136. doi:10.1074/jbc.M109.019059

92. Gjorevski N, Piotrowski AS, Varner VD, Nelson CM (2015) Dynamic tensile forces drive collective cell migration through three-dimensional extracellular matrices. Sci Rep 5:11458. doi:10.1038/srep11458

93. Mierke CT, Rosel D, Fabry B, Brabek J (2008) Contractile forces in tumor cell migration. Eur J Cell Biol 87(8–9):669–676. doi:10.1016/j.ejcb.2008.01.002

94. Augsten M (2014) Cancer-associated fibroblasts as another polarized cell type of the tumor microenvironment. Front Oncol 4:62. doi:10.3389/fonc.2014.00062

95. Stanisavljevic J, Loubat-Casanovas J, Herrera M, Luque T, Pena R, Lluch A, Albanell J, Bonilla F, Rovira A, Pena C, Navajas D, Rojo F, Garcia de Herreros A, Baulida J (2015) Snail1-expressing fibroblasts in the tumor microenvironment display mechanical properties that support metastasis. Cancer Res 75(2):284–295. doi:10.1158/0008-5472.CAN-14-1903

96. Calvo F, Ege N, Grande-Garcia A, Hooper S, Jenkins RP, Chaudhry SI, Harrington K, Williamson P, Moeendarbary E, Charras G, Sahai E (2013) Mechanotransduction and YAP-dependent matrix remodelling is required for the generation and maintenance of cancer-associated fibroblasts. Nat Cell Biol 15(6):637–646. doi:10.1038/ncb2756

97. Goetz JG, Minguet S, Navarro-Lerida I, Lazcano JJ, Samaniego R, Calvo E, Tello M, Osteso-Ibanez T, Pellinen T, Echarri A, Cerezo A, Klein-Szanto AJ, Garcia R, Keely PJ, Sanchez-Mateos P, Cukierman E, Del Pozo MA (2011) Biomechanical remodeling of the microenvironment by stromal caveolin-1 favors tumor invasion and metastasis. Cell 146(1):148–163. doi:10.1016/j.cell.2011.05.040

98. Erez N, Truitt M, Olson P, Arron ST, Hanahan D (2010) Cancer-associated fibroblasts are activated in incipient neoplasia to orchestrate tumor-promoting inflammation in an NF-kappaB-dependent manner. Cancer Cell 17(2):135–147. doi:10.1016/j.ccr.2009.12.041

99. Karagiannis GS, Poutahidis T, Erdman SE, Kirsch R, Riddell RH, Diamandis EP (2012) Cancer-associated fibroblasts drive the progression of metastasis through both paracrine and mechanical pressure on cancer tissue. Mol Cancer Res (MCR) 10(11):1403–1418. doi:10.1158/1541-7786.MCR-12-0307

100. Hellstrom M, Phng LK, Hofmann JJ, Wallgard E, Coultas L, Lindblom P, Alva J, Nilsson AK, Karlsson L, Gaiano N, Yoon K, Rossant J, Iruela-Arispe ML, Kalen M, Gerhardt H, Betsholtz C (2007) Dll4 signalling through Notch1 regulates formation of tip cells during angiogenesis. Nature 445(7129):776–780. doi:10.1038/Nature05571

101. Zeng Q, Li S, Chepeha DB, Giordano TJ, Li J, Zhang H, Polverini PJ, Nor J, Kitajewski J, Wang CY (2005) Crosstalk between tumor and endothelial cells promotes tumor angiogenesis by MAPK activation of Notch signaling. Cancer Cell 8(1):13–23. doi:10.1016/j.ccr.2005.06.004

102. Gjorevski N, Boghaert E, Nelson CM (2012) Regulation of epithelial-mesenchymal transition by transmission of mechanical stress through epithelial tissues. Cancer Microenviron (Official Journal of the International Cancer Microenvironment Society) 5(1):29–38. doi:10.1007/s12307-011-0076-5

103. Gomez EW, Chen QK, Gjorevski N, Nelson CM (2010) Tissue geometry patterns epithelial-mesenchymal transition via intercellular mechanotransduction. J Cell Biochem 110(1):44–51. doi:10.1002/jcb.22545

104. Sewell-Loftin MK, Delaughter DM, Peacock JR, Brown CB, Baldwin HS, Barnett JV, Merryman WD (2014) Myocardial contraction and hyaluronic acid mechanotransduction in epithelial-to-mesenchymal transformation of endocardial cells. Biomaterials. doi:S0142-9612(13)01535-4 [pii] 10.1016/j.biomaterials.2013.12.051

105. Chien S (2008) Role of shear stress direction in endothelial mechanotransduction. Mol Cell Biomech (MCB) 5(1):1–8

106. Li YS, Haga JH, Chien S (2005) Molecular basis of the effects of shear stress on vascular endothelial cells. J Biomech 38(10):1949–1971. doi:10.1016/j.jbiomech.2004.09.030

107. Galie PA, Nguyen DH, Choi CK, Cohen DM, Janmey PA, Chen CS (2014) Fluid shear stress threshold regulates angiogenic sprouting. Proc Natl Acad Sci U S A 111(22):7968–7973. doi:10.1073/pnas.1310842111

108. Vickerman V, Kamm RD (2012) Mechanism of a flow-gated angiogenesis switch: early signaling events at cell-matrix and cell-cell junctions. Integr Biol-Uk 4(8):863–874. doi:10.1039/c2ib00184e

109. Buchanan CF, Verbridge SS, Vlachos PP, Rylander MN (2014) Flow shear stress regulates endothelial barrier function and expression of angiogenic factors in a 3D microfluidic tumor vascular model. Cell Adhes Migr 8(5):517–524. doi:10.4161/19336918.2014.970001

110. Buchanan CF, Voigt EE, Szot CS, Freeman JW, Vlachos PP, Rylander MN (2014) Three-dimensional microfluidic collagen hydrogels for investigating flow-mediated tumor-endothelial signaling and vascular organization. Tissue Eng Part C Methods 20(1):64–75. doi:10.1089/ten.TEC.2012.0731

111. Ingber DE (2008) Tensegrity-based mechanosensing from macro to micro. Prog Biophys Mol Biol 97(2–3):163–179. doi:S0079-6107(08)00015-1 [pii] 10.1016/j.pbiomolbio.2008.02.005

112. Lehoux S, Castier Y, Tedgui A (2006) Molecular mechanisms of the vascular responses to haemodynamic forces. J Intern Med 259(4):381–392. doi:10.1111/j.1365-2796.2006.01624.x

113. Ngu H, Feng Y, Lu L, Oswald SJ, Longmore GD, Yin FC (2010) Effect of focal adhesion proteins on endothelial cell adhesion, motility and orientation response to cyclic strain. Ann Biomed Eng 38(1):208–222. doi:10.1007/s10439-009-9826-7

114. Avraamides CJ, Garmy-Susini B, Varner JA (2008) Integrins in angiogenesis and lymphangiogenesis. Nat Rev Cancer 8(8):604–617. doi:10.1038/Nrc2353

115. Weinbaum S, Zhang X, Han Y, Vink H, Cowin SC (2003) Mechanotransduction and flow across the endothelial glycocalyx. Proc Natl Acad Sci U S A 100(13):7988–7995. doi:10.1073/pnas.1332808100

116. Reitsma S, Slaaf DW, Vink H, van Zandvoort MA, oude Egbrink MG (2007) The endothelial glycocalyx: composition, functions, and visualization. Pflugers Arch 454(3):345–359. doi:10.1007/s00424-007-0212-8

117. Pelham RJ Jr, Wang YL (1998) Cell locomotion and focal adhesions are regulated by the mechanical properties of the substrate. Biol Bull 194(3):348–349. discussion 349–350

118. Pelham RJ Jr, Wang Y (1997) Cell locomotion and focal adhesions are regulated by substrate flexibility. Proc Natl Acad Sci U S A 94(25):13661–13665

119. Dong Y, Xie X, Wang Z, Hu C, Zheng Q, Wang Y, Chen R, Xue T, Chen J, Gao D, Wu W, Ren Z, Cui J (2014) Increasing matrix stiffness upregulates vascular endothelial growth factor expression in hepatocellular carcinoma cells mediated by integrin beta1. Biochem Biophys Res Commun 444(3):427–432. doi:10.1016/j.bbrc.2014.01.079

120. Kojima T, Moraes C, Cavnar SP, Luker GD, Takayama S (2015) Surface-templated hydrogel patterns prompt matrix-dependent migration of breast cancer cells towards chemokine-secreting cells. Acta Biomater 13:68–77. doi:10.1016/j.actbio.2014.11.033

121. Fraley SI, Feng Y, Krishnamurthy R, Kim DH, Celedon A, Longmore GD, Wirtz D (2010) A distinctive role for focal adhesion proteins in three-dimensional cell motility. Nat Cell Biol 12(6):598–604. doi:10.1038/ncb2062

122. Zebda N, Dubrovskyi O, Birukov KG (2012) Focal adhesion kinase regulation of mechanotransduction and its impact on endothelial cell functions. Microvasc Res 83(1):71–81. doi:10.1016/j.mvr.2011.06.007

123. Kim DH, Khatau SB, Feng Y, Walcott S, Sun SX, Longmore GD, Wirtz D (2012) Actin cap associated focal adhesions and their distinct role in cellular mechanosensing. Sci Rep 2:555. doi:10.1038/srep00555

124. Nagelkerke A, Bussink J, Sweep FC, Span PN (2013) Generation of multicellular tumor spheroids of breast cancer cells: how to go three-dimensional. Anal Biochem 437(1):17–19. doi:10.1016/j.ab.2013.02.004

125. Timmins NE, Nielsen LK (2007) Generation of multicellular tumor spheroids by the hanging-drop method. Methods Mol Med 140:141–151

126. Skardal A, Devarasetty M, Rodman C, Atala A, Soker S (2015) Liver-tumor hybrid organoids for modeling tumor growth and drug response in vitro. Ann Biomed Eng 43(10):2361–2373. doi:10.1007/s10439-015-1298-3

127. Fong EL, Wan X, Yang J, Morgado M, Mikos AG, Harrington DA, Navone NM, Farach-Carson MC (2015) A 3D in vitro model of patient-derived prostate cancer xenograft for

controlled interrogation of in vivo tumor-stromal interactions. Biomaterials 77:164–172. doi:10.1016/j.biomaterials.2015.10.059

128. Bates RC, Buret A, van Helden DF, Horton MA, Burns GF (1994) Apoptosis induced by inhibition of intercellular contact. J Cell Biol 125(2):403–415

129. Takebe T, Enomura M, Yoshizawa E, Kimura M, Koike H, Ueno Y, Matsuzaki T, Yamazaki T, Toyohara T, Osafune K, Nakauchi H, Yoshikawa HY, Taniguchi H (2015) Vascularized and complex organ buds from diverse tissues via mesenchymal cell-driven condensation. Cell Stem Cell 16(5):556–565. doi:10.1016/j.stem.2015.03.004

130. Takebe T, Sekine K, Enomura M, Koike H, Kimura M, Ogaeri T, Zhang RR, Ueno Y, Zheng YW, Koike N, Aoyama S, Adachi Y, Taniguchi H (2013) Vascularized and functional human liver from an iPSC-derived organ bud transplant. Nature 499(7459):481–484. doi:10.1038/nature12271

131. Takebe T, Zhang RR, Koike H, Kimura M, Yoshizawa E, Enomura M, Koike N, Sekine K, Taniguchi H (2014) Generation of a vascularized and functional human liver from an iPSC-derived organ bud transplant. Nat Protoc 9(2):396–409. doi:10.1038/nprot.2014.020

132. Verbridge SS, Choi NW, Zheng Y, Brooks DJ, Stroock AD, Fischbach C (2010) Oxygen-controlled three-dimensional cultures to analyze tumor angiogenesis. Tissue Eng Part A 16(7):2133–2141. doi:10.1089/ten.TEA.2009.0670

133. Kilarski WW, Samolov B, Petersson L, Kvanta A, Gerwins P (2009) Biomechanical regulation of blood vessel growth during tissue vascularization. Nat Med 15(6):657–U145. doi:10.1038/Nm.1985

134. Liang Y, Jeong J, DeVolder RJ, Cha C, Wang F, Tong YW, Kong H (2011) A cell-instructive hydrogel to regulate malignancy of 3D tumor spheroids with matrix rigidity. Biomaterials 32(35):9308–9315. doi:10.1016/j.biomaterials.2011.08.045

135. Hsu YH, Moya ML, Abiri P, Hughes CC, George SC, Lee AP (2013) Full range physiological mass transport control in 3D tissue cultures. Lab Chip 13(1):81–89. doi:10.1039/c2lc40787f

136. Hsu YH, Moya ML, Hughes CC, George SC, Lee AP (2013) A microfluidic platform for generating large-scale nearly identical human microphysiological vascularized tissue arrays. Lab Chip 13(15):2990–2998. doi:10.1039/c3lc50424g

137. Moya ML, Alonzo LF, George SC (2014) Microfluidic device to culture 3D in vitro human capillary networks. Methods Mol Biol 1202:21–27. doi:10.1007/7651_2013_36

138. Chung S, Sudo R, Mack PJ, Wan CR, Vickerman V, Kamm RD (2009) Cell migration into scaffolds under co-culture conditions in a microfluidic platform. Lab Chip 9(2):269–275. doi:10.1039/B807585a

139. Park YK, Tu TY, Lim SH, Clement IJM, Yang SY, Kamm RD (2014) In vitro microvessel growth and remodeling within a three-dimensional microfluidic environment. Cell Mol Bioeng 7(1):15–25. doi:10.1007/s12195-013-0315-6

140. Sudo R, Chung S, Zervantonakis IK, Vickerman V, Toshimitsu Y, Griffith LG, Kamm RD (2009) Transport-mediated angiogenesis in 3D epithelial coculture. FASEB J 23(7):2155–2164. doi:10.1096/fj.08-122820

141. Cross MJ, Claesson-Welsh L (2001) FGF and VEGF function in angiogenesis: signalling pathways, biological responses and therapeutic inhibition. Trends Pharmacol Sci 22(4):201–207. doi:10.1016/S0165-6147(00)01676-X

142. Lee H, Kim S, Chung M, Kim JH, Jeon NL (2014) A bioengineered array of 3D microvessels for vascular permeability assay. Microvasc Res 91:90–98. doi:10.1016/j.mvr.2013.12.001

143. Alizadeh AM, Shiri S, Farsinejad S (2014) Metastasis review: from bench to bedside. Tumour Biol (The Journal of the International Society for Oncodevelopmental Biology and Medicine) 35(9):8483–8523. doi:10.1007/s13277-014-2421-z

144. Blazejczyk A, Papiernik D, Porshneva K, Sadowska J, Wietrzyk J (2015) Endothelium and cancer metastasis: perspectives for antimetastatic therapy. Pharmacol Rep (PR) 67(4):711–718. doi:10.1016/j.pharep.2015.05.014

145. Chang J, Erler J (2014) Hypoxia-mediated metastasis. Adv Exp Med Biol 772:55–81. doi:10.1007/978-1-4614-5915-6_3

146. Irmisch A, Huelsken J (2013) Metastasis: new insights into organ-specific extravasation and metastatic niches. Exp Cell Res 319(11):1604–1610. doi:10.1016/j.yexcr.2013.02.012

147. Garcia-Roman J, Zentella-Dehesa A (2013) Vascular permeability changes involved in tumor metastasis. Cancer Lett 335(2):259–269. doi:10.1016/j.canlet.2013.03.005

148. Miles FL, Pruitt FL, van Golen KL, Cooper CR (2008) Stepping out of the flow: capillary extravasation in cancer metastasis. Clin Exp Metastasis 25(4):305–324. doi:10.1007/s10585-007-9098-2

149. Reymond N, d'Agua BB, Ridley AJ (2013) Crossing the endothelial barrier during metastasis. Nat Rev Cancer 13(12):858–870. doi:10.1038/nrc3628

150. van Zijl F, Krupitza G, Mikulits W (2011) Initial steps of metastasis: cell invasion and endothelial transmigration. Mutat Res 728(1–2):23–34. doi:10.1016/j.mrrev.2011.05.002

151. Bersini S, Jeon JS, Moretti M, Kamm RD (2014) In vitro models of the metastatic cascade: from local invasion to extravasation. Drug Discov Today 19(6):735–742. doi:10.1016/j.drudis.2013.12.006

152. Kaplan RN, Riba RD, Zacharoulis S, Bramley AH, Vincent L, Costa C, MacDonald DD, Jin DK, Shido K, Kerns SA, Zhu Z, Hicklin D, Wu Y, Port JL, Altorki N, Port ER, Ruggero D, Shmelkov SV, Jensen KK, Rafii S, Lyden D (2005) VEGFR1-positive haematopoietic bone marrow progenitors initiate the pre-metastatic niche. Nature 438(7069):820–827. doi:10.1038/nature04186

153. Ghajar CM, Peinado H, Mori H, Matei IR, Evason KJ, Brazier H, Almeida D, Koller A, Hajjar KA, Stainier DYR, Chen EI, Lyden D, Bissell MJ (2013) The perivascular niche regulates breast tumour dormancy. Nat Cell Biol 15(7):807–817. doi:10.1038/ncb2767. http://www.nature.com/ncb/journal/v15/n7/abs/ncb2767.html#supplementary-information

154. Lee H, Park W, Ryu H, Jeon NL (2014) A microfluidic platform for quantitative analysis of cancer angiogenesis and intravasation. Biomicrofluidics 8(5):054102. doi:10.1063/1.4894595

155. Zervantonakis IK, Hughes-Alford SK, Charest JL, Condeelis JS, Gertler FB, Kamm RD (2012) Three-dimensional microfluidic model for tumor cell intravasation and endothelial barrier function. Proc Natl Acad Sci U S A 109(34):13515–13520. doi:10.1073/pnas.1210182109

156. Camerer E, Qazi AA, Duong DN, Cornelissen I, Advincula R, Coughlin SR (2004) Platelets, protease-activated receptors, and fibrinogen in hematogenous metastasis. Blood 104(2):397–401. doi:10.1182/blood-2004-02-0434

157. Coupland LA, Chong BH, Parish CR (2012) Platelets and P-selectin control tumor cell metastasis in an organ-specific manner and independently of NK cells. Cancer Res 72(18):4662–4671. doi:10.1158/0008-5472.CAN-11-4010

158. Reymond N, Im JH, Garg R, Vega FM, Borda d'Agua B, Riou P, Cox S, Valderrama F, Muschel RJ, Ridley AJ (2012) Cdc42 promotes transendothelial migration of cancer cells through beta1 integrin. J Cell Biol 199(4):653–668. doi:10.1083/jcb.201205169

159. Shirure VS, Liu T, Delgadillo LF, Cuckler CM, Tees DF, Benencia F, Goetz DJ, Burdick MM (2015) CD44 variant isoforms expressed by breast cancer cells are functional E-selectin ligands under flow conditions. Am J Physiol Cell Physiol 308(1):C68–C78. doi:10.1152/ajpcell.00094.2014

160. Jeon JS, Zervantonakis IK, Chung S, Kamm RD, Charest JL (2013) In vitro model of tumor cell extravasation. PLoS One 8(2):e56910. doi:10.1371/journal.pone.0056910

161. Heyder C, Gloria-Maercker E, Entschladen F, Hatzmann W, Niggemann B, Zanker KS, Dittmar T (2002) Realtime visualization of tumor cell/endothelial cell interactions during transmigration across the endothelial barrier. J Cancer Res Clin Oncol 128(10):533–538. doi:10.1007/s00432-002-0377-7

162. Nolan DJ, Ginsberg M, Israely E, Palikuqi B, Poulos MG, James D, Ding BS, Schachterle W, Liu Y, Rosenwaks Z, Butler JM, Xiang J, Rafii A, Shido K, Rabbany SY, Elemento O, Rafii S (2013) Molecular signatures of tissue-specific microvascular endothelial cell heterogeneity in organ maintenance and regeneration. Dev Cell 26(2):204–219. doi:10.1016/j.devcel.2013.06.017

163. Moya ML, George SC (2014) Integrating organ-specific function with the microcirculation. Curr Opin Chem Eng 3:103–111. doi:10.1016/j.coche.2013.12.004

Microfluidics in Cell and Tissue Studies

Shiny Amala Priya Rajan, Parker Hambright, Rosemary Clare Burke, and Adam R. Hall

Abstract The central challenge inherent to conventional cell culture systems in general and tumor systems in particular is that any but the most rudimentary studies requires an enormous amount of infrastructure and handling capabilities to investigate numerous, interdependent variables in discrete samples. In addition, analysis of outcomes is both separate and potentially challenging. Significant strides have been made to address both of these challenges through the use of microfluidic technologies and cell culture techniques toward the goal of an integrated delivery and assessment platform that recapitulates in vivo conditions. Here, we review microfluidic approaches that enable the study of cells and cell culture, with specific applications to cancer cells and tumor organoids.

Keywords Microfluidics • Single-cell • Cell culture • Organoids • Lab-on-a-chip • 3D culture

S.A.P. Rajan
Virginia Tech-Wake Forest School of Biomedical Engineering and Sciences,
Wake Forest University School of Medicine, Winston-Salem, NC, USA

P. Hambright
Virginia Tech-Wake Forest School of Biomedical Engineering and Sciences,
Wake Forest University School of Medicine, Winston-Salem, NC, USA

Department of Biology, Wake Forest University, Winston-Salem, NC, USA

R.C. Burke
Virginia Tech-Wake Forest School of Biomedical Engineering and Sciences,
Wake Forest University School of Medicine, Winston-Salem, NC, USA

Department of Biomedical Engineering, University of Texas Austin, Austin, TX, USA

A.R. Hall (✉)
Virginia Tech-Wake Forest School of Biomedical Engineering and Sciences,
Wake Forest University School of Medicine, Winston-Salem, NC, USA

Comprehensive Cancer Center, Wake Forest University School of Medicine,
Winston-Salem, NC, USA
e-mail: arhall@wakehealth.edu

© Springer International Publishing AG 2018
S. Soker, A. Skardal (eds.), *Tumor Organoids*, Cancer Drug Discovery
and Development, DOI 10.1007/978-3-319-60511-1_8

149

1 Introduction

The structures, functions, responses, remodeling, and interactions of complex tissues are represented most accurately in vivo. This fact has made the use of animal models a constant in biological research since before the formal inception of the field, but the modern use of animals also presents a variety of challenges, including ethical concerns, expense and infrastructure requirements for maintenance, and limitations in analytical diagnostics of living systems. Perhaps most critically to biomedical research, there is also often only poor association between animal models and humans, meaning that even successful findings in a mouse or primate may not necessarily translate to success in patients.

In response to these challenges, and in balancing the need to protect human subjects with the need for experimentation, cell culture emerged as a critical technology in the early to mid twentieth century. Pioneering work using explanted tissue [36] and the later identification of nutrient requirements for growth media [19] laid a foundation for the approach. However, only upon the report of the first human cell line [28] did the full potential impact of cell culture in relation to biomedical research become clear. Since that time, a wide range of human cell lines have been produced and used to bolster fields like oncology, virology, and pharmaceutics. Nonetheless, working with plate-, dish-, or media-based cell culture brings with it challenges in implementation. For example, systematic delivery of drugs and analysis of response must conventionally be done either manually or through the use of robotic handling equipment that can entail significant infrastructural requirements and costs.

For these reasons, miniaturization, integration, and automation have long been a central goal in the field, and microfluidic devices have been a major focus of this drive due to their strong potential to touch on each of the cogent factors. In this chapter, we aim to describe the use of microfluidics in probing cell behavior, either independently, in culture, or in pseudo-tissue 3D constructs (organoids), with a specific focus on cancer. We will first review fabrication methods commonly used to realize the microfluidic architectures themselves, specifically to highlight the capabilities available to researchers in the discipline. Then, we will discuss strategies for interfacing cells within devices, moving from single cells to traditional 2D cell cultures and finally to the integration of 3D cell culture for in situ study. Finally, we will describe an assortment of analytical techniques available for assessing cells and their behaviors when they are in microfluidic structures.

2 Microfluidic Devices

Broadly, microfluidic devices are fabricated, chip-based fluid handling systems that use microchannels with dimensions in the hundreds of μm or less to achieve low fluid volume. Microfluidics can in principle be produced at low cost and

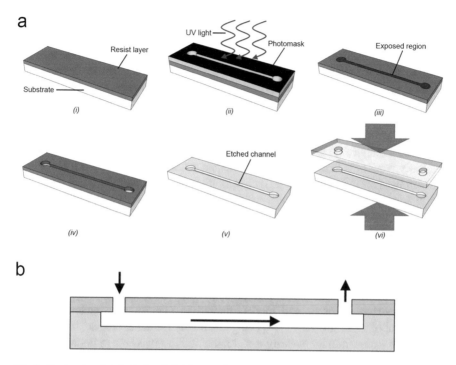

Fig. 1 Basic microfluidic device definition. (**a**) Scheme for photolithographic device definition. A substrate coated with photoresist (*i*) is exposed with UV light through a photomask (*ii*) to define an exposed region (*iii*) that is soluble in developer. Following development to remove exposed resist (*iv*), remaining resist can be used as an etch mask to remove substrate material (*v*). A flat substrate with inlet/outlets can then be bonded to the structured surface to enclose the device (*vi*). (**b**) Cross-section of the device, showing fluid flow pathway (*arrows*)

high-throughput to enable potential widespread use of what Manz, *et al.* first referred [47] to as a *micro total analysis system*: miniaturized fluid manipulation, mixing, and delivery to an integrated sensor for self-contained analytical assessment. Beyond reduced fluid volume and automated handling, such systems can also offer increased sensitivity, massively parallel processing, and portability, making obvious their potential utility in fields like biodefense, molecular analysis, and cellular biology. Just some of the biological assays integrated with microfluidic structures include polymerase chain reaction (PCR) amplification of DNA [58, 86], sequence analysis [1], and immunoassays [34]. These capabilities can be realized using devices produced through a variety of techniques, each varying in applicable materials, attainable resolution, and degree of difficulty to perform.

Microfluidic structures have traditionally been made using techniques originating from the production of electronic devices, and these methods continue to be common to several of the most widely used fabrication approaches. Briefly, photolithography can be performed by first coating a substrate with a thin film of photosensitive polymer (photoresist) and then defining channel shapes with UV light through either a direct contact shadow mask or patterned exposure (Fig. 1a, *i–iii*).

More rarely, an electron beam can also be used to expose certain types of resist, yielding exceptionally high-resolution features. Typically, resist exposure solubilizes it to a developer solution (i.e. negative lithography), which is subsequently used to remove patterned regions selectively, leaving access to the underlying substrate (Fig. 1a, *iv*). The resulting structured resist layer can subsequently be used as an etch mask, followed by total removal of the resist layer to leave a monolithic substrate with defined topological structures (Fig. 1a, *v*). Bonding of a second flat substrate to this surface and supplying inlet/outlet ports (Fig. 1a, *vi*) results in an enclosed channel structure with no intrinsic dead volume (Fig. 1b).

Early work [48] defined devices in silicon substrates in this way. The use of silicon brought specific advantages, including high planarity and the availability of a large selection of etching modalities, especially isotropic (unidirectional) ones. However, the disadvantages were numerous. First, silicon is expensive, setting a high potential cost of resulting devices. Second, it is opaque, making any optics-based analytical approaches impossible. Third, it is a stiff material, making it not only unsuitable for biological applications like direct integration with mechanosensitive cells, but also limiting overall devices to being passive in nature. Without actuating elements, integrated manipulation was made challenging, with flow requiring external pumps and mixing limited to feature-based techniques [44]. Integration of glass substrates [74] using essentially the same process, while bringing with it a reduction in planarity and etching options, was able to improve devices in terms of cost and optical transparency. However, its own inflexibility did little to address the issues inherent to silicon stiffness.

In response, the Whitesides group introduced [18] an alternative approach for patterning elastomeric polymers referred to as soft lithography. Fundamentally, the technique involves using topographically-patterned solid substrates (Fig. 2a, top), fabricated as described above or as the direct products of high aspect ratio photolithography, as negative molds (Fig. 2a, middle) for heat-curable polymers like polydimethyl siloxane (PDMS). The relief structure is subsequently removed from the mold (Fig. 2a, bottom) and bonded to glass slides or other PDMS components to be used as channel elements. This advancement brought with it numerous advantages. For example, process costs were reduced, with PDMS being relatively inexpensive and the structured mold itself becoming reusable. The materials were transparent and considerably easier to integrate with biological systems, being gas permeable and having mechanical properties that could in principle be adjusted, at least to some degree. And perhaps most significantly, the intrinsic flexibility of PDMS lent itself to actuation. This latter idea was elegantly demonstrated by the Quake lab [79] when they showed that patterned thin films of PDMS layered atop one another could be used to form active control elements. By forming independent channels that cross each other's path, hydraulic pressure in one chamber (control line) could be used to deform the elastomeric barrier separating them, causing obstruction of the other chamber (flow line) (Fig. 2b). Additionally, alignment and alternating actuation of several series valves of this kind could produce peristaltic pumping of fluid. Crucially, the bottom-up, parallel production of these structures

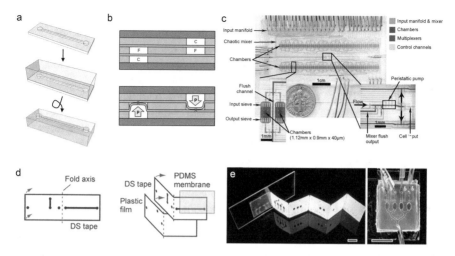

Fig. 2 PDMS and tape microfluidics. (**a**) PDMS replica molding scheme, wherein an etched substrate (see Fig. 1) is coated in PDMS, which is then cured and removed to yield a relief structure. (**b**) Schematic cross-section of Quake-style microfluidic valves. *Top*: Beginning, multi-layer structure featuring a centralized layer for flow lines ('F') and control lines ('C') above and below (channel direction is into the page). *Bottom*: Hydraulic pressure ('P') actuates the flexible layers, closing the flow lines. Each valve is individually addressable. (**c**) Example of a complex microfluidic device incorporating structures like those in (**b**) as valves and pumps (Adapted with permission from [29], Copyright © 2007, American Chemical Society). (**d**) Basic scheme of self-alignment to form a tape microfluidic device, in which patterned adhesive films are folded around a flexible actuation layer. (**e**) Example of multilayer self-alignment pattern (*left*) and the resulting, multichannel device (*right*). (**d, e**) Adapted with permission from [12], Copyright © 2014, Royal Society of Chemistry

make them capable of supporting systems of nearly arbitrary complexity [3] (c.f. Fig. 2c).

Due to these advantages, PDMS-based microfluidics continues to be the dominant approach, but some challenges do remain. One pertains to the infrastructure required to operate active microfluidics, including those described above. Hydraulic pressure control of valves and pumps typically requires either an external pressure supply [79] or vacuum [51], depending on the actuation approach taken. This necessitates potentially bulky equipment to support a given device. In addition, each actuating element can require an independent pressure control, making all but the most basic device architectures complex to control. In the laboratory setting, this may not be an issue, but it does negatively impact some of the overarching goals of the technology; namely true miniaturization, portability, and even accessibility. While alternative actuation approaches are being pursued [32], an off-shoot of traditional microfluidics has emerged that instead operates based on the principle of capillary action to produce flow, using paper as a central component [49, 50]. Paper microfluidics are built on chromatographic or filter papers and are usually fabricated using photolithography as above, but towards the goal of defining hydrophilic channels through which fluids can flow. These devices typically – but not always [77]

–incorporate no internal control elements and are inherently a unidirectional flow, single-use system. In addition, the analytical capabilities integrated into paper microfluidics are largely confined to colorimetric ones. However, the advantages include extreme low cost of materials as well as ease of use and interpretation, all of which are important factors, especially in low resource settings.

A second challenge with conventional PDMS microfluidics concerns the use of multiple layers to form control and flow channel combinations in complex device architectures. Microscopic interlayer registration is essential in such structures, and is made more relevant as the number of elements increases, where even a slight lateral or rotational shift can cause severe misalignment. Here, the usually advantageous flexibility of PDMS layers can create problems in handling while its transparency can make visual inspection difficult. An approach that specifically responds to this challenge is the emerging technique of tape microfluidics [12], wherein an overall structure resembling PDMS microfluidics is made by layering patterned adhesive films. The layers themselves – essentially double-sided tape – are typically produced either by razor plotter or laser etching. Multiple, computer-designed layers can be fabricated as a monolithic film featuring perforations to promote directed folding, enabling self-alignment of the overall structure (Fig. 2d). Because the tapes themselves are usually not particularly elastomeric, flexible polymeric films like PDMS or polyvinyl chloride can be inserted between strata to act as actuating layers. Crucially, however, these layers are unpatterned, require no alignment, and are bonded to the surrounding layers by the adhesive intrinsic to the tapes. Stacked layers can be sandwiched between solid substrates (e.g. glass or polystyrene slides with inlets/outlets) or even between non-adhesive elastomeric films to produce an overall device with high flexibility and potential complexity [12] (c.f. Fig. 2e).

The main disadvantage with tape microfluidics as compared to conventional PDMS is feature resolution, which is typically hundreds of micrometers laterally and limited by tape thickness vertically (also typically 100–200 μm). While these values can be improved, they are already sufficiently sized to house small numbers of cells, which is the most pertinent factor for our present discussion. In addition, these devices also typically still rely on external infrastructure for hydraulic actuation, much like PDMS microfluidics. However, the advantages brought on by the approach include easy, rapid prototyping of devices and extremely low cost of materials, making them attractive for a range of potential applications.

3   Interfacing Single Cells with Microfluidic Systems

A basic notion for integrating cells, including cancer cells, with microfluidics is to introduce a cell suspension to a device and retain one or more for subsequent probing. The most straightforward method of accomplishing this utilizes the valve elements that can be incorporated in modern microfluidic devices, especially PDMS and tape-based devices. Here, a dilute suspension of cells is introduced to a microfluidic device and when a cell enters a target region, valves on either side of it are

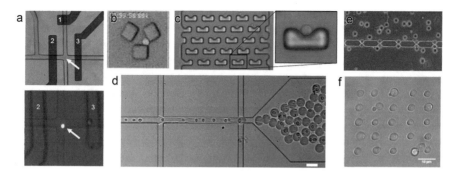

Fig. 3 Single cell studies in microfluidic devices. (**a**) Isolation of a single cell using microfluidic valve actuation. *Top*: device layout with valves labeled 1–3. *Bottom*: fluorescent micrograph of captured Jurkat cell labeled with calcein AM (Reprinted with permission from [65], Copyright © 2006, Springer). (**b**) A single yeast cell (*green*) trapped sterically by a microfabricated structure in a microfluidic device (Adapted with permission from [66], Copyright © 2006 John Wiley & Sons, Ltd). (**c**) A microfabricated array of structured posts for hydrodynamic capture of individual human cervical carcinoma cells. Flow direction for capture is from top. Inset: micrograph of typical captured cell (Reprinted with permission from [17], Copyright © 2006, Royal Society of Chemistry). (**d**) Cell encapsulation device, showing cells flowing in from left and being captured in single droplets to right (Reprinted from [60] and licensed under a Creative Commons Attribution 3.0 Unported License). (**e**) Dielectrophoretic capture of mouse fibroblasts at the high field regions (gaps) of a microfabricated structure inside a microfluidic device (Adapted with permission from [27], Copyright © 2010 American Institute of Physics). (**f**) Demonstration of positioning of individual cells (yeast) by optical tweezer in a microfluidic channel (Adapted with permission from [22], Copyright © 2009, Royal Society of Chemistry)

closed to prevent its escape [63, 65] (Fig. 3a). A cell can in principle be held in this state for an arbitrary time, but a major challenge is that the closed valves may limit delivery of nutrients and oxygen and the removal of waste products via the main channel, reducing cell viability. While many cancer cells are robust, this must be accounted for in most cases, potentially through side channels and/or perfusion elements.

Another fundamental approach to achieve cellular isolation is the use of mechanical or structural components for capture. For example, because of the layer-by-layer structure of microfluidic devices, porous thin films can be easily incorporated as barriers between layers, and thus can be organized such that fluid flow is directed through the pores. By engineering the pore size, cells larger than the size cutoff can be sterically captured [8, 31]. Besides incorporation of alternative extrinsic materials like porous membranes, the same microfabrication approaches used to define the channels and control elements in a microfluidic device can also themselves be used to define physical barriers *within* the chamber. This approach can be utilized in a number of ways. First, discrete structures can be formed around a region that hinder passage of target cells within them sterically, forming essentially 'jail bars' around a cell [66] (Fig. 3b). In this case, a cell must enter the region either by squeezing through the gaps via applied pressure or other forces, or enter when it is of a small enough size to pass and then grow inside the constriction. In a related method, microwells [62] can be fabricated in a microfluidic chamber [33, 42], sized to allow only one target cell to fit within them. By introducing cells in suspension, simple sedimentation can be used to fill the wells, after which excess materials can be easily flowed away, leaving individual isolates. This approach has been applied to the study of myelomonocytic leukemia cells, for example [42]. Inversely, arrays of pillars can be fabricated along a chamber to act as continuous size-exclusion for flowing cells. This approach can capture cells too large to pass through the constrictions, retaining them for further assessment, and has the further advantage of being inherently selective by size. This enables, for example, the capture and study of circulating tumor cells [16, 38], which are large compared to other components of blood.

Similar to but distinct from size-exclusion is the use of microfabricated structures to isolate cells via hydrodynamic capture. In this approach, a combination of structure conformation and a continuous flow work to hold a single cell in place, and elements are included to make the seeding process self-limiting. An early example of this concept [82] used a lateral microwell. Incorporated into the walls of this well were drain channels to allow fluid flow. Using adjacent fluidics, Jurkat cells (used to probe T cell leukemia) could be delivered to the trap using a steerable flow focus, and once there, the presence of the cell occluded the small drain channel, thus preventing additional cells from entering. While pioneering, this approach was serial, only allowing assessment of a single cell at a time. A subsequent technique [17] addressed this by instead utilizing a large array of discrete structures, each of which was capable of capturing a single cell (Fig. 3c). Here, rectangular pillars with a concave feature on one face were constructed in a microfluidic device. With flow direction into the structured surface, fluid would be drawn into the concave feature and stagnate, thus drawing objects like cells to that point. However, when filled, the flow pattern was altered such that fluid was directed around the pillar, keeping a cell statically trapped. In this way, thousands of individual HeLa (human cervical carcinoma) cells could be isolated and studied in situ within an active device. Many other clever variations on a similar theme have likewise been demonstrated, including devices for repeatable trap and release of individual cells [76].

A separate approach to single-cell isolation is the concept of microencapsulation, wherein cells are compartmentalized into droplets in a device [4, 60, 83] (Fig. 3d). The introduction of aqueous solution into hydrophobic fluid such as mineral oil produces an immiscible phase. Within a microfluidic environment, the result can be a series of discrete droplets formed by periodic pinched flow. Crucially, the dispensing of the aqueous solution can be regulated by differential pressures and channel dimensions, allowing droplet dimensions to be tailored. By suspending dilute cells in the aqueous solution and engineering sufficiently small droplets, individual cells can be isolated. Through condition optimization, a high yield of droplets containing only a single cell can be achieved, though there are statistically many empty droplets and likely some featuring more than one. Although this approach is very effective and has been applied to the study of cancer cells ranging from lymphoma [4] to carcinoma [83], there are specific aspects that must be taken into account when using it. For instance, captured cells are confined to very small volumes with no exchange, and therefore viability may again be a concern. Furthermore, while cells are isolated form one another, they are also isolated from the device environment, which can present challenges for some analytical assessments.

Finally, there is the potential of incorporating electromagnetic forces for the capture of individual cells in a microfluidic device. A common example of this is dielectrophoresis (DEP), or the use of alternating current electric fields to attract cells to a given location [27, 84]. This effect refers to the force induced on dielectric materials in a non-uniform alternating electric field. By patterning electrodes within a microfluidic device, such a field can be produced to attract individual cells (Fig. 3e). Unlike electrophoresis, DEP does not act only on charged materials, but instead acts on all dielectrics to varying degrees. What's more, the force and indeed its direction depend strongly on variables like the electrical permittivity of the object and its surrounding media, object size and shape, and the frequency at which the field alternates. Notably, these factors give DEP a great deal of potential selectivity, through which a subset of cells could be isolated and probed from within a mixture and then replaced by another based on differential properties.

A second example of electromagnetic capture in single cell isolation is the use of optical tweezers [30]. In this technique, dielectric objects like cells can be attracted to the focus of an incident laser beam in solution via a gradient force created by the refractive index mismatch between the object and its surrounding media. Because modern microfluidic systems are both optically transparent and thin enough to support the short working distances required for most optical tweezers, integration of such technologies is relatively straightforward. Once combined, the optical trap can be used to temporarily arrest cells, either individually or in arrays [81] (Fig. 3f), and direct target cells into neighboring flows [21] or chambers [22, 52, 59] for analysis. Importantly, despite the high power lasers used for these applications, heating damage inflicted on trapped cells has been found to be negligible [54].

4   Interfacing 2D Cell Culture with Microfluidic Systems

While approaches for interfacing single cells with microfluidics are effective for many applications, a central limitation is that such an arrangement does not reflect the environment cells usually encounter in vivo, where they are only rarely isolated from neighboring cells and cell signals – an exception being circulating tumor cells, for example – and are normally interfaced with extracellular matrix (ECM). As an iteration of complexity, we now discuss the incorporation of 2D cultures.

Most methods of achieving 2D culture on a chip resemble conventional dish- and plate-based culture studies, only reduced in size. In general, this means that target substrates within a microfluidic device are coated with a surface relevant to cell adhesion, cells are seeded onto that surface, nutrients and other factors are provided, and cells allowed to grow to confluency (Fig. 4a). The coatings used in this process are inspired by those used in conventional culture, typically involving components of the ECM like fibronectin [29], collagen [10, 56], and gelatin [80]. One factor that must be considered in a microfluidic environment, however, is that these coatings

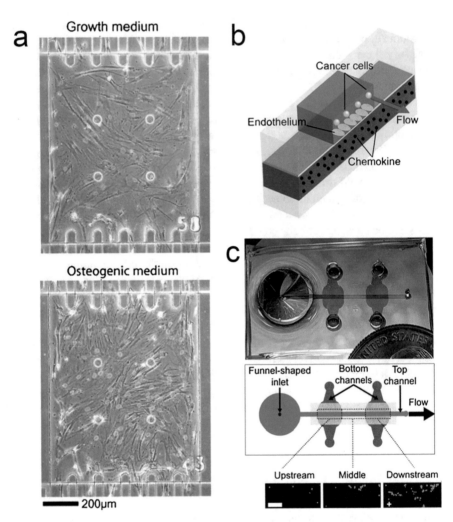

Fig. 4 2D cell culture in microfluidic environments. (**a**) Example 2D cell cultures from individual growth chambers in the device shown in Fig. 2c, showing (phase contrast images with superimposed false color DAPI stain) stem cells grown in normal growth media (*left*) and under osteogenic conditions. Differentiation can be observed (Adapted with permission from [29], Copyright © 2007, American Chemical Society) (**b**) Rendering of device architecture for studying interactions of metastatic breast cancer cells with pseudo endothelium grown on a porous membrane. (**c**) *Top*: an optical image and corresponding diagram of the total device. *Bottom*: example fluorescent micrographs of metastatic breast cells in three regions. (**b, c**) Adapted from [73] under the terms of the Creative Commons Attribution License

should be introduced only to a designated growth chamber and not indiscriminately throughout all channels, as cells seeded in control elements, for example, are likely to interfere with proper functioning of the device. This patterning can be accomplished through a variety of approaches, including use of passivation layers and strategic valving during introduction of coating solutions.

Another consideration is the reduction in fluid volume, the result of which is that nutrients and oxygen must be refreshed and waste products expelled at a higher rate than in conventional culture. This is typically achieved via perfusion and/or constant flow to the chamber through the microfluidic network surrounding it. One approach that directly responds to this need is the use of porous membranes, similar to but distinct from what was described above for single cell capture. In this case, flow is not directed though the membrane, but instead cells are seeded and cultured on top of it. The result is access of cells to a neighboring channel via the pores, which can be used not only for supplying nutrients, but also for recapitulating specific physiological conditions necessary for the study of certain cells, including adhesion of metastatic breast cancer cells to microvascular endothelia [73] (Fig. 4b, c) and others [23, 39].

The strongest advantage in performing 2D cell culture in a microfluidic system is the potential for studying many cultures in parallel [29], especially under varying conditions. The automation, and individual addressability offered by microfluidics enables complex screening of cellular response to differential stimuli in a compact format that would require significant infrastructure.

5 Interfacing 3D Cell Culture with Microfluidic Systems

Conventional 2D cell culture on a dish or plate is limited in its ability to reproduce the 3D microenvironment in which cells normally reside. 3D in vitro cell culture techniques ensure that cells experience unbiased 3D motility and interact not only with each other, but also with factors in the ECM. Consisting largely of glycoproteins, the ECM serves as the primary facilitator of cellular communication, and interactions with it are known to regulate cell migration, differentiation, and tissue organization in vivo. This suggests that cells in 3D environments are more representative of normal cell behavior; a concept that is supported by numerous studies evaluating the functionality of cells in each. For example, colon cancer cells in 2D plated culture have been found to display an epithelial phenotype and did not metastasize while the same cells in a hydrogel-based 3D microenvironment did metastasize [71].

Numerous techniques exist to produce 3D culture, but among the simplest conceptually is the use of hanging drops to form self-assembled structures. Here, cells suspended in a nutrient rich fluid are pipetted into a well or onto a concave plate such that a droplet is formed and held in place by surface tension. The cells naturally collect at the bottom of the drop where they self-assemble into a spheroid. The resulting structures feature cellular organization, a self-produced scaffold, and exhibit intracellular communication [78]. Furthermore, hanging drop spheroid formation is a relatively simple technique, and provides consistent geometry with easily accessed constructs. However, incorporating this technique within a microfluidic device presents a variety of challenges. The chamber in which the cells reside must support pipetting of fluid to form the suspended drop and thus cannot be embedded in a closed system like a sealed microfluidic device. More importantly, the process is not typically suitable for a continuous flow environment, as the approach relies on a single, discrete droplet of liquid to promote spheroid formation, which is normally incongruent with a fluid-filled network. Nonetheless, integration of microfluidics into the system has been demonstrated, wherein a device was used as a delivery vehicle for cell suspension to open-air hanging drops and a means of network interconnectivity [25] (Fig. 5a). Much like the conventional approach, the microfluidic form enables reproducible spheroid production with different cell types, including colon carcinoma (HCT-116). Unlike the conventional technique, multiple cell types can be utilized in parallel on the same chip, are interconnected via an active fluidic network that features a route for continuous nutrient supply for long-term experiments.

Another distinct method that resembles hanging drop spheroid production conceptually, but is more easily compatible with microfluidics, is so-called "gel free" 3D construct formation [57] (Fig. 5b). Here, cells are introduced to a chamber featuring microfabricated pillars for steric capture of conglomerations. Incubated with these cells is a polymeric intercellular linker that induces cell-cell adhesion. Crucially, this linker is transient, with a half-life on the order of days, and so does not remain within the final construct, but does enable extended cell-cell interaction that ultimately promotes the native formation of ECM. In this way, a final construct featuring interconnected and reasonably self-organized cells is produced, similar to a spheroid. In addition, the structure in which it resides is separated from the wider microfluidic environment only by a porous barrier of micropillars, enabling nutrient supply as above and potential for interconnectivity between discrete constructs.

While these approaches enable the use of ECM produced natively by the cells themselves, alternative scaffolds may also provide a similar microenvironment and facilitate communication between cells. Natural materials like agarose and gelatin can serve as scaffolding, as can synthetic polymers, but purified components of biological ECM are among the most important materials for this task since they intrinsically possess qualities of in vivo matrices. To this end, some of the most widely used biomaterials include collagen, fibronectin, vitronectin, laminin, and hyaluronic acid [61]. Each of these materials can in principle provide an environment for cell support by using cross-linkers to induce hydrogel formation.

Cell laden hydrogels are central to one of the most promising 3D culture technologies, 3D bioprinting [53], in which artificial tissue constructs over a large range of sizes and with nearly arbitrary shape are produced through layer-by-layer manufacturing (Fig. 5c). This approach has tremendous potential and various modalities of it have been developed to form multi-domain [68] and complex, organ-like structures [75], but its integration with microfluidics is particularly problematic. This is because, as a nozzle-based technology, open access to the deposition chamber is required, rendering biofabriaction in situ in a closed mcirofluidic environment

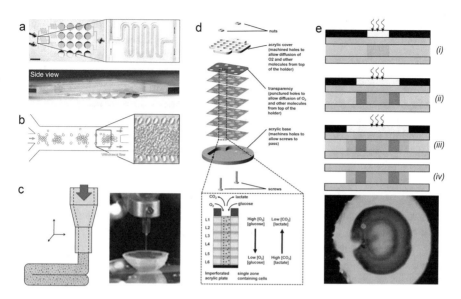

Fig. 5 3D cell cultures in microfluidic devices. (**a**) A microfluidic embodiment of the hanging drop method of spheroid formation. *Top*: overall device design, featuring discrete open-air chambers for droplet formation. *Bottom*: side view showing sixteen individual hanging drops under varying conditions (Reprinted with permission from [25], Copyright © 2014, Macmillan Publishers Limited) (**b**) Schematic of a gel-free culturing technique using microfabricated barriers and a polymeric intercellular linker to promote adhesion. Inset shows optical micrograph of actual device with cell culture (Adapted with permission from [57], Copyright © 2008, Elsevier Ltd.) (**c**) Cartoon depicting (extrusion based) 3D bioprinting, in which cell laden gel precursor is deposited by pressure (*red arrow*) as a nozzle is manipulated in three dimensions to yield predetermined structures. Right: Image of bioprinter in use (Adapted with permission from [53], Copyright © 2014, Macmillan Publishers Limited). (**d**) Schematic representation of paper microfluidic 3D cell culture built up from patterned paper layers (Reprinted with permission from [69], Copyright © 2016, Elsevier BV). (**e**) In situ photopatterning of multidomain constructs, showing successive introduction of hydrogel precursors, exposure through progressively larger photomasks (mask is *black* and exposed regions are darkened), and flushing (*i–iii*) to yield a multicomponent structure (*iv*). *Bottom*: Optical micrograph of an example total structure, with layers labeled by colored dyes

impossible. It is feasible in principle to manufacture a bioprinted structure prior to sealing of a microfluidic device, but even then, the resolution of the technique – typically [67] 100–300 μm – is such that stresses may be induced or large fluidic devices may be necessitated.

Several approaches are able to address this integration challenge, one of which utilizes a paper-based matrix to support the 3D cell culture [14]. Here, hydrogel precursor with cells mixed in can be loaded into a patterned paper substrate (Fig. 5d) that can be integrated with a wider paper microfluidic infrastructure. Crucially, these patterned layers can be stacked to form interconnected gel-laden networks of like or diverse cell types [15], reminiscent of the bottom-up manufacturing of 3D bioprinting. Just one example application of this paper-based solution examined the effect of radiation on a 3D model of lung cancer [69]. However, one possible challenge for this platform in general was discussed above: because fluids are delivered via capillary action, it is not trivial to change those conditions in situ with paper microlfuidics in general, requiring other means of control [13].

A second approach used to overcome the bioprinter integration problem is the patterned gelation of cell-loaded hydrogel precursor in predetermined locations within an assembled microfluidic device, with the most promising route being photopatterning [2, 41, 72]. The use of a photoinitiator can allow a hydrogel to cross-link rapidly under UV exposure, very similar to the photolithography methods used in making several types of microfluidics. By delivering a mixture of hydrogel precursor, photoinitiator, and target cells throughout a device chamber, gelation can be induced at discrete locations via patterned exposure through the transparent support substrate. Subsequent washing of unexposed precursor and cells yield a monolithic construct with properties similar to those of 3D bioprinted structures, but in a microfluidic architecture. One limitation of this approach relative to bioprinting is that the UV exposure affects the precursor in a columnar fashion, reducing the ability to include multiple discrete domains in the vertical direction. However, the use of sequential exposures does enable the building of complex, multi-domain polymerized structures in the lateral dimension. An example of this type of additive manufacturing is shown in Fig. 5e, where a series of photomasks are used to form multiple interfaces. The same technique can be used with cell mixtures to produce tissue-like organoids as well, including with cancer cells. Crucially, in situ photopatterning of (cell-laden) hydrogels, much like photolithography, can be performed massively in parallel to produce a large number of nearly identical, multifaceted structures simultaneously. When combined with the potential addressability of complex microfluidic design, this enables the realization of large numbers of discrete 3D cell cultures with individual control of conditions to support systematic studies of qualities like drug response.

6 Analytical Approaches Interfaced with Microfluidics

Having discussed techniques for interfacing cells and cell culture with microfluidics, we now review an assortment of analytical approaches that enable quantitative and qualitative assessment in situ; a critical component in the development of a *micro total analytical system*. Many, but not all, of these approaches involve the miniaturization and/or integration of techniques established in larger systems like conventional cell culture, slides, or microarrays. The most common analytical approach in this vein is optical microscopy, aided by the thin, transparent substrate layers utilized in most devices that make optical access easy. Optical microscopy can be used for the examination of the viability, motility, and signaling through the use of fluorescent reporters. While microscopy requires external infrastructure to perform and is therefore not strictly on-chip, we discuss it here because of both its analytical power and the potential for integration with mobile devices [46] that could maintain portability.

Simple vitality is among the most important metrics for cells, reporting on both the suitability of growth conditions and the response to changing stimuli in a given system. Optical assessment can probe this with relative ease using LIVE/DEAD staining [40] (Fig. 6a). Briefly, cells are exposed to two compounds: calcein ace-toxymethyl ester, a membrane permeable molecule that is activated to fluoresce by esterase activity in living cells, and ethidium homodimer 1, an intercalating nucleic acid dye that is not membrane permeable, but can enter the permeabilized membranes of dead cells. The result is that living cells are stained with one color, and dead cells with another, enabling quantification of overall cell viability. One limitation to this approach is that it is irreversible, offering only a snapshot of cell vitality. But, especially when conducted in microfluidic devices where multiple cell culture structures could be probed independently and at different time points, LIVE/DEAD assessment is critical for measuring not only environmental or chemical effects on cell health, but also in determining the fundamental ability of the culturing technique to support cells in the first place.

Direct live cell imaging with fluorescent tags is also extremely valuable. For example, dyes with low toxicity, such as Hoecst 33,258, which binds the minor groove in A-T dense areas of duplex DNA [43], or cells designed to produce fluorescent proteins allow cells to be imaged dynamically with fluorescent microscopy. This capability can be used, for example, to monitor cancer cell motility in the study of chemotaxis [45, 85] and metastasis [70]. The analysis of cellular migration is particularly well-studied in a microfluidic environment due to its thin (quasi-1D) nature and the ability to control factors like hydrostatic pressure. Alternatively, fluorescent reporters can also be activated by common signaling pathways, allowing aspects like metabolism and cell signaling to be studied. A variety of approaches enable components of many different pathways to be probed in this way [11, 64].

There are of course a large number of non-imaging techniques that can be integrated with microfluidics to assess cells and cell behavior as well. One that is very specific to the microfluidic environment is flow-based mechanical testing of individual cells, in which a channel with one or more restrictions smaller than the diameter of a cell is used to determine the moduli of passing cells. In general, flow forces are used to squeeze a cell through the constriction, during which either deformation associated with the translocation (Fig. 6b) or the additional time required for passage is monitored and used to determine fundamental properties of each cell. Mechanical testing is not viable for cells in culture *per se*, due to the interconnectedness of the cells under those conditions, but individual cells can be assessed rapidly. This approach is particularly valuable for screening cancer cells [6], for which mechanical properties are known to change relative to their non-cancer counterparts, but it can be applied to other types of cells as well [37].

Biochemical assays are a driving force in cell and cell culture analytics for the quantification of specific analytes in solution. Such assessments are akin to fluorescent reporters as described above, but encompassing a wider range of targets and enabling more multiplexed detection. The major example of this type of assay is the enzyme-linked immunosorbent assay, or ELISA [20]. Broadly, ELISA encompasses techniques that use a combination of antibodies for a target antigen and (most

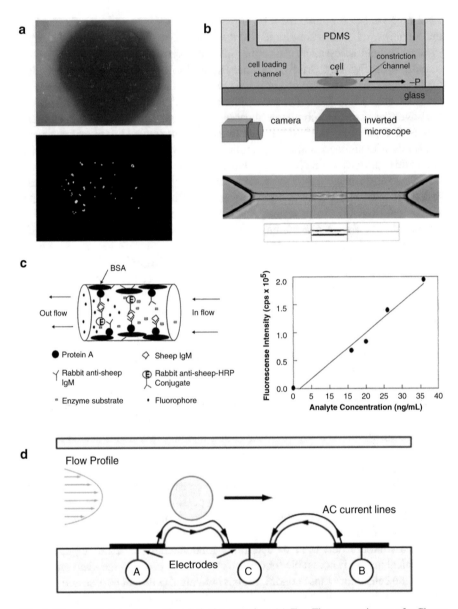

Fig. 6 Microfluidic integration of analytical approaches. (**a**) *Top*: Fluorescent image of mCherry (nuclear stain) colorectal carcinoma cells in central region of a concentric, bi-region construct in a microfluidic device (overlaid on brightfield; outer layer dyed green). *Bottom*: LIVE/DEAD of cells after 72 h (~75% viability). (**b**) *Top*: schematic of flow-based mechanical testing device. *Bottom*: micrograph of a cell in a microfabricated constriction. *Red lines* indicate cell length (Reprinted with permission from [6], Copyright © 2011, Royal Society of Chemistry) (**c**) *Top*: diagram of in situ microfluidic ELISA assay. *Bottom*: calibration plot between target analyte concentration and ELISA fluorescent signal (Reprinted with permission from [24], Copyright © 2001, Elsevier BV). (**d**) Mechanism of on-chip impedance measurement for probing cell motion, showing the transient presence of a cell distorting AC field lines between electrodes. (Reprinted with permission from [26], Copyright © 2001, Royal Society of Chemistry)

typically) a chemiluminescent, fluorescent, or colorimetric reporter enzyme to produce a quantifiable signal. The most powerful variety of this is the sandwich assay, in which unlabeled primary antibodies are immobilized to a solid substrate and secondary antibodies with a bound reporter are introduced. In the presence of the antigen, the reporter becomes linked to the substrate as well. ELISA has been integrated with various forms of microfluidics, wherein antibodies may be linked to either the walls and support substrates of a fluidic chamber in a conventional device [24] (PDMS or tape, for example; see Fig. 6c) or within the porous structure of a paper microfluidic device [5]. In either case, a major advantage can be found in the ultra-low fluid volumes attainable in the reduced environments, which can enable extremely sensitive detection and quantification. Additionally, immobilization in small area regions can potentially enable screening of a large number of independent targets simultaneously.

Finally, a range of electrical measurements have been integrated with microfluidics through the use of fabricated electrodes positioned within the device. One major example of this is impedance spectroscopy, in which pairs of electrodes are used to probe cells that pass between them [26] (Fig. 6d). The approach can be used to determine cellular migration, including in tumor models [55], and also yields frequency-dependent measurements of single-cell dielectric properties, which vary dramatically based on cell type and activity. This is true, for instance, with cancer cells having varying metastatic potential [9], suggesting possible routes to sorting and detailed study of subpopulations.

Another typical form of in situ electrical detection is electrochemical assessment, which can be used to probe chemical analytes in solution through three common means: potentiometry (measurement of potential differences between electrodes), coulometry (measurement of induced current as a function of time), and voltammetry (measurement of current as a function of voltage). This family of methods is especially powerful in determining enzymatic kinetics in closed systems [35], but has two significant limitations: first, only chemical reactions that involve an electrochemically active substrate or product can be probed, and second, it can be challenging to differentiate multiple analytes in the same system. For these reasons, electrochemical detection is also frequently used along with antibodies coupled to enzymes that produce electrochemically-active elements, enabling electrical readout of ELISA-like signals [7].

7   Conclusions

With an ability to support cellular growth and proliferation in a controlled environment and a potential for direct assessment of outcomes, microfluidic technology enables extensive experiments to be performed in a miniaturized format. In a general sense, the technology therefore supports measurements that might in principle be pursued at a larger scale, but with a requirement for considerably less infrastructure and manual preparation. Here, we have discussed the fundamentals of microfluidic technology, methods for coupling cells and cell culture to them, and major techniques for determining responses. While the platform is powerful for many applications beginning from fundamental studies of single cell behavior, we believe one of its most important applications will be in the study of tumor behavior in the form of complex organoids. Few techniques are capable of recapitulating the three-dimensional, multidomain structures of in vivo tumors, and fewer still are both at a scale that avoids necrosis and are easily integrated with control and analytical elements. As a result, microfluidic measurement of tumor organoids will enable a better understanding of cancer biology through in vitro observation and offer a route to study cancer drug responses through combinatorial processing.

References

1. Abate AR, Hung T, Sperling RA et al (2013) DNA sequence analysis with droplet-based microfluidics. Lab Chip 13:4864–4869. doi:10.1039/c3lc50905b
2. Albrecht DR, Tsang VL, Sah RL, Bhatia SN (2005) Photo- and electropatterning of hydrogel-encapsulated living cell arrays. Lab Chip 5:111–118. doi:10.1039/b406953f
3. Anderson JR, Chiu DT, Jackman RJ et al (2000) Fabrication of topologically complex three-dimensional microfluidic systems in PDMS by rapid prototyping. Anal Chem 72:3158–3164. doi:10.1021/ac9912294
4. Brouzes E, Medkova M, Savenelli N et al (2009) Droplet microfluidic technology for single-cell high-throughput screening. Proc Natl Acad Sci 106:14195–14200. doi:10.1073/pnas.0903542106
5. Cheng C-M, Martinez AW, Gong J et al (2010) Paper-based ELISA. Angew Chem Int Ed 49:4771–4774. doi:10.1002/anie.201001005
6. Chen J, Zheng Y, Tan Q et al (2011) Classification of cell types using a microfluidic device for mechanical and electrical measurement on single cells. Lab Chip 11:3174–3181. doi:10.1039/C1LC20473D
7. Chikkaveeraiah BV, Mani V, Patel V et al (2011) Microfluidic electrochemical immunoarray for ultrasensitive detection of two cancer biomarker proteins in serum. Biosens Bioelectron 26:4477–4483. doi:10.1016/j.bios.2011.05.005
8. Choi D-H, Yoon G-W, Park JW et al (2015) Fabrication of a membrane filter with controlled pore shape and its application to cell separation and strong single cell trapping. J Micromech Microeng 25:105007. doi:10.1088/0960-1317/25/10/105007
9. Cho Y, Kim HS, Frazier AB et al (2009) Whole-cell impedance analysis for highly and poorly metastatic cancer cells. J Microelectromech Syst 18:808–817. doi:10.1109/JMEMS.2009.2021821
10. Chung S, Sudo R, Mack PJ et al (2009) Cell migration into scaffolds under co-culture conditions in a microfluidic platform. Lab Chip 9:269–275. doi:10.1039/b807585a
11. Clayton AHA, Tavarnesi ML, Johns TG (2007) Unligated epidermal growth factor receptor forms higher order oligomers within microclusters on A431 cells that are sensitive to tyrosine kinase inhibitor binding. Biochemistry (Mosc) 46:4589–4597. doi:10.1021/bi700002b
12. Cooksey GA, Atencia J (2014) Pneumatic valves in folded 2D and 3D fluidic devices made from plastic films and tapes. Lab Chip 14:1665–1668. doi:10.1039/c4lc00173g
13. Deiss FT, Derda R, Mazzeo A, et al (2013) 96-well, paper-based platform for high-throughput testing of the effect of soluble compounds on 3D cell cultures.
14. Derda R, Laromaine A, Mammoto A et al (2009) Paper-supported 3D cell culture for tissue-based bioassays. Proc Natl Acad Sci 106:18457–18462. doi:10.1073/pnas.0910666106

15. Derda R, Tang SKY, Laromaine A et al (2011) Multizone paper platform for 3D cell cultures. PLoS One 6:e18940. doi:10.1371/journal.pone.0018940

16. Dharmasiri U, Njoroge SK, Witek MA et al (2011) High-throughput selection, enumeration, electrokinetic manipulation, and molecular profiling of low-abundance circulating tumor cells using a microfluidic system. Anal Chem 83:2301–2309. doi:10.1021/ac103172y

17. Di Carlo D, Wu LY, Lee LP (2006) Dynamic single cell culture array. Lab Chip 6:1445–1449. doi:10.1039/b605937f

18. Duffy DC, McDonald JC, Schueller OJA, Whitesides GM (1998) Rapid prototyping of microfluidic systems in poly(dimethylsiloxane). Anal Chem 70:4974–4984. doi:10.1021/ac980656z

19. Eagle H (1955) Nutrition needs of mammalian cells in tissue culture. Science 122:501–514

20. Engvall E, Perlmann P (1971) Enzyme-linked immunosorbent assay (ELISA) quantitative assay of immunoglobulin-G. Immunochemistry 8:871. doi:10.1016/0019-2791(71)90454-X

21. Eriksson E, Enger J, Nordlander B et al (2006) A microfluidic system in combination with optical tweezers for analyzing rapid and reversible cytological alterations in single cells upon environmental changes. Lab Chip 7:71–76. doi:10.1039/B613650H

22. Eriksson E, Sott K, Lundqvist F et al (2010) A microfluidic device for reversible environmental changes around single cells using optical tweezers for cell selection and positioning. Lab Chip 10:617–625. doi:10.1039/b913587a

23. Esch MB, Sung JH, Yang J et al (2012) On chip porous polymer membranes for integration of gastrointestinal tract epithelium with microfluidic "body-on-a-chip" devices. Biomed Microdevices 14:895–906. doi:10.1007/s10544-012-9669-0

24. Eteshola E, Leckband D (2001) Development and characterization of an ELISA assay in PDMS microfluidic channels. Sens Actuators B-Chem 72:129–133. doi:10.1016/S0925-4005(00)00640-7

25. Frey O, Misun PM, Fluri DA et al (2014) Reconfigurable microfluidic hanging drop network for multi-tissue interaction and analysis. Nat Commun. doi:10.1038/ncomms5250

26. Gawad S, Schild L, Renaud P (2001) Micromachined impedance spectroscopy flow cytometer for cell analysis and particle sizing. Lab Chip 1:76–82. doi:10.1039/b103933b

27. Gel M, Kimura Y, Kurosawa O et al (2010) Dielectrophoretic cell trapping and parallel one-to-one fusion based on field constriction created by a micro-orifice array. Biomicrofluidics. doi:10.1063/1.3422544

28. Gey GO (1954) Some aspects of the constitution and behavior of normal and malignant cells maintained in continuous culture. Harvey Lect 50:154–229

29. Gómez-Sjöberg R, Leyrat AA, Pirone DM et al (2007) Versatile, fully automated, microfluidic cell culture system. Anal Chem 79:8557–8563. doi:10.1021/ac071311w

30. Grier DG (2003) A revolution in optical manipulation. Nature 424:810–816. doi:10.1038/nature01935

31. Guo P, Hall EW, Schirhagl R et al (2012) Microfluidic capture and release of bacteria in a conical nanopore array. Lab Chip 12:558–561. doi:10.1039/c2lc21092d

32. Gu W, Zhu X, Futai N et al (2004) Computerized microfluidic cell culture using elastomeric channels and Braille displays. Proc Natl Acad Sci U S A 101:15861–15866. doi:10.1073/pnas.0404353101

33. Han C, Zhang Q, Ma R et al (2010) Integration of single oocyte trapping, in vitrofertilization and embryo culture in a microwell-structured microfluidic device. Lab Chip 10:2848–2854. doi:10.1039/C005296E

34. Han KN, Li CA, Seong GH (2013) Microfluidic chips for immunoassays. Annu Rev Anal Chem 6:119–141. doi:10.1146/annurev-anchem-062012-092616

35. Han Z, Li W, Huang Y, Zheng B (2009) Measuring rapid enzymatic kinetics by electrochemical method in droplet-based microfluidic devices with pneumatic valves. Anal Chem 81:5840–5845. doi:10.1021/ac900811y

36. Harrison RG, Greenman MJ, Mall FP, Jackson CM (1907) Observations of the living developing nerve fiber. Anat Rec 1:116–128. doi:10.1002/ar.1090010503

37. Herricks T, Antia M, Rathod PK (2009) Deformability limits of Plasmodium falciparum-infected red blood cells. Cell Microbiol 11:1340–1353. doi:10.1111/j.1462-5822.2009.01334.x
38. Hosokawa M, Hayata T, Fukuda Y et al (2010) Size-selective microcavity array for rapid and efficient detection of circulating tumor cells. Anal Chem 82:6629–6635. doi:10.1021/ac101222x
39. Jang K-J, Suh K-Y (2010) A multi-layer microfluidic device for efficient culture and analysis of renal tubular cells. Lab Chip 10:36–42. doi:10.1039/b907515a
40. Kaneshiro ES, Wyder MA, Wu Y-P, Cushion MT (1993) Reliability of calcein acetoxy methyl ester and ethidium homodimer or propidium iodide for viability assessment of microbes. J Microbiol Methods 17:1–16. doi:10.1016/S0167-7012(93)80010-4
41. Koh W-G, Pishko MV (2006) Fabrication of cell-containing hydrogel microstructures inside microfluidic devices that can be used as cell-based biosensors. Anal Bioanal Chem 385:1389–1397. doi:10.1007/s00216-006-0571-6
42. Kovac JR, Voldman J (2007) Intuitive, image-based cell sorting using optofluidic cell sorting. Anal Chem 79:9321–9330. doi:10.1021/ac071366y
43. Latt SA, Stetten G, Juergens LA et al (1975) Recent developments in the detection of deoxyribonucleic acid synthesis by 33258 Hoechst fluorescence. J Histochem Cytochem 23:493–505. doi:10.1177/23.7.1095650
44. Lee C-Y, Chang C-L, Wang Y-N, Fu L-M (2011) Microfluidic mixing: a review. Int J Mol Sci 12:3263–3287. doi:10.3390/ijms12053263
45. Liao C-L, Lai K-C, Huang A-C et al (2012) Gallic acid inhibits migration and invasion in human osteosarcoma U-2 OS cells through suppressing the matrix metalloproteinase-2/–9, protein kinase B (PKB) and PKC signaling pathways. Food Chem Toxicol 50:1734–1740. doi:10.1016/j.fct.2012.02.033
46. Liu X, Lin T-Y, Lillehoj PB (2014) Smartphones for cell and biomolecular detection. Ann Biomed Eng 42:2205–2217. doi:10.1007/s10439-014-1055-z
47. Manz A, Graber N, Widmer HM (1990) Miniaturized total chemical analysis systems: a novel concept for chemical sensing. Sens Actuators B Chem 1:244–248. doi:10.1016/0925-4005(90)80209-I
48. Manz A, Harrison DJ, Verpoorte EMJ et al (1992) Planar chips technology for miniaturization and integration of separation techniques into monitoring systems. J Chromatogr A 593:253–258. doi:10.1016/0021-9673(92)80293-4
49. Martinez AW, Phillips ST, Butte MJ, Whitesides GM (2007) Patterned paper as a platform for inexpensive, low-volume, portable bioassays. Angew Chem Int Ed 46:1318–1320. doi:10.1002/anie.200603817
50. Martinez AW, Phillips ST, Whitesides GM (2008) Three-dimensional microfluidic devices fabricated in layered paper and tape. Proc Natl Acad Sci U S A 105:19606–19611. doi:10.1073/pnas.0810903105
51. Mohan R, Schudel BR, Desai AV et al (2011) Design considerations for elastomeric normally closed microfluidic valves. Sens Actuators B Chem 160:1216–1223. doi:10.1016/j.snb.2011.09.051
52. Munce NR, Li J, Herman PR, Lilge L (2004) Microfabricated system for parallel single-cell capillary electrophoresis. Anal Chem 76:4983–4989. doi:10.1021/ac0496906
53. Murphy SV, Atala A (2014) 3D bioprinting of tissues and organs. Nat Biotechnol 32:773–785. doi:10.1038/nbt.2958
54. Nève N, Kohles SS, Winn SR, Tretheway DC (2010) Manipulation of suspended single cells by microfluidics and optical tweezers. Cell Mol Bioeng 3:213–228. doi:10.1007/s12195-010-0113-3
55. Nguyen TA, Yin T-I, Reyes D, Urban GA (2013) Microfluidic chip with integrated electrical cell-impedance sensing for monitoring single cancer cell migration in three-dimensional matrixes. Anal Chem 85:11068–11076. doi:10.1021/ac402761s
56. O'Neill AT, Monteiro-Riviere NA, Walker GM (2009) Microfabricated curtains for controlled cell seeding in high throughput microfluidic systems. Lab Chip 9:1756–1762. doi:10.1039/b819622b

57. Ong S-M, Zhang C, Toh Y-C et al (2008) A gel-free 3D microfluidic cell culture system. Biomaterials 29:3237–3244. doi:10.1016/j.biomaterials.2008.04.022
58. Ottesen EA, Hong JW, Quake SR, Leadbetter JR (2006) Microfluidic digital PCR enables multigene analysis of individual environmental bacteria. Science 314:1464–1467. doi:10.1126/science.1131370
59. Probst C, Grünberger A, Wiechert W, Kohlheyer D (2013) Microfluidic growth chambers with optical tweezers for full spatial single-cell control and analysis of evolving microbes. J Microbiol Methods 95:470–476. doi:10.1016/j.mimet.2013.09.002
60. Ramji R, Wang M, Bhagat AAS et al (2014) Single cell kinase signaling assay using pinched flow coupled droplet microfluidics. Biomicrofluidics 8:034104. doi:10.1063/1.4878635
61. Ravi M, Paramesh V, Kaviya SR et al (2015) 3D cell culture systems: advantages and applications. J Cell Physiol 230:16–26. doi:10.1002/jcp.24683
62. Rettig JR, Folch A (2005) Large-scale single-cell trapping and imaging using microwell arrays. Anal Chem 77:5628–5634. doi:10.1021/ac0505977
63. Rho HS, Yang Y, Hanke AT et al (2016) Programmable v-type valve for cell and particle manipulation in microfluidic devices. Lab Chip 16:305–311. doi:10.1039/C5LC01206F
64. Roelse M, de Ruijter NCA, Vrouwe EX, Jongsma MA (2013) A generic microfluidic biosensor of G protein-coupled receptor activation-monitoring cytoplasmic Ca^{2+} changes in human HEK293 cells. Biosens Bioelectron 47:436–444. doi:10.1016/j.bios.2013.03.065
65. Roman GT, Chen Y, Viberg P et al (2006) Single-cell manipulation and analysis using microfluidic devices. Anal Bioanal Chem 387:9–12. doi:10.1007/s00216-006-0670-4
66. Ryley J, Pereira-Smith OM (2006) Microfluidics device for single cell gene expression analysis in Saccharomyces cerevisiae. Yeast 23:1065–1073. doi:10.1002/yea.1412
67. Seol Y-J, Kang H-W, Lee SJ et al (2014) Bioprinting technology and its applications. Eur J Cardio-Thorac Surg Off J Eur Assoc Cardio-Thorac Surg 46:342–348. doi:10.1093/ejcts/ezu148
68. Shim J-H, Lee J-S, Kim JY, Cho D-W (2012) Bioprinting of a mechanically enhanced three-dimensional dual cell-laden construct for osteochondral tissue engineering using a multi-head tissue/organ building system. J Micromech Microeng 22:085014. doi:10.1088/0960-1317/22/8/085014
69. Simon KA, Mosadegh B, Minn KT et al (2016) Metabolic response of lung cancer cells to radiation in a paper-based 3D cell culture system. Biomaterials 95:47–59. doi:10.1016/j.biomaterials.2016.03.002
70. Skardal A, Devarasetty M, Forsythe S et al (2016) A reductionist metastasis-on-a-chip platform for in vitro tumor progression modeling and drug screening. Biotechnol Bioeng. doi:10.1002/bit.25950
71. Skardal A, Devarasetty M, Rodman C et al (2015a) Liver-tumor hybrid organoids for modeling tumor growth and drug response in vitro. Ann Biomed Eng 43:2361–2373. doi:10.1007/s10439-015-1298-3
72. Skardal A, Devarasetty M, Soker S, Hall AR (2015b) In situ patterned micro 3D liver constructs for parallel toxicology testing in a fluidic device. Biofabrication 7:031001. doi:10.1088/1758-5090/7/3/031001
73. Song JW, Cavnar SP, Walker AC et al (2009) Microfluidic endothelium for studying the intravascular adhesion of metastatic breast cancer cells. PLoS One. doi:10.1371/journal.pone.0005756
74. Stjernstrom M, Roeraade J (1998) Method for fabrication of microfluidic systems in glass. J Micromech Microeng 8:33–38. doi:10.1088/0960-1317/8/1/006
75. Tabriz AG, Hermida MA, Leslie NR, Shu W (2015) Three-dimensional bioprinting of complex cell laden alginate hydrogel structures. Biofabrication 7:045012. doi:10.1088/1758-5090/7/4/045012
76. Tan W-H, Takeuchi S (2007) A trap-and-release integrated microfluidic system for dynamic microarray applications. Proc Natl Acad Sci U S A 104:1146–1151. doi:10.1073/pnas.0606625104
77. Toley BJ, Wang JA, Gupta M et al (2015) A versatile valving toolkit for automating fluidic operations in paper microfluidic devices. Lab Chip 15:1432–1444. doi:10.1039/C4LC01155D

78. Tung Y-C, Hsiao AY, Allen SG et al (2011) High-throughput 3D spheroid culture and drug testing using a 384 hanging drop array. Analyst 136:473–478. doi:10.1039/C0AN00609B
79. Unger MA, Chou HP, Thorsen T et al (2000) Monolithic microfabricated valves and pumps by multilayer soft lithography. Science 288:113–116. doi:10.1126/science.288.5463.113
80. Wang Z, Kim M-C, Marquez M, Thorsen T (2007) High-density microfluidic arrays for cell cytotoxicity analysis. Lab Chip 7:740–745. doi:10.1039/b618734j
81. Werner M, Merenda F, Piguet J et al (2011) Microfluidic array cytometer based on refractive optical tweezers for parallel trapping, imaging and sorting of individual cells. Lab Chip 11:2432–2439. doi:10.1039/c1lc20181f
82. Wheeler AR, Throndset WR, Whelan RJ et al (2003) Microfluidic device for single-cell analysis. Anal Chem 75:3581–3586
83. Wu L, Chen P, Dong Y et al (2013) Encapsulation of single cells on a microfluidic device integrating droplet generation with fluorescence-activated droplet sorting. Biomed Microdevices 15:553–560. doi:10.1007/s10544-013-9754-z
84. Xu J, Wu L, Huang M et al (2001) Dielectrophoretic separation and transportation of cells and bioparticles on microfabriacted chips. In: Ramsey JM, van den Berg A (eds) Micro total analysis systems. Springer, Netherlands, pp 565–566
85. Zhang C, Jang S, Amadi OC, et al (2013) A sensitive chemotaxis assay using a novel microfluidic device. BioMed Res Int. doi: http://dx.doi.org/10.1155/2013/373569
86. Zhang C, Xu J, Ma W, Zheng W (2006) PCR microfluidic devices for DNA amplification. Biotechnol Adv 24:243–284. doi:10.1016/j.biotechadv.2005.10.002

Stiffness-Tuned Matrices for Tumor Cell Studies

Amanda M. Smelser, Manuel M. Gomez, Scott Smyre,
Melissa L. Fender Pashayan, and Jed C. Macosko

Abstract The stiffness of a cell's microenvironment influences its behavior. Testing the effect of stiffness, or elasticity, on tumor cell behavior requires a matrix that provides the integrin binding sites that are found in stroma. Collagen I is a major component of stroma and allows integrin binding, but when it is reconstituted after extraction and solubilization, it is difficult to work with and too soft to model tumor tissue. Although the stiffness of collagen I matrices can be adjusted by changing collagen concentration, doing so also affects the number of integrin binding sites available to cells, confounding experimental variables. The goal of this work was to tune collagen I matrices over a range of elasticities (1–6 kPa) relevant for modeling normal and tumorous breast tissue, without altering the density of cell-matrix ligands. This was accomplished by functionalizing collagen I with glycidyl methacrylate (GMA), and using lithium acylphosphinate (LAP) as a photoinitiator of GMA cross-linking. Cross-links were photoactivated by irradiating the GMA-functionalized collagen at 365 nm for 2 min or less (4.4 mW/cm^2). Breast cancer cells (MDA-MB-231) survived and migrated on these matrices. Collagen I-GMA gels can be used to ascertain how varying extracellular matrix elasticity affects breast cancer cell behavior.

Keywords Collagen • 3D matrix • Cross-linking • Methacrylate • Photoactivation • Migration • Tumor model • Stiffness • Elastic modulus

This chapter was adapted from a dissertation:
Smelser, AM (2016) Breast Cancer Cell Mechanical Properties and Migration on Collagen I Matrices with Tunable Elasticity. Dissertation, Wake Forest University

A.M. Smelser (✉)
Department of Cancer Biology, Wake Forest Baptist Medical Center, Medical Center Boulevard, Winston-Salem, NC 27157, USA
e-mail: asmelser@wakehealth.edu

M.M. Gomez • S. Smyre • M.L. Fender Pashayan • J.C. Macosko
Department of Physics, Wake Forest University, 100 Olin Physical Laboratory, Wake Forest University, Winston-Salem, NC 27109-7507, USA
e-mail: gomemm14@wfu.edu; smyresa@wfu.edu; pashml15@wfu.edu; macoskjc@wfu.edu

© Springer International Publishing AG 2018
S. Soker, A. Skardal (eds.), *Tumor Organoids*, Cancer Drug Discovery and Development, DOI 10.1007/978-3-319-60511-1_9

171

1   Matrix Stiffness Regulates Cell Behavior

The stiffness of cell matrices is an important consideration in tumor cell studies because human tissues exhibit a wide range of characteristic stiffnesses, or elasticities, according to type; neurons experience an elastic modulus less than 100 Pa, but osteoblasts experience an elastic modulus of 20,000 Pa [1]. Similarly, normal and diseased states of the same tissue type confer a significant difference in stiffness, for example in breast tumors. While the elastic modulus of normal breast tissue ranges in the low hundreds of Pascals, average breast tumor stiffness is ~4000 Pa [2].

A cancer cell leaving a tumor is thus descending a stiffness gradient. A few reasons for this higher stiffness in tumors have been suggested. Breast tumor development is accompanied by increased extracellular matrix (ECM) deposition, and particularly, an increase in collagen V content from less than 0.1% to 10% of stromal collagens [3, 4]. Proliferation of mutated cells in acinus lumens and an increase in interstitial fluid from leaky vasculature in tumors also increase pressure [1].

Furthermore, cells respond to variations in ECM stiffness. When mammary epithelial cells (MECs) were cultured on polyacrylamide of varying stiffnesses crosslinked with ECM, they retained a polarized, acinar structure on stiffnesses comparable to normal breast tissue, but this structure was lost at higher stiffnesses comparable to breast tumor tissue (Fig. 1) [2]. Vidi et al. demonstrated that polarized tissue architecture regulates the maintenance of genome integrity in MECs, suggesting that the properties of a cell's microenvironment affect processes in the nucleus and the genome [5].

A remarkable demonstration of the degree to which ECM stiffness can regulate gene expression was the observation that mesenchymal stem cells differentiated into entirely different cell types, neurons vs. osteoblasts, when cultured on soft and stiff substrates, respectively [6]. The substrate used in this experiment was polyacrylamide coated with collagen I; the stiffness was adjusted by altering the concentrations of acrylamide and bis-acrylamide cross-linker. In this way biochemical signals (e.g. ligand density, growth factors) were kept constant while the stiffness was varied, demonstrating that the mechanical property was responsible for the change.

ECM stiffness is conveyed into the cell as a force across integrins into focal adhesions, which can convert force into a biochemical signal and cellular response. Integrins themselves respond to force by clustering and conformational changes. Other mechanotransducers in focal adhesions, such as α-actinin, vinculin, talin, and p130Cas respond to forces to, for example, allow binding of signaling molecules, like MAPK1 [7, 8]. The folded up p130Cas substrate domain demonstrates a striking example of one way a mechanical force can be converted to a biochemical signal; cell stretching unfolds it, exposing phosphorylation sites for Src family kinases and leading to activation of other signaling molecules [9]. Forces transduced via integrins can also signal a contractile response in the actomyosin cytoskeletal network via ERK and ROCK activation [2].

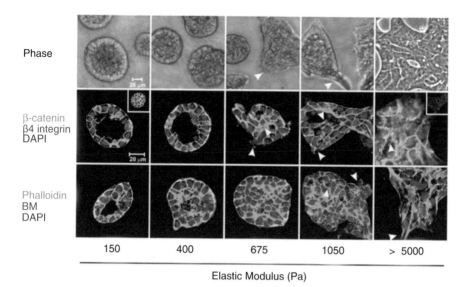

Phase

β-catenin
β4 integrin
DAPI

Phalloidin
BM
DAPI

| 150 | 400 | 675 | 1050 | > 5000 |

Elastic Modulus (Pa)

Fig. 1 Matrix stiffness modulates integrin adhesions to regulate MEC growth and behavior [2]

It has been suggested that cells have "tensional homeostasis", or respond to the stiffness of their surroundings by altering their internal mechanics in response to the mechanics of their microenvironment [2]. One effort to provide evidence for this hypothesis used a model system of MEC cell lines transformed by overexpression of ErbB2, a breast cancer biomarker, and/or 14-3-3ζ, which confers resistance to apoptosis upon extracellular ligand detachment. These were seeded on collagen I gels of increasing concentration, and thus stiffness. The effective G', or stiffness, within cells was measured by passive particle tracking microrheology. The G' of cells overexpressing ErbB2 appeared to increase when cultured on collagen I gels of increased stiffness [10]. However, because ligand density, and not just stiffness, increases with increasing collagen I concentration, the effect could have been the result of either property.

2 Ideal Properties of a Stiffness Model

Many cell culture models have been developed with variable stiffness for determining cell responses. Some of these are synthetic (polyacrylamide, PEG-diacrylate), and some are based on extracellular matrix proteins. Ideally, a 3D cell culture model for assessing cell responses to microenvironment stiffness should allow for (1) cell integrin binding, (2) cell migration in 3D, and (3) tunable stiffness (independent of ligand density). Cell culture matrices ought to represent an optimal balance between physiological relevance and simplicity. The natural cell microenvironment is too complex to recreate exactly at this point and have full control of relevant

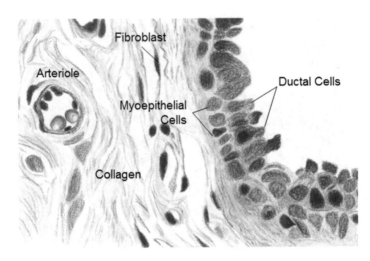

Fig. 2 Normal histology of breast tissue. Stromal collagen is *pink*. Sketch is based on microscopy from [11]

biochemical and physical variables. Figure 2 shows the normal histology of breast tissue. Epithelial cells form a mammary duct, or acinus, which is lined by myoepithelial cells and the basal lamina [11]. The basal lamina is composed primarily of laminin and collagen IV [12]. A number of proteins make up the breast stromal tissue, including collagens I, III, and V, proteoglycans, glycoproteins, and fibronectin [3, 12, 13]. Metastastic cells from an acinus en route to nearby arterioles, for example, would traverse this matrix.

Collagen I, one of the fibrillar collagens (fibrillar collagens include I, II, III, V, XI, XXIV, and XXVII), is the most abundant protein in interstitial and stromal tissues. As such, it is a physiologically relevant choice of matrix for studying invasive behaviors of breast cancer cells.

3   Collagen I Structure and Mechanics

Collagen I fibrils form porous matrices in vivo that mechanically support tissue structure. The basic unit of a collagen I fibril is a right-handed triple helix composed of three left-handed polypeptide helices, two $\alpha 1$ and one $\alpha 2$, held together by hydrogen bonds between prolines and glycines. These triple helices, called tropocollagens, are secreted by cells and then self-assemble into staggered bundles with 4–5 tropocollagens per cross-section, to form microfibrils. Microfibrils are cross-linked with each other via the oxidation of lysines by lysyl oxidase to form fibrils which are hundreds of nanometers in diameter [14].

To use collagen matrices for cell culture, the cross-links in native collagen are broken down by acid extraction to produce monomeric, soluble collagen [15]. Upon neutralization of this solution at 37 °C, fibrils reform in vitro. Temperature, pH, ionic strength of the solution, and collagen concentration all affect the kinetics of fibril formation as well as the fibril diameters [16–18]. Confocal reflectance microscopy images of 2 mg/ml collagen gels formed at 32, 27, and 22 °C show pore size increases from 7 to 12 μm, and fibril diameter increases from 51 to 65 nm with decreasing temperature [17]. Pore sizes of collagen matrices at 1.2 mg/ml and 2.4 mg/ml concentrations were approximately 3 μm and 2 μm, respectively, when measured from reconstructed CRM images [19]. Based on this data, the predicted pore size for the 8.8 mg/ml collagen gels in this work would be less than 1 μm.

The compressive elastic modulus of individual collagen I fibrils ranges from 2 to 200 MPa, depending on pH and ionic strength of the buffer in which they are measured [20, 21]. These numbers are 3–4 orders of magnitude larger than the compressive elastic moduli of collagen gels determined by indentation. These moduli range from 300–3000 Pa, depending on collagen concentration (3–9 mg/ml) [22].

4 Stiffening Collagen I Matrices

Although collagen I matrices are frequently used in cell culture, in vitro they have a limited range of stiffness and unstable mechanical properties, which lead to inconsistent reproducibility. Compression of collagen I has been used to increase its elasticity and mechanical stability, but this also results in increased cell-collagen ligand density [23]. Collagen I matrices have also been stiffened by mixing with agarose, but agarose fills the pores between collagen fibrils and thus slows cell invasion [24]. A number of chemical and enzymatic methods for cross-linking collagen I have been used, including EDC/NHS, methacrylate, glutaraldehyde, genipin, riboflavin, and transglutaminase [25–30]. Synthetic matrices like polyacrylamide and PEG hydrogels have more easily tunable elasticity, and can be cross-linked with ECM proteins for integrin binding. Polyacrylamide gels can be tuned to E values, or stiffnesses, ranging from the low hundreds to hundreds of thousands of Pascals simply by changing the concentrations of acrylamide and bis-acrylamide, making them particularly suitable for mimicking tissue stiffnesses [31]. One well-established protocol for 3D culture is to seed cells on polyacrylamide coated with ECM proteins, then overlay with a layer of collagen I [32, 33]. A disadvantage of this system is that it is mechanically non-homogeneous above and below cells, and ligand density-independent tuning of the stiffness of the matrix is only possible in the layer below the cells.

For 3D culture matrices, cross-linkers also should be cytocompatible before and during matrix cross-linking, since the cells are usually embedded in the matrix prior to the cross-linking process. Glutaraldehyde, for example, is cytotoxic and thus not ideal for cross-linking collagen matrices after embedding cells. Genipin, naturally found in gardenia fruit extract, is less cytotoxic but must be used at low concentrations (<5 mM) if cells are embedded in the gel during cross-linking. Genipin cross-linked collagen also turns a dark purple color, and fluoresces when excited with 590 nm light with intensities dependent on the degree of cross-linking [27].

Some of the above cross-linking methods, riboflavin and methacrylate, are photoactivatable with UV light. One advantage of photoactivation is the capability for post hoc stiffness tuning, as well as the possibility for precise patterning of varying stiffnesses within gels. Photomasks could potentially be designed to create stiffness gradients for studying durotaxis, for example. One potential disadvantage includes cytotoxicity of the photoinitiators, which form free radicals upon photoactivation. Riboflavin generates superoxide radicals in the presence of 465 nm light, and the photoactivated riboflavin and superoxide radicals both enable cross-linking of collagen [34]. Tronci et al. functionalized collagen I with the organic cross-linkers glycidyl methacrylate (GMA) and 4-vinylbenzyl chloride (4VBC) [35]. A nucleophilic reaction functionalized the methacrylate or vinylbenzyl groups to the ε-amino groups of collagen lysines. Functional groups on lysines of neighboring collagen molecules are linked together when they interact with free radicals produced by photoactivation of Irgacure 2959® (I2959) with UV light. Any free radical-forming initiator can be used in this system to form cross-links between the functional groups.

5   Measuring Stiffness with Atomic Force Microscopy (AFM)

Although there are a number of methods for determining mechanical properties of collagen, atomic force microscopy is one that can be used to determine the compressive elastic modulus of a material at the approximate scale that a cell would be exerting force. The primary components of an atomic force microscope (AFM) include a cantilever with a probe (which can vary in shape and size), a laser which reflects off the top of the cantilever at an angle determined by the extent of cantilever deflection, and a photodiode which registers a voltage based on the extent of deflection of the laser (Fig. 3). The voltage is converted back to units of deflection using the calibrated sensor response in nm/V for each cantilever.

The deflection vs. indentation curve can then be converted to a force vs. indentation curve using the cantilever spring constant, and this curve is fitted using the Hertz model,

$$F = \frac{3}{4}\frac{E}{\left(1-v^2\right)}R^{1/2}d^{3/2} \tag{1}$$

where F is force, E is the Young's modulus (elastic modulus), v is the Poisson's ratio of the material, R is the radius of the spherical probe on the cantilever, and d is the indentation depth of the sphere in the material [36]. The Hertz model assumes that the medium is elastic and fills an infinitely large half-space, the contact surfaces are "even", and the surfaces are frictionless [37].

Neither collagen I nor polyacrylamide is a purely elastic material, but the Hertz model still fits their force vs. indentation curves well [38, 39]. Furthermore, because

Fig. 3 Schematic of contact atomic force microscopy (AFM) for determination of the elastic modulus of a sample

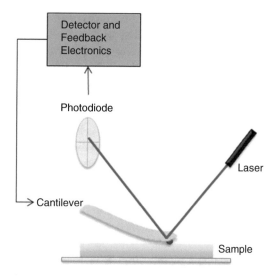

the contribution of the viscous component depends on the relaxation time of the gel, if the indentation curves are acquired at the same indentation speed for all measurements, comparison of these elastic moduli is still valid. Adhesion is also an issue when indenting collagen I, particularly, but probes can be coated to reduce this effect.

6 Method for Tuning Collagen I Stiffness

6.1 Functionalization of Collagen I

To functionalize rat tail collagen I (Corning Life Sciences, Inc) with 4-vinylbenzyl chloride or glycidyl methacrylate, high concentration collagen I in 0.02 M acetic acid was diluted to 0.25 wt% in deionized water, stirred on ice, and neutralized with 1 M NaOH. Based on a trinitrobenzene sulfonic acid (TNBS) assay it was previously determined there were 6×10^{-4} mol lysines per gram of collagen I. This is a reasonable result given a tenuous theoretical value of 4×10^{-4} mol lysines per gram (~91 lysines in triple helix of MW ~250 kDa), calculated from the amino acid composition of the alpha-1 and alpha-2 chains of collagen I from *Rattus norvegicus*, for which 11% of amino acids are unspecified [40]. Either 4-vinylbenzyl chloride or glycidyl methacrylate was added at a 75 molar ratio relative to the collagen lysines. Triethylamine was added as a catalyst for the substitution reaction at an amount equimolar with the cross-linker, and 1% Tween-20 was added to solubilize the cross-linker in solution. The reaction mixture was stirred at RT overnight. The functionalized collagen was precipitated out of solution by stirring in at least 10 volumes of 200 proof ethanol overnight, then centrifuging at 5000 rpm for 30 min in a Sorvall

RC-5B Superspeed Refrigerated Centrifuge. The ethanol was decanted, and pellets were re-dissolved in 0.02 M acetic acid. Re-dissolved functionalized collagen I was dialyzed in at least 10 volumes of 0.02 M acetic acid overnight to dilute out any remaining ethanol, then lyophilized. Lyophilized collagen I-GMA or -4VBC was re-dissolved in 0.02 M acetic acid at 8–13 mg/ml as needed for use.

To determine the concentration of re-dissolved, functionalized collagen I, the Bicinchoninic Acid (BCA) Protein Assay (Pierce) was used because it yielded more consistent absorbance readings between repeats and more linear standard curves than the Bradford Protein Assay (Bio-Rad). Absorbances of the functionalized collagen I solutions at 280 nm were not used for concentration determination because one of the cross-linkers, 4VBC, contains a benzene ring, which would absorb at this wavelength.

The concentration of stock collagen I used for producing standard curve dilutions had been determined by pyrochemiluminescence by Corning® and was reported on the product label. The Pierce protocol for the BCA assay was followed with the major modification being the addition of 0.0035% sodium dodecyl sulfate (SDS) to the BCA reagent. SDS was added based on work by López et al. which showed that the addition of 0.0035% SDS increased the sensitivity of the Bradford assay to collagen relative to non-collagen proteins, possibly by altering conformational structure of collagen molecules to increase their binding capacity [41].

The trinitrobenzene sulfonic acid (TNBS) colorimetric assay for determination of free ε-amino groups was used to determine the percentage of collagen lysines that were functionalized with cross-linker [35, 42]. The percent functionalization was determined from the moles of free lysine per gram collagen for functionalized and non-functionalized collagen samples as follows:

$$\%F = 1 - \frac{mol(Lys)_{Funct.\ Collagen}}{mol(Lys)_{Collagen}} \qquad (2)$$

In initial experiments, functionalization of collagen with GMA was achieved by addition of GMA at a molar ratio of 50 relative to collagen lysines. The percent lysine functionalization for these batches varied between 20–60%. The final batch, however, was made using a GMA/lysine molar ratio of 75, and percent functionalization increased to 80%. The percent functionalization achieved with 4VBC was generally lower, ranging between 4 and 30%, even when the molar ratio of 4VBC relative to collagen lysines was increased from 50 to 75.

6.2 Photoinitiator Synthesis

Initially, Irgacure® 2959, or 2-hydroxy-1-[4-(2-hydroxyethoxy) phenyl]-2-methyl-1-propanone, was used as a photoinitiator for cross-linking of functionalized collagen, since it is commonly used for biological applications [35]. The molar absorptivity of I2959 at 365 nm was not sufficient to induce cross-linking by irra-diation with 8 W bulbs in a UVP transilluminator for up to 1 h. Even at 302 nm, for which its molar absorptivity is higher, sufficient cross-linking required at least 30 minutes of irradiation. Collagen I-GMA solutions of approximately 5 mg/ml (determined by Bradford, rather than BCA Assay) were mixed with 1.0% I2959 by irradiating 30, 60, and 90 min at 302 nm, and the elastic moduli of resulting gels were determined by AFM. The elastic moduli averaged 480 ± 93 Pa, 908 ± 200 Pa, and 1024 ± 203 Pa, respectively.

These times required for adequate cross-linking (30–90 min) were too long for 3D culture applications with cells embedded in gels, because cell exposure to UV light should be minimal. Additionally, the shorter wavelength required for cross-linking, 302 nm, is more likely to induce DNA damage than 365 nm UV. In a cyto-toxicity experiment, 30 min of irradiation at 302 nm resulted in less than 50% survival of breast cancer (MDA-MB-231) cells (no collagen, no photoinitiator), when inspected using Trypan Blue exclusion dye three days later.

For these reasons, an alternative photoinitiator was tested. Fairbanks et al. showed that lithium acylphospinate (LAP) had a higher efficiency as a photoinitia-tor than I2959 when PEG-diacrylate was irradiated with 365 nm UV light (2009). The use of this longer wavelength UV light for irradiation is advantageous because it reduces the potential for DNA damage in cells that may be embedded in the col-lagen gels during cross-linking. LAP was synthesized according to the literature [43, 44]. The crystallized, washed lithium acylphosphinate was dissolved in deion-ized water at 4 mM to acquire an absorption spectrum and determine if it showed peak absorption near 365 nm as expected. Figure 4a shows the confirming absorp-tion spectrum. In a direct comparison between 2.2 mM (0.07%) LAP, 2.2 mM (0.05%) I2959, and water as a control, the collagen I-GMA gel (3.8 mg/ml) with LAP remained flat and intact when tipped after 10 min of irradiation (365 nm), but the I2959 and control gels did not. LAP was a more efficient photoinitiator for cross-linking collagen I with 365 nm irradiation, and was used in subsequent experiments.

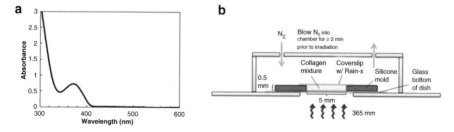

Fig. 4 (**a**) Absorbance spectrum of 4 mM lithium acylphosphinate from 300 to 600 nm, confirm-ing a peak in absorbance near 365 nm. Cuvette path length is 1 cm (**b**) Setup for cross-linking of functionalized collagen gels

6.3   Photoactivation of Cross-Links in Collagen

Photo-crosslinkable collagen gels were made by mixing functionalized collagen with NaOH and 10X Dulbecco's Phosphate Buffered Saline (DPBS) for neutralization, phenol red for confirmation of neutralization, and LAP for photoactivation. Collagen I-4VBC differed from collagen I-GMA in that it gelled rapidly upon neutralization, interfering with thorough mixing, so it was mixed only with LAP and was cross-linked at acidic pH. A positive displacement pipet (Gilson) was used for pipetting high concentration functionalized collagen, to prevent loss of sample due to adhesion within the tip. After mixing by pipetting ~20X, the mixture was briefly centrifuged to remove air bubbles. This mixture (20 μL) was added to a 5 × 5 well cut out of 0.5 mm thick cell culture grade silicone sheet (Electron Microscopy Sciences) in a glass-bottom culture dish coated with 3-aminopropyltriethoxysilane and glutaraldehyde for protein adhesion. Coverslips coated with Rain-X were placed on top to flatten the gel surface.

Once the mixture was formed in the dish, it was placed in an N_2 environment for at least 2 min to prevent formation of reactive oxygen species (ROS) that could interfere with the cross-linking reaction (Fig. 4b). It was then irradiated by a Blak-Ray® B-100A High Intensity UV lamp (100 W, 365 nm) for 60–120 s. The intensity of irradiation was 4.4 mW/cm². Gels were stored in DPBS or cell culture medium.

6.4   Calibrating the AFM for Stiffness Measurements

To ascertain the precision and accuracy of elastic measurements made with a new AFM, polyacrylamide gels, which are well-characterized in the literature in the appropriate range of stiffness, were used as a standard. Polyacrylamide gels were made to target an elastic modulus of 6000 Pa, which is near the high end of the range of elastic moduli relevant to this study [1]. The weight percents of acrylamide and bis-acrylamide were chosen based on work by Yeung et al. showing how the elastic shear modulus, G', varies with these amounts [31]. We assumed G' is related to the Young's modulus, E, by a ratio of 1/3, because the Poisson's ratio (v) of poly-acrylamide gels is ~0.5 [45, 46], and because,

$$E = 2G(1+v) \qquad (3)$$

To make the polyacrylamide gels, 7.5% acrylamide was mixed with 0.08% bis-acrylamide, 0.1% ammonium persulfate, and 0.003% N,N,N′,N′-tetramethylethylenediamine. Thick gels were made by pipetting mixtures into cylindrical molds with radii of 6 mm and heights of 5 mm on glass-bottom dishes coated with 3-aminopropyltriethoxysilane and glutaraldehyde for adhesion. Rain-X®-coated coverslips and 50 g weights were placed on top to ensure flat surfaces.

Thin gels were made by pipetting into 10 x 10 x 1 mm square silicone wells. Gels were stored in PBS and transported the same day for measurement on the AFM.

An MFP-3D-BIO AFM (Asylum Research) was used to acquire force vs. indentation curves. Silicon cantilevers were gold-coated and tipless (AppNano). A 6 µm carboxylate-coated polystyrene bead (PolyBead®) was glued to the end of the cantilever with marine epoxy (Loctite®). The beads were subsequently coated with poly-L-lysine-PEG (PLL-PEG, SuSos) or Rain-X to reduce adherence to the substrate. Cantilever spring constants were determined by the Sader method in air [47]. The Sader method uses the cantilever's resonance frequency, which is determined by recording the cantilever's thermal oscillations in air. From these thermal oscillations, the angular resonance frequency, ω_0, and quality factor, Q, were calculated by the software to determine the spring contant as follows:

$$k = 0.1906 \rho_f b^2 L Q \Gamma \left(\omega_0 \right) \omega_0^2 \tag{4}$$

where ρ_f is the density of the medium (air), b and L are the width and length of the cantilever, and $\Gamma(\omega_0)$ is the hydrodynamic function [47]. Using this method, the spring constant of the cantilever used for the calibration experiments was determined to be ~55 pN/nm. The cantilever sensitivity (nm/V) was determined by indenting a glass coverslip in water or buffer; from a linear fit of this deflection vs. indentation curve and from the spring constant, the sensitivity could be calculated by the software. For measurements of polyacrylamide, the force distance used was 1 µm, velocity was 1 µm/s, and the trigger voltage was 1 V. The resulting force vs. indentation curves were fit with the Hertz model (Eq. 1).

The same polyacrylamide gels were also measured by an ElectroForce indenter (Bose®) to confirm the AFM measurements. The indenter system determines the elastic modulus by compression, like the AFM, but at a larger scale and with a more direct readout. The gel is compressed at a user-determined rate of displacement between two flat platens (larger in diameter than the gel) as shown in Fig. 5a, and a load cell in line with one of the platens yields a force readout. Platens were coated with dodecane to reduce the adherence of gels to the platen for unconfined compression.

True stress, σ, and true strain, ε, were determined as follows,

$$\sigma = \frac{F\left(H_0 - \Delta H\right)}{\pi \left(\dfrac{d}{2}\right)^2 H_0} \tag{5}$$

$$\varepsilon = \ln\left(\frac{H_0 - \Delta H}{H_0}\right) \tag{6}$$

where σ is true stress, ε is true strain, F is the force exerted on the gel, H_0 is the initial height of the gel, ΔH is the resulting change in height after a given time

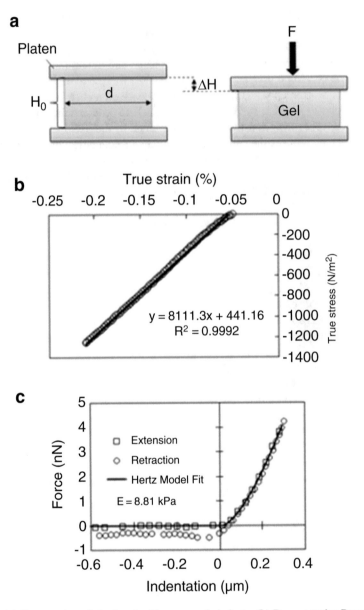

Fig. 5 (**a**) Compression of elastic gel with macroscale indenter (**b**) Representative Bose® macroscale indenter true stress vs. true strain curve (*circles*) with linear regression fit (*line*) for a polyacrylamide (0.75% acrylamide, 0.08% bis-acrylamide) gel. Slope of linear regression is the elastic modulus (**c**) Representative AFM force vs. indentation curves for the same polyacrylamide gel shown in **b**, showing extension curve (*squares*), retraction curve (*circles*), and Hertz model fit (*line*). The retraction curve dips below the extension curve, indicating some adhesion between probe and substrate

interval, and d is the initial diameter of the gel [48]. True stress and true strain differ from engineering stress and strain by accounting for the increasing diameter of the material as it is compressed. The elastic modulus, E, was determined as the slope of the linear fit of true stress plotted against true strain, according to the relation,

$$\sigma = E\varepsilon \tag{7}$$

On separate days, three polyacrylamide gels were made up with the same composition targeting 6 kPa, and on the same day each was made it was measured twice at each of three random locations by AFM. The average elastic modulus for the three gels was 9.11 ± 0.87 kPa, 9.39 ± 0.55 kPa, and 8.84 ± 0.16 kPa, which shows good consistency despite differences in thickness (1 and 5 mm), as there was no significant difference between average elastic moduli of these gels by the ANOVA test, $p = 0.31$. These elastic moduli are higher than expected according to the literature, so one gel was made and measured on the AFM, then measured on the macroscale indenter on the same day. The average modulus for this gel as measured by the AFM was 8.99 ± 0.12 kPa, and by the indenter was 8.53 ± 0.37 kPa. Example data for the indenter and AFM are shown in Fig. 5b, c, respectively.

The agreement between measurements from the two different instruments supports the accuracy of both. The expected modulus from the literature, however, was much lower, which could be explained by differences in storage time prior to measurement. When a gel was made according to the same method but stored in PBS for 4 days prior to measurement, the average elastic modulus was 5.92 ± 0.58 kPa, in agreement with the literature, so it is possible that swelling by storage in buffer could be responsible for the difference. Polyacrylamide gel swelling over time by storage in water causes Poisson's Ratio to drop from 0.50 to 0.26, indicating that storage conditions affect their mechanical properties [46]. These results demonstrate the consistency of the measurements made using the atomic force microscope and the described cantilever calibration method. The good agreement with measurements made by the macroscale indenter supports their accuracy. The discrepancy with literature values could be explained by different degrees of swelling.

6.5   Collagen I-GMA Spanned the Range of Breast Cancer-Relevant Stiffnesses

The elastic moduli of 6.5 mg/ml collagen-GMA gels irradiated for durations from 5 to 120 s increased from ~300 Pa (5 s) to ~1000 Pa (90 s). When irradiated for 120 s, the modulus dropped back to 500 Pa. These results demonstrate that the elastic moduli of collagen I-GMA gels cross-linked using LAP increase with irradiation time, up to a maximum. The maximum elastic modulus here, ~1000 Pa, was achieved after 90 s, whereas the original protocol using I2959 required 90 min of irradiation. Collagen I-4VBC gels (6.5 mg/ml) had higher elastic moduli than collagen I-GMA for up to 30 s of irradiation, which was expected since 4VBC is a shorter cross-linker [49]. For both cross-linkers, elastic moduli of gels appeared to drop when irradiation times were prolonged beyond a certain time. This drop in modulus could be due to alteration of collagen structure by the accumulation of superoxide radicals [50]. Additionally, the peak time could be changed; gels made from a different batch of collagen I-GMA and at higher concentrations had higher moduli at longer irradiation times. This change in irradiation time for the peak modulus could be explained by the higher percent functionalization in the second batch.

Work with collagen I-4VBC was discontinued because elastic moduli of these gels cross-linked at neutral pH were inconsistent. These solutions gelled inconsistently because, unlike collagen I-GMA, they formed fibrils rapidly upon neutralization, which impeded proper mixing. For example, a gel mixed at acidic pH had an elastic modulus of 757 ± 54 Pa, but for another gel mixed at neutral pH, the elastic modulus had a much higher standard deviation, 682 ± 319 Pa. Another cause for inconsistency in these functionalized collagen gels may have been degradation of the functionalized collagen stock over time. For example, 5 mg/ml collagen I-4VBC gels made 3 months apart from the same stock had elastic moduli of 1307 ± 51 Pa versus 675 ± 372 Pa.

To stiffen collagen gels further to suitably represent tumorous breast tissue, collagen I-GMA gels were prepared at a higher concentration of collagen I-GMA (8.8 m/gml vs. 6.5 m/gml) and a lower concentration of LAP (1.1 mM vs. 2.2 mM). To represent normal breast tissue, non-functionalized collagen I gels were mixed according to the same recipe, except without LAP, then allowed to gel for 2–3 h in a 37 °C, 5% CO_2 incubator. All collagen gels were stored in DPBS overnight prior to measurement of elastic moduli.

Figure 6 shows the elastic moduli of 8.8 mg/ml collagen I-GMA gels irradiated for 60 and 120 s compared to the elastic modulus of 8.8 mg/ml non-functionalized collagen. The elastic modulus of 8.8 mg/ml collagen I-GMA gels is higher than non-functionalized collagen gelled by neutralization and 37 °C temperature. These high concentration cross-linked collagen I- GMA gels can be tuned to stiffnesses ranging from the stiffness of normal breast tissue to the stiffnesses of breast tumors by irradiating gels with 365 nm UV for 2 min. or less.

7   Matrix Stiffness Affects Invasive Behavior

Certain cell types respond to the stiffness of their environments by altering their migration. Lo et al. demonstrated that 3T3 fibroblasts preferentially migrate toward the stiff end of a stiffness gradient [51]. This behavior is termed "durotaxis". Vascular smooth muscle cells also undergo durotaxis in 2D on collagen-coated polyacrylamide [52]. Raab et al. observed durotaxis in mesenchymal stem cells in a semi-3D system; cells were seeded on collagen I-coated polyacrylamide with a stiffness gradient ranging from 1 to 34 kPa, and then after adherence, cells were overlaid with more collagen I [33]. Ovarian cancer cells, on the other hand, tend to metastasize to soft tissues, so different cell types may respond differently to environment stiffness. McGrail et al. compared metastatic characteristics between these

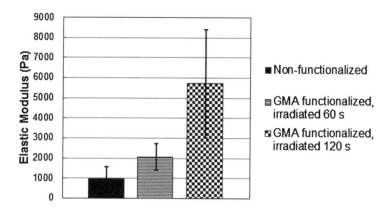

Fig. 6 Elastic moduli of non-functionalized collagen I gels and collagen I-GMA gels (8.8 mg/ml) irradiated 60 and 120 s. *Error bars* represent standard deviation of 15 total measurements on 3 gels, 5 per gel

cells on soft and hard substrates and demonstrated that they migrate more, have higher traction stress, elongate to the mesenchymal phenotype, and express lower levels of cytokeratin on the soft substrates [53].

Increased breast tissue stiffness does not seem to be solely an effect of cancer, as was described in section 1, but may also contribute to its progression. Increased stiffness and mammographic density, which correlates with increased stromal collagen content relative to fat, are also risk factors for breast cancer [54–57]. Furthermore, cross-linking of collagen in mammary fat pads of mice by injecting fibroblasts with heightened lysyl oxidase expression led to breast tumor progression. In vitro, stiffening by addition of ribose (150 Pa vs 110 Pa) led to clustering of cell integrins and increased invasion in a model breast cancer cell line [58]. On the other hand, Fenner et al. observed that more metastases occurred after cutting out compliant tumors from mice than occurred after cutting out stiff tumors [59]. Thus, the effect of stiffness on the invasiveness of breast cancer cells is not yet clear. Collagen I matrices tuned by GMA cross-linking provide a ligand density-controlled, biomimetic system with an appropriate stiffness range for determining the effect of stiffness on breast cancer cell migration. The MDA-MB-231 breast cancer cell line survived and migrated on these gels and can be assayed by measuring speeds of individual cells. The following work is a proof of concept for conducting such experiments.

8 Migration Assay on Stiffness-Tuned Collagen I

Collagen I and collagen I-GMA gels (8.8 mg/ml) were prepared according to the method described in section 6.5, but as thin layers (≤90 μm). Polystyrene beads (90 μm) were mixed into the collagen, and 10 μL of mixture was added to the center

Fig. 7 Schematic of setup
for making thin collagen
gels [60]

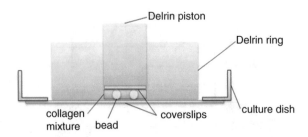

of a delrin ring on a 50 mm glass-bottom dish that was coated with APTES and
glutaraldehyde for gel adherence. A delrin piston with a Rain-X®-coated coverslip
glued to the end was dropped onto the droplet to make a thin gel with a flat surface
(Fig. 7). Collagen I-GMA gels were irradiated with 365 nm UV for 120 s, with an
intensity of 4.4 mW/cm^2.

MDA-MB-231 cells (100,000–200,000) were seeded on the surface of the gels in
complete mammary epithelial growth medium (MEGM) with bovine pituitary extract
(BPE), and 1–3 days later, stained with CellTracker™ Green CMFDA. Fluorescent
cells were imaged with a 20X objective for 20 h with a Nikon Eclipse Ti inverted
epifluorescence microscope equipped with a FITC fluorescence cube, while maintained at 37 °C and 5% CO$_2$ atmosphere. A scientific CMOS camera (pco.edge, PCO,
Kelheim, Germany, 6.5 μm × 6.5 μm pixel size) acquired one image every 10 min. An
automated shutter (Uniblitz VS25, Vincent Associates) in the fluorescence excitation
path prevented bleaching of the fluorophore between images.

An ImageJ bandpass filter was applied to images to eliminate features larger or
smaller than cells for ease of tracking. Contrast-limited adaptive histogram equal-
ization was performed with a window half size of 100 × 100, and slope of 2. Icy
bioimage analysis software (Quantitative Image Analysis Unit, Institut Pasteur) was
used for tracking cell migration. The Active Contours plug-in was used to outline
the cells and track these over time; it allows user-defined ROI to be drawn around
individual cells, then the borders snap on to the outline of the cell automatically. Ten
to twenty isolated cells were selected for each gel, avoiding those that appeared to
be floating or likely to be difficult to track. Track manager yielded the center coordinates each frame. Figure 8 shows the initial image of a video with Active Contours
outlines and tracks.

Average frame-to-frame speed (μm/h) was acquired for each cell track from the
coordinates of the centers of the cells as follows:

$$\overline{s} = \frac{\sum_{n=1}^{N} \dfrac{\sqrt{\left(x_{n+1} - x_n\right)^2 + \left(y_{n+1} - y_n\right)^2}}{t_{n+1} - t_n}}{N-1} \tag{8}$$

where N is the total number of images in the track, x_n and y_n are the coordinates of
the centers of the cell in each image, and t is the time when each image was taken,
0.17 h (10 min) apart. The average frame-to-frame speeds of all cell tracks were
averaged together for three collagen I gels and for three collagen I-GMA gels.

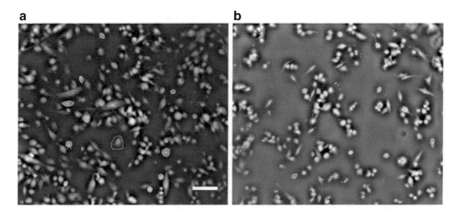

Fig. 8 Bandpass-filtered fluorescence images of MDA-MB-231 cells seeded on thin layers of collagen I (8.8 mg/ml). Figure also shows Icy software Active Contours outlines (multi-colored) and tracks (*yellow*). Scale bar is 100 μm. (**a**) is non-functionalized collagen I, and (**b**) is collagen I-GMA cross-linked by irradiation for 120 s

MDA-MB-231 s survived on both collagen I and collagen I-GMA gels. The average frame-to-frame speed of cells seeded on non-functionalized collagen I was 0.88 μm/h, and on collagen I-GMA irradiated for 120 s was 0.67 μm/h. None of the cells on the cross-linked gels had average speeds that exceeded 2.5 μm/h, while some reached nearly 4 μm/h on regular collagen I. Because the seeding densities were not controlled across these two stiffness conditions, it is not possible to conclude from these data whether stiffness or seeding density is responsible for these differences. These results demonstrate the feasibility of future migration experiments and analysis, in which cell seeding density will be controlled.

9   Conclusions

Photoactivated cross-linking of collagen I-GMA using LAP as a photoinitiator provides a way to tune collagen I stiffnesses from 1 to 6 kPa, matching that of normal breast tissue and that of breast tumors, without changing the concentration of collagen I. This provides a way to assess whether breast tumor cells respond to stiffness in their environment independently of ligand density and fibril alignment. Photoactivation also provides the potential for creation of stiffness gradients and patterns by using easily produced photomasks. The concentration of collagen I-GMA necessary to achieve this range in these studies, however, is higher than ideal for invasion studies with embedded tumor cells in 3D culture. Migration of MDA-MB-231 cells in collagen I matrices of density 5 mg/ml or higher is significantly impeded (private communication, Dr. Nicholas Kurniawan). In future, development of less dense collagen I gels with equivalent stiffnesses, and lower doses of UV would be beneficial to development of invasion assays in 3D.

However, MDA-MB-231 cells survive and migrate on the surface of these collagen I-GMA gels. Average migration speeds for cells on both non-functionalized collagen I and UV-crosslinked, collagen I-GMA gels were less than 1 μm/h. The methods here provide a way to determine whether matrix stiffness, independently of ligand density, influences speeds of MDA-MB-231 cells in 2D. In combination with photomasks, it may be possible to create stiffness gradients for durotaxis assays within these UV-crosslinked collagen I gels. Stiffness gradients have already been made in synthetic hydrogels by using photoactivated cross-linking; Yeung et al. and Sunyer et al. used transparency masks with printed gradients and a sliding mask, respectively, to create stiffness gradients [31, 61]. Although stiffness gradients in collagen and gelatin matrices have also been achieved by non-photoactivating methods, the use of photoactivation in conjunction with patterned photomasks may open the door for precise and varied stiffness patterns that would not be feasible using these other methods [62, 63].

As a final note for future work toward development of 3D tumor models and invasion assays, in early experiments cross-linking 3.8 mg/ml collagen I-GMA, MDA-MB-231 cells were embedded into the gels by mixing them into the collagen mixture prior to irradiation. Irgacure 2959® was used as a photoinitiator, and a UVP transilluminator was used to irradiate gels at 302 nm for 5 min. Cells were stained with calcein AM and fluoresced, indicating they survived the irradiation and cross-linking of collagen. Furthermore, they visibly migrated inside the gel. These results suggest the potential for using collagen I-GMA gels for performing durotaxis assays inside 3D matrices, not just by tracking the motion of cells on the surface of these gels.

Acknowledgements The authors would like to thank Dr. Xinyi Guo for performing the initial AFM measurements of collagen I-GMA gels with Irgacure 2959. We would also like to thank Dr. Kristi Anseth (University of Colorado) for providing us with an initial sample of LAP, and Dr. Paul Jones (Wake Forest University) for assistance in synthesizing LAP from the Anseth protocol.

References

1. Butcher DT, Alliston T, Weaver VM (2009) A tense situation: forcing tumour progression. Nat Rev Cancer 9:108–122. doi:10.1038/nrc2544
2. Paszek MJ, Zahir N, Johnson KR et al (2005) Tensional homeostasis and the malignant phenotype. Cancer Cell 8:241–254. doi:10.1016/j.ccr.2005.08.010
3. Barsky SH, Rao CN, Grotendorst GR, Liotta LA (1982) Increased content of Type V Collagen in desmoplasia of human breast carcinoma. Am J Pathol 108:276–283
4. Schedin P, Keely PJ (2011) Mammary gland ECM remodeling, stiffness, and mechanosignaling in normal development and tumor progression. Cold Spring Harb Perspect Biol 3:a003228. doi:10.1101/cshperspect.a003228
5. Vidi P-A, Chandramouly G, Gray M et al (2012) Interconnected contribution of tissue morphogenesis and the nuclear protein NuMA to the DNA damage response. J Cell Sci 125:350–361. doi:10.1242/jcs.089177
6. Engler AJ, Sen S, Sweeney HL, Discher DE (2006) Matrix elasticity directs stem cell lineage specification. Cell 126:677–689. doi:10.1016/j.cell.2006.06.044

7. Holle AW, Del Alamo JC, Engler AJ (2013) Focal adhesion mechanotransduction regulates stiffness-directed differentiation. ASME 2013 Summer Bioengineering Conference. doi:10.1115/SBC2013-14676

8. Janoštiak R, Pataki AC, Brábek J, Rösel D (2014) Mechanosensors in integrin signaling: the emerging role of p130Cas. Eur J Cell Biol 93:445–454. doi:10.1016/j.ejcb.2014.07.002

9. Sawada Y, Tamada M, Dubin-Thaler BJ et al (2006) Force sensing by mechanical extension of the Src family kinase substrate p130Cas. Cell 127:1015–1026. doi:10.1016/j.cell.2006.09.044

10. Baker EL, Lu J, Yu D et al (2010) Cancer cell stiffness: integrated roles of three-dimensional matrix stiffness and transforming potential. Biophys J 99:2048–2057. doi:10.1016/j.bpj.2010.07.051

11. Wilson R (2006) Normal Histology of the Breast. http://robbiewilson.50webs.com/Breast%20act%202.htm. Accessed 10 Jun 2016

12. Maller O, Martinson H, Schedin P (2010) Extracellular matrix composition reveals complex and dynamic stromal-epithelial interactions in the mammary gland. J Mammary Gland Biol Neoplasia 15:301–318. doi:10.1007/s10911-010-9189-6

13. Lu P, Weaver VM, Werb Z (2012) The extracellular matrix: a dynamic niche in cancer progression. J Cell Biol 196:395–406. doi:10.1083/jcb.201102147

14. Shoulders MD, Raines RT (2009) Collagen structure and stability. Annu Rev Biochem 78:929–958. doi:10.1146/annurev.biochem.77.032207.120833

15. Chandrakasan G, Torchia DA, Piez KA (1976) Preparation of intact monomeric collagen from rat tail tendon and skin and the structure of the nonhelical ends in solution. J Biol Chem 251:6062–6067

16. Williams BR, Gelman RA, Poppke DC, Piez KA (1978) Collagen fibril formation. Optimal in vitro conditions and preliminary kinetic results. J Biol Chem 253:6578–6585

17. Yang Y, Leone LM, Kaufman LJ (2009) Elastic moduli of collagen gels can be predicted from two-dimensional confocal microscopy. Biophys J 97:2051–2060. doi:10.1016/j.bpj.2009.07.035

18. Achilli M, Mantovani D (2010) Tailoring mechanical properties of collagen-based scaffolds for vascular tissue engineering: the effects of pH, temperature and ionic strength on gelation. Polymers 2:664–680. doi:10.3390/polym2040664

19. Lang NR, Münster S, Metzner C et al (2013) Estimating the 3D pore size distribution of biopolymer networks from directionally biased data. Biophys J 105:1967–1975. doi:10.1016/j.bpj.2013.09.038

20. Grant CA, Brockwell DJ, Radford SE, Thomson NH (2009) Tuning the elastic modulus of hydrated collagen fibrils. Biophys J 97:2985–2992. doi:10.1016/j.bpj.2009.09.010

21. Baldwin SJ, Quigley AS, Clegg C, Kreplak L (2014) Nanomechanical mapping of hydrated rat tail tendon collagen I fibrils. Biophys J 107:1794–1801. doi:10.1016/j.bpj.2014.09.003

22. Raub C, Putnam A, Tromberg B, George S (2010) Predicting bulk mechanical properties of cellularized collagen gels using multiphoton microscopy. Acta Biomater 6:4657–4665. doi:10.1016/j.actbio.2010.07.004

23. Hadjipanayi E, Mudera V, Brown RA (2009) Guiding cell migration in 3D: a collagen matrix with graded directional stiffness. Cell Motil Cytoskeleton 66:121–128. doi:10.1002/cm.20331

24. Ulrich TA, Jain A, Tanner K et al (2010) Probing cellular mechanobiology in three-dimensional culture with collagen–agarose matrices. Biomaterials 31:1875–1884. doi:10.1016/j.biomaterials.2009.10.047

25. Orban JM, Wilson LB, Kofroth JA et al (2004) Crosslinking of collagen gels by transglutaminase. J Biomed Mater Res A 68:756–762. doi:10.1002/jbm.a.20110

26. Ibusuki S, Halbesma GJ, Randolph MA et al (2007) Photochemically cross-linked collagen gels as three-dimensional scaffolds for tissue engineering. Tissue Eng 13:1995–2001. doi:10.1089/ten.2006.0153

27. Sundararaghavan HG, Monteiro GA, Lapin NA et al (2008) Genipin-induced changes in collagen gels: correlation of mechanical properties to fluorescence. J Biomed Mater Res A 87A:308–320. doi:10.1002/jbm.a.31715

28. Nichol JW, Koshy S, Bae H et al (2010) Cell-laden microengineered gelatin methacrylate hydrogels. Biomaterials 31:5536–5544. doi:10.1016/j.biomaterials.2010.03.064

29. Haugh MG, Murphy CM, McKiernan RC et al (2011) Crosslinking and mechanical properties significantly influence cell attachment, proliferation, and migration within collagen glycosaminoglycan scaffolds. Tissue Eng Part A 17:1201–1208. doi:10.1089/ten.TEA.2010.0590

30. Mullen CA, Vaughan TJ, Billiar KL, McNamara LM (2015) The effect of substrate stiffness, thickness, and cross-linking density on osteogenic cell behavior. Biophys J 108:1604–1612. doi:10.1016/j.bpj.2015.02.022

31. Yeung T, Georges PC, Flanagan LA et al (2005) Effects of substrate stiffness on cell morphology, cytoskeletal structure, and adhesion. Cell Motil Cytoskeleton 60:24–34. doi:10.1002/cm.20041

32. Tse JR, Engler AJ (2010) Preparation of hydrogel substrates with tunable mechanical properties. Curr Protoc Cell Biol Editor Board Juan Bonifacino Al Chapter 10:Unit 10.16. doi:10.1002/0471143030.cb1016s47

33. Raab M, Swift J, Dingal PCDP et al (2012) Crawling from soft to stiff matrix polarizes the cytoskeleton and phosphoregulates myosin-II heavy chain. J Cell Biol 199:669–683. doi:10.1083/jcb.201205056

34. Rich H, Odlyha M, Cheema U et al (2014) Effects of photochemical riboflavin-mediated crosslinks on the physical properties of collagen constructs and fibrils. J Mater Sci Mater Med 25:11–21. doi:10.1007/s10856-013-5038-7

35. Tronci G, Russell SJ, Wood DJ (2013) Photo-active collagen systems with controlled triple helix architecture. J Mater Chem B 1:3705–3715. doi:10.1039/c3tb20720j

36. Popov V, Heß M (2014) Method of dimensionality reduction in contact mechanics and friction, 1st edn. Springer, Berlin Heidelberg, Berlin

37. Popov V (2010) Contact mechanics and friction: physical principles and applications, 1st edn. Springer, Berlin Heidelberg, Berlin, Heidelberg

38. Xu B, Li H, Zhang Y (2013) Understanding the viscoelastic behavior of collagen matrices through relaxation time distribution spectrum. Biomatter. doi:10.4161/biom.24651

39. Abidine Y, Laurent VM, Michel R et al (2013) Probing the viscoelastic properties of polyacrylamide polymer gels in a wide frequency range. Comput Methods Biomech Biomed Engin 16:15–16

40. Bolboaca DSD, Jäntschi DL (2007) Amino acids sequences analysis on collagen. In: Bull. Univ. Agric. Sci. Vet. Med. – Anim. Sci. Biotechnol. http://cogprints.org/5748/. Accessed 20 Jun 2016

41. López J, Imperial S, Valderrama R, Navarro S (1993) An improved bradford protein assay for collagen proteins. Clin Chim Acta 220:91–100. doi:10.1016/0009-8981(93)90009-S

42. Bubnis WA, Ofner CM (1992) The determination of epsilon-amino groups in soluble and poorly soluble proteinaceous materials by a spectrophotometric method using trinitrobenzenesulfonic acid. Anal Biochem 207:129–133

43. Majima T, Schnabel W, Weber W (1991) Phenyl-2,4,6-trimethylbenzoylphosphinates as watersoluble photoinitiators – generation and reactivity of O=p(c6h5)(o-) radical-anions. Macromol Chem Phys 192:2307–2315

44. Fairbanks BD, Schwartz MP, Bowman CN, Anseth KS (2009) Photoinitiated polymerization of PEG-diacrylate with lithium phenyl-2,4,6-trimethylbenzoylphosphinate: polymerization rate and cytocompatibility. Biomaterials 30:6702–6707. doi:10.1016/j.biomaterials.2009.08.055

45. Takigawa T, Morino Y, Urayama K, Masuda T (1996) Poisson's ratio of polyacrylamide (PAAm) gels. Polym Gels Netw 4:1–5. doi:10.1016/0966-7822(95)00013-5

46. Pritchard RH, Lava P, Debruyne D, Terentjev EM (2013) Precise determination of the Poisson ratio in soft materials with 2D digital image correlation. Soft Matter 9:6037–6045. doi:10.1039/C3SM50901J

47. Sader JE, Chon JWM, Mulvaney P (1999) Calibration of rectangular atomic force microscope cantilevers. Rev Sci Instrum 70:3967–3969. doi:10.1063/1.1150021

48. Normand V, Lootens DL, Amici E et al (2000) New insight into agarose gel mechanical properties. Biomacromolecules 1:730–738. doi:10.1021/bm005583j
49. Smelser AM (2016) Breast cancer cell mechanical properties and migration on collagen I matrices with tunable elasticity. Dissertation, Wake Forest University
50. Greenwald RA, Moy WW (1979) Inhibition of collagen gelation by action of the superoxide radical. Arthritis Rheum 22:251–259. doi:10.1002/art.1780220307
51. Lo C-M, Wang H-B, Dembo M, Wang Y (2000) Cell movement is guided by the rigidity of the substrate. Biophys J 79:144–152. doi:10.1016/S0006-3495(00)76279-5
52. Wong JY, Velasco A, Rajagopalan P, Pham Q (2003) Directed movement of vascular smooth muscle cells on gradient-compliant hydrogels. Langmuir 19:1908–1913
53. McGrail DJ, Kieu QMN, Dawson MR (2014) The malignancy of metastatic ovarian cancer cells is increased on soft matrices through a mechanosensitive Rho-ROCK pathway. J Cell Sci 127:2621–2626. doi:10.1242/jcs.144378
54. McCormack VA, Silva I dos S (2006) Breast density and parenchymal patterns as markers of breast cancer risk: a meta-analysis. Cancer Epidemiol Biomark Prev 15:1159–1169. doi:10.1158/1055-9965.EPI-06-0034
55. Boyd NF, Martin LJ, Yaffe MJ, Minkin S (2011) Mammographic density and breast cancer risk: current understanding and future prospects. Breast Cancer Res (BCR) 13:223. doi:10.1186/bcr2942
56. Huo CW, Chew G, Hill P et al (2015) High mammographic density is associated with an increase in stromal collagen and immune cells within the mammary epithelium. Breast Cancer Res 17:79. doi:10.1186/s13058-015-0592-1
57. Pang J-MB, Byrne DJ, Takano EA et al (2015) Breast tissue composition and immunophenotype and its relationship with mammographic density in women at high risk of breast cancer. PLoS One 10:e0128861. doi:10.1371/journal.pone.0128861
58. Levental KR, Yu H, Kass L et al (2009) Matrix crosslinking forces tumor progression by enhancing integrin signaling. Cell 139:891–906. doi:10.1016/j.cell.2009.10.027
59. Fenner J, Stacer AC, Winterroth F et al (2014) Macroscopic stiffness of breast tumors predicts metastasis. Sci Rep. doi:10.1038/srep05512
60. Kreutzfeldt TW (2014) Development of mechanically soft gels for use in wide-field microscopy of live cells. Honors Thesis, Wake Forest University
61. Sunyer R, Jin AJ, Nossal R, Sackett DL (2012) Fabrication of hydrogels with steep stiffness gradients for studying cell mechanical response. PLoS One 7:e46107. doi:10.1371/journal.pone.0046107
62. Gorgone C, Hambright C, Hock L, Wiater M (2014) 3D hydrogel system with continuous stiffness gradient. Project Report, Worcester Polytechnic Institute
63. Sundararaghavan HG, Monteiro GA, Firestein BL, Shreiber DI (2009) Neurite growth in 3D collagen gels with gradients of mechanical properties. Biotechnol Bioeng 102:632–643. doi:10.1002/bit.22074

Mathematical Modeling of Tumor Organoids: Toward Personalized Medicine

Aleksandra Karolak and Katarzyna A. Rejniak

Abstract Three-dimensional organoid and organoidal cell cultures can recreate certain aspects of in vivo tumors and tumor microenvironments, and thus can be used to test intratumoral interactions and tumor response to treatments. In silico organoid models, when based on biological or clinical data, are an invaluable tool for hypothesis testing, and provide an opportunity to explore experimental conditions beyond what is feasible experimentally. In this chapter, three different approaches to building in silico organoids are described together with methods for integration with experimental or clinical data. The first model will be used to determine the mechanisms of development of breast tumor acini, based on their in vitro morphology. The second model will be used to predict conditions for the most effective cellular uptake of therapies targeting pancreatic cancers that incorporate intravital microscopy data. The third model will provide a procedure for assessing patients' response to chemotherapeutic treatments, based on the biopsy data. For each of the models, a protocol will be proposed indicating how it can be used to generate testable hypotheses or predictions. These models can help biologists in determining what experiments should be performed in the laboratory. They can also assist clinicians in assessing cancer patients' response to a given therapy and their risk of tumor recurrence.

Keywords In silico organoids • Digitized tissue • Organotypic cultures • Mammary acini • Drug penetration • Single-cell delivery • Targeted therapy • Personalized medicine • Mathematical modeling

A. Karolak
Integrated Mathematical Oncology Department, H. Lee Moffitt Cancer Center & Research Institute, Tampa, FL, USA
e-mail: Aleksandra.Karolak@moffitt.org

K.A. Rejniak (✉)
Integrated Mathematical Oncology Department, H. Lee Moffitt Cancer Center & Research Institute, Tampa, FL, USA

Department of Oncologic Sciences, College of Medicine, University of South Florida, Tampa, FL, USA
e-mail: Kasia@rejniak.net

© Springer International Publishing AG 2018
S. Soker, A. Skardal (eds.), *Tumor Organoids*, Cancer Drug Discovery and Development, DOI 10.1007/978-3-319-60511-1_10

193

1 Introduction

With the recent advances in three-dimensional (3D) culture technology, there is increased interest in utilizing such multicellular systems to investigate how they develop, how the transition from non-tumorigenic to malignant colonies takes place, to examine how they respond to various therapies, and to test different treatment options. While these in vitro models are obviously a simplification of an in vivo tissue structure and function, they mimic in vivo physiology better than 2D cell cultures, and are much easier to handle than in vivo models.

In the 3D organotypic cultures, the individual cells derived from immortalized cell lines are grown in the extracellular matrix (ECM) constructs, such as Matrigel, and self-assemble into 3D multicellular architectures. These cultures recapitulate the structure of the tissue from which they are derived: either a hollow epithelial acinus resembling the normal cyst or duct [5, 7, 14, 35, 48, 50] or the fully filled spheroid that has tumor-like features [4, 6, 7, 13, 21, 46]. However, these cultures usually contain only one type of cells, and thus are a very simplified representation of the in vivo tissues. The ultimate experimental goal is to grow an organoid, a multicellular system that is complex enough to attain the morphology, cellular heterogeneity, stromal composition, and some functionality of the in vivo organ, but that is still amenable to control and analysis [17, 34, 49]. Nevertheless, both organotypic cultures and tissue organoids need to be kept in the 3D culture for a significant length of time to either reach a size comparable to in vivo tumors (organotypic cultures) or to observe the results of anti-cancer therapies (organoids). Integrating laboratory experiments with in silico approaches can reduce the time and amount of experimental work.

Mathematical modeling in silico of organoids can provide a platform for systematically testing how perturbations in individual components of the complex organoid system influence their emerging properties. Computer simulations can be performed on a high-throughput scale that is not feasible in a laboratory setting. A large number of parameters can be varied in these simulations simultaneously and over a wide range of values that allows the factors that are essential for answering the investigated question to be identified. Such broad and multiparametrical studies can generate various experimentally testable hypotheses and point toward directions that are worth pursuing experimentally. Moreover, they can also indicate which potential experiments will not show any promising results and thus may be omitted. This will provide a cost-effective tool for selecting which experiments should be carried on.

In this chapter, we present examples of mathematical modeling of tumor organoids and organotypic cultures. In the first example, we discuss how the mathematical model *IBCell* (Immersed Boundary model of the Cell) can be used to delineate cell-intrinsic properties that lead to perturbations of the structure of normal mammary acini and result in the development of tumor multicellular spheroids. Mammary acini are one of the first organotypic cultures to have been grown in 3D microenvironments. While they are composed of epithelial cells only, they arise due to local interactions between non-tumorigenic cells by repeated proliferation, cell differentiation, and self-organization into a shell of cells enclosing the hollow lumen. The *IBCell* is an in silico organoid, a computational analog of the 3D in vitro organotypic cultures. In the second example, we present a mathematical model *microPK/PD* (microscale pharmacokinetics/pharmacodynamics) that utilizes the tumor tissue architecture digitized from an experimental sample. Our focus of interest here is the tumor microenvironment on the microscopic scale, and simulating drug or imaging agent transport through the tissue. This model is a simplification of the in vivo tissue, but it includes tumor cells, stroma, interstitial fluid, and tumor vasculature. As such, it takes into consideration a section of the whole tumor organoid. We finish by putting forward the idea of a Virtual Clinical Trials model that can be used to simulate how a cohort of tumors (based on either mice or human histology) will respond to a particular treatment. This will provide a way to formulate a personalized treatment based on the tissue sample acquired from a patient's biopsy.

2   In Silico Organoid Model of Mammary Acini

Epithelial tissues are one of the most abundant tissues in the human body. They cover cavities and the surfaces of many organs, including breast ducts and lobules, the bronchi and alveoli of the lungs, and the endocrine glands. They form well-organized, multicellular systems consisting of a layer of tightly packed epithelial cells enclosing a lumen cavity and surrounded by the basement membrane and by other types of cells. The maintenance of epithelial structure and function depends on physical interactions and chemical signals shared locally between individual neighboring cells. For example, epithelial cells develop specialized cell–cell connections, such as adherens junctions, which mechanically attach cells to one another. Similarly, cell surface receptors, such as integrins, transmit forces from the external environment. Additionally, cells develop gap junctions that mediate the passage of chemical and electrical signals between neighboring cells and provide a mechanism for coordinating the activities of individual cells in the tissue. Thus, mechanical signals sensed by the cell result in activation of intracellular biochemical signaling pathways, which in turn regulate cell behavior [2, 16, 24].

To preserve the integrity of the epithelial tissue, most of the cellular processes, such as initiation of cell growth, selection of the axis of cell division, or the induction of cell death, must also be correlated with the actions of neighboring cells and the dynamically evolving microenvironment [12, 27]. The disruption of the normal epithelial tissue architecture, such as filling the lumen with malignant cells observed in ductal carcinomas in situ (DCIS), is one of the initial symptoms of progression to epithelial tumors [3, 45]. From this perspective, the emergence of pre-invasive cancers can be viewed as tissue homeostatic imbalance, in which the natural symbiosis between cellular and microenvironmental components is perturbed [36].

Mammary acini are 3D organotypic cultures that are in vitro models of breast epithelia. The most commonly used mammary acini cell lines are the non-tumorigenic human MCF10A cells. When these cells are cultured on top of Matrigel, they undergo several rounds of divisions, forming first a multicellular spheroid, before the cells in an outer layer differentiate and self-organize into a shell of epithelially polarized cells. This epithelial cell layer surrounds the hollow lumen that arises from inner cells' death by apoptosis [4, 5, 37]. Such 3D organotypic cultures provide a useful tool for dissecting cell–cell interactions that are important in mammary gland development and its homeostatic maintenance. They are also used to study the impact of different physical and chemical microenvironments on mammary cell transformations that lead to MCF10A malignant mutants [20, 21, 31, 46, 51].

To delineate differences in the development of normal and tumorigenic mammary acini and to identify which intrinsic or extrinsic cues can lead to the development of malignant spheroids, we created a computational analog of the acini organotypic culture: the *IBCell* model [38]. *IBCell* was calibrated to quantitatively reconstruct the development of both the MCF10A acini and the MCF10A-HER2 mutant. The exploration of differences in model parameter values and model rules suggested that the observed acinar morphology distortion may result from the loss of negative feedback from secreted ECM proteins responsible for acinus stabilization.

2.1 Outline of Our Approach

Here, we present a general framework in which *IBCell* is used to identify core alternations between normal and malignant cells by integrating the in silico model with 3D experimental acinar morphologies. We use confocal images of multicellular spheroids arising from non-tumorigenic cell lines grown in 3D cultures as hollow acini, and employ them to calibrate *IBCell*. This *IBCell*-tuned model is subsequently used for the double-tuning process with morphologies from 3D cultures of specific acinar mutants. By quantitatively reproducing morphologies and growth dynamics of both experimental systems, we can determine which model features must be set up differently. Thereafter, these differences in parameter values are used to suggest potential mechanisms that lead to such morphological (and molecular) distortions arising in mutant cells as compared to non-tumorigenic cells. The proposed procedure is outlined in Fig. 1.

2.2 The IBCell Model

In the *IBCell* model, the cells are represented as deformable bodies filled with a viscous, incompressible fluid and equipped with a set of cell membrane pseudo-receptors. For the application to MCF10A cells, we considered receptors responsible for the initiation of cell growth, death, adhesion to other cells or to the ECM, and epithelial polarization (Fig. 1a, top row). Based on the cell receptor composition

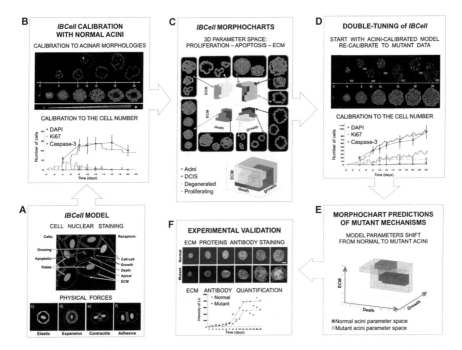

Fig. 1 *IBCell* model—in silico analog of mammary acini organotypic culture. The *IBCell* model of individual deformable cells (**a**) is tuned to fluorescent data collected from non-tumorigenic mammary acini morphologies (**b**). By exploring the *IBCell* Morphochart—the parameter space of cellular processes thresholds—different mutant morphologies can be identified (**c**). The Morphocharts are used for double-tuning of *IBCell* to match morphologies and cell counts for acinar mutants (**d**). This allows for identification of model parameters that differentiate between the two simulation sets (**e**), and suggests experiments to test molecular differences between normal and mutant cells (**f**)

(the percentage of each kind of receptors) and the specific receptor thresholds, the cell can undergo one of the following processes: growth, proliferation, division, epithelial polarization, or apoptosis. The morphologies of multicellular structures emerge spontaneously as a function of interacting cell processes and the prescribed threshold levels for active receptors. For example, the cell can grow only if a certain percentage of all cell pseudo-receptors take on the function of growth receptors, or the cell becomes epithelially polarized if the percentage of cell adhesive and ECM receptors reaches the prescribed thresholds. These receptor threshold levels define how sensitive the cell is to the given cues. Therefore, when the cues change, the cells undergo spontaneous state-switching (e.g., from growing to resting or to dying), as the receptors become engaged in particular processes. Model mechanical aspects are defined by the introduction of physical forces to enable cell membrane elasticity and expansion during cell growth, formation of a contractile ring during cell division, and a dynamic assembly and disassembly of adhesive contacts between neighboring cells (Fig. 1a, bottom row). More details on the model mathematical framework are included in Appendix A and [38, 40].

2.3   IBCell Calibration

The *IBCell* calibration process is based on confocal images of central cross-sections from MCF10A spheroids, stained with nuclear markers for cell nuclei (DAPI), apoptosis (antibodies against cleaved caspase-3), and proliferation (Ki-67). The acini grown in Matrigel culture were collected every four days during a 20-day period, fixed, and stained. The confocal images of the central cross-section of each acinus (Fig. 1b, top row) were segmented, cellular nuclei delineated, and the intensities of red (for caspase-3) and green (for Ki67) wavelengths used for determining the counts of growing, dying, and the total number of cells (Fig. 1b, bottom row). The goal was to reproduce the acinar shapes, averaged cell counts, and spatial locations of proliferating and dying cells at each time point at which the experimental data were collected. For example, initially, the proliferating cells were detectable in the whole cluster; at the later stages, the growing cells were mostly confined to the outer layer; in contrast, the dying cells were located inside the cluster only. As a result of this tuning process, we identified a set of model parameters that reproduced an acinar morphology and growth dynamics in good quantitative agreement with the experimental cellular baseline of MCF10A cells. More detailed description of this calibration process can be found in [44].

2.4   IBCell Morphocharts

Once the model is calibrated with data from a non-tumorigenic cell line, the three thresholds for growth, death, and ECM receptor ratio constitute a baseline parameter set for producing an acinus of normal morphology. This combination of thresholds can then be utilized as the initial seed for a suite of simulations that systematically examine model outcomes when all three thresholds are varied simultaneously and produce a Morphochart—a multidimensional parameter space of acinar morphologies (Fig. 1c, top set of images). These outcomes can then be grouped into similarity classes depending on their morphologies (Fig. 1c, bottom row). A broad region in this parameter space that consists only of hollow acini of various areas, cell counts, and luminal sizes is indicated by red color. A smaller subregion, shown in blue, contains morphologies of partially or fully filled lumina (corresponding to ductal carcinomas in situ, DCIS). Another region, colored yellow, represents acini of degenerated, non-circular shapes. Finally, the green area outside the indicated regions contains multicellular morphologies that are not stabilized and are still growing. Interestingly, each of these morphological classes corresponds to experimental acinar mutants (compare [43, 39]).

2.5   Double-Tuning of IBCell

In order to delineate differences between a non-tumorigenic cell line and its specific mutant, an *IBCell* double-tuning technique was developed. This method is presented here using an example of the MCF10A-HER2 mutant [44]. The double-tuning process requires an adjustment of the receptor thresholds (for cell growth, death, and ECM-dependent inhibition of cell growth) to match qualitatively and quantitatively experimental data from 3D cultures of both MCF10A and MCF10A-HER2 cells. The model already calibrated with the MCF10A data has to be readjusted to match MCF10-HER2-derived data (Fig. 1d, top row). As in the case of model calibration, the confocal images of spheroids derived from the mutant cell line were collected at various stages of their development and quantified by counting the number of cells stained with DAPI (blue), Ki67 (green), and caspase-3 (red). Visually, these MCF10A and MCF10A-HER2 data sets differ in the size of generated spheroids, in the lack of lumen in the mutant spheroids, and in numerous proliferative events observed even at the latest stages of the mutant development. By inspecting the Morphochart for the MCF10A-calibrated model, changes can be foreseen in *IBCell* pseudo-receptor thresholds that lead to reproduction of the structural and temporal sequences of MCF10A-HER2 development (Fig. 1d, bottom row). These new receptor threshold values (for cell growth, death, and ECM) constitute the baseline for reproduction of the growth dynamics and morphology of the MCF10A-HER2 mutant.

2.6   Identification of Potential Mechanisms of Mutant Development

The double-tuning procedure determines the parameter ranges for which *IBCell* generates morphologies that quantitatively reproduce experimental data from either the MCF10A acini (red region in Fig. 1e) or MCF10A-HER2 spheroids (dark green region in Fig. 1e). Interestingly, the tuned and double-tuned regions highlight that there is a degree of variability in the cellular processes that match the experimental data. These two parameter subspaces define how the processes need to be shifted in order to generate the MCF10A-HER2 mutant spheroid and not the MCF10A hollow acinus. These subspaces also indicate that, consistent with experimental observations, the growth threshold is upregulated and the apoptotic threshold is downregulated (dark green region occupies higher thresholds for death and lower for proliferation, when compared to red MCF10A region). However, *IBCell* simulations revealed also upregulation of the ECM threshold (the green region is above the red one), suggesting that either the ECM protein level is lower around the MCF10A-HER2 spheroids, preventing the cells from becoming growth-arrested, or that the

MCF10A-HER2 cells require higher concentrations of ECM proteins for entering into the growth-arrested state that subsequently would result in stabilization of the whole structure. These differently set up model parameters provide two potential mechanisms of acinar morphology distortion and testable hypotheses about the mechanisms of the absence of growth arrest in the mutant spheroids.

2.7 Experimental Validation

The *IBCell* parameter corresponding to ECM density was treated in the model in a quite generic way. However, experimentally, it may be matched with density of ECM proteins, such as collagen, elastin, fibronectin, or laminin. In our case, the ECM proteins that accumulated around both the MCF10A and MCF10A-HER2 structures were treated with an antibody against the laminin (Ln-332), a basement membrane component required for proper polarization of mammary epithelial acini. As expected, Ln-332 was present along the perimeter of both structures, MCF10A and MCF10A-HER2 (Fig. 1f, top rows). Nonetheless, their intensities at the later stages of development saturated on different levels with significantly lower and irregularly distributed intensities around the MCF10A-HER2 cells (Fig. 1f, bottom row). This confirmed the hypothesis that the loss of negative feedback from secreted ECM proteins is responsible for the defect in acinus stabilization.

2.8 Genotype-to-Phenotype Bridging with IBCell

One of the major challenges in biology is the mapping of genotypic changes to phenotypic outcomes. Molecular alterations in individual cells lead to complex emergent tissue phenotypes, such as distorted tissue architecture or unsuppressed cellular growth. However, the way in which oncogenic mutations and other molecular changes lead to tumorigenesis and, especially, how molecular alterations lead to specific alterations of epithelial architecture are not yet fully understood. This is a challenging problem because it requires integration across several scales: from genes, to molecules, to cellular core traits, to multicellular organization. Our model of epithelial morphogenesis is able to link molecular alterations to epithelial morphology through cellular core processes. With the *IBCell* double-tuning procedure and the construction of the Morphocharts, we can investigate the mapping between molecular and cellular processes via multicellular organization by projecting morphologies of experimental multicellular culture systems onto the model parameter space and identify which cellular processes are altered. Since the dysmorphic *IBCell*-generated mammospheres reproduce observed abnormal morphologies caused by changes in cancer-related genes, our model establishes a multiscale link between molecular and cell/tissue scales.

3 In Silico Organotypic Model for Drug Delivery in Tumors

One of the most critical issues limiting the effectiveness of chemotherapy is inefficient drug delivery to each individual cell within the tumor tissue. There are several barriers impacting the transvascular, interstitial, and transmembrane transport of drug particles. These include high interstitial fluid pressure inside tumors, tumor and stromal cellular architecture, fiber alignment and composition of the extracellular space biochemical milieu, charges on the cell membranes, and tissue metabolic landscape [1, 22, 28, 41]. Additionally, the tumor tissue is highly heterogeneous, which is manifested on various levels, from irregular tumor vasculature to non-homogeneous spatial locations and sizes of tumor cells, to variable levels of receptors expressed on cell membranes, to diverse genetic profiles among the neighboring tumor cells [47]. Furthermore, many tumors contain regions with highly irregular gradients of metabolites or severely low levels of nutrients, in which tumor cells often become resistant to drugs. These cell- and tissue-related aspects of tumor heterogeneity that lead to disturbed drug delivery and to failure of chemotherapeutic treatments are difficult to test in animal experiments in their entire complexity. The systematic manipulations of tumor microenvironment or drug properties that would allow for development of more specific and deeply penetrating drugs capable of reaching the regions of densely packed cells or hypoxic cells distant from the vessels, while minimizing toxic effects on normal cells, are still not experimentally achievable. Therefore, experimentally-informed mathematical models of tumor tissues are vital for in-depth exploration of microenvironmental barriers to drug delivery, even if, by their nature, these models are a simplified representation of the biological systems.

In order to explore and quantify the spatio-temporal dynamics of the imaging or therapeutic agents that diffuse through the interstitial space and bind to the tumor cell membrane receptors, we developed a computational tissue-based model, *microPK/PD*, which represents the tumor organoid. This model has been used to test how modulation of drug biophysical and biochemical properties or adjustment of drug release schemes can improve the delivery of therapeutic agents to a tissue and their efficacy at single-cell level. Such computational models not only allow for the broad exploration of the drug properties beyond experimental limits, but also can reduce the experimental costs.

3.1 Outline of Our Approach

Here, we illustrate how to identify the optimal conditions for the maximum receptor saturation and binding in an in silico multicellular model of a heterogeneous tumor tissue that has been informed by the 3D data from dorsal window chamber experiments. In our approach, the *microPK/PD* model was first calibrated based on experimental data, and a set of parameters that characterize the imaging agent was used for in vivo studies. This allowed us to represent faithfully the key components of the biological system. Next, we explored the model parameter space beyond what was done in laboratory experiments by sampling the values of biochemical and biophysical properties of the agent. We also considered two different agent release schemes. The outcomes of our studies revealed which combinations of the considered factors—the agent properties (diffusion, affinity), tissue topology (density, cellular loci), agent concentrations and/or extravasation rates—are critical for agent optimal delivery and cellular uptake on the level of individual cells. This approach can be adjusted to represent different ligand–receptor interactions and various tumor tissue architectures, including digitization of the patients' biopsy samples and/or resected tumors for the assessment of personalized treatment procedures. The schematic of our approach is summarized in Fig. 2.

3.2 The Image-Based microPK/PD Model

In order to build an in silico organoid that would be representative of a slice of a tumor tissue, we included in the *microPK/PD* model a segment of tumor vasculature from which the agent molecules are released, the explicitly defined individual tumor cells and the extracellular matrix that fills the interstitial space and is interpenetrated by the diffusive agent molecules. The biological base for our model is provided by the intravital dorsal window chamber experiments (Fig. 2a). In these experiments, the tumor construct containing the Su.86.86 human pancreatic cancer cells expressing the membrane-bound toll-like receptor 2 (TLR2) was exposed to the fluorescent, cyanine-5-marked ligand (TLR2L-Cy5), which bound to these cell receptors with high affinity and specificity. The confocal images acquired from these experiments at several time points during the period of 30 days have captured the spatiotemporal transport of the imaging agent molecules and their uptake by the tumor cells. Therefore, in the in silico model, the molecules of a fluorescent imaging agent were modeled as individual particles slowly extravasating from blood capillaries and spreading through the tumor (Fig. 2b).

To define the topology of a computational tissue, we used a set of confocal images that included a bright field image and a fluorescent red channel image (Fig. 2c) of a tumor tissue interpenetrated by the imaging agent. The cell sizes and shapes, as well as the location of active receptors on each cell boundary, were identified from the intensity of the emission wavelength of Cy-5 probe (red channel) along cell surfaces. The TLR2-Cy5 extravasation was modeled as a continuous constant-rate influx of ligand particles to mimic the intravenous injection and match the experimental observations. The virtual ligand transport through the interstitial space utilizes Brownian motion, and ligand–receptor binding affinity is assumed high to agree with the experimental data. The transport of the virtual agent particles takes place from the capillary located along the left boundary of the computational domain into the explicitly defined tissue architecture, and the tissue clearance takes place along the right boundary. Details of the mathematical framework of this model are given in Appendix B.

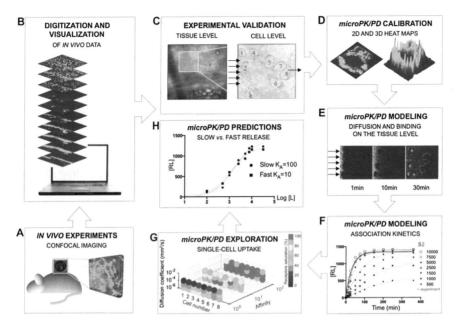

Fig. 2 *microPK/PD* model—in silico analog of tumor tissue organoid. Data images from dorsal window chamber experiments (**a**) were digitized for visualization and quantification (**b**). Image-based tissue architecture was explicitly reproduced in the model (**c**), and the process of ligand–receptor binding was quantified spatially (**d**). The progression of imaging particles' transport through the tissue (**e**) generated by *microPK/PD* allowed for calculations of the association kinetics for various ligand concentrations (**f**). Exploration of model parameter space: diffusion, affinity, and particle release schemes (**g**) led to scientific predictions (**h**)

3.3 *microPK/PD Model Calibration*

Quantification of the binding process between agent molecules and the membrane-bound receptors, together with bound complex internalization within the cell cytoplasm, was determined from the red channel images collected at different time points of the experiment. Digitization of experimental data allowed for assessment of the minimum residence time on the cell membrane (Fig. 2d), before the endocytosis process of the entire complex into cell cytoplasm took place. *microPK/PD* simulations permit tracing the agent dynamics in space and in time (Fig. 2e) for multiple ligand concentrations. A total of six experimental time points were used for model calibration and for quantitative reconstruction of the experimental time-dependent association kinetics curve (red line in Fig. 2f) by fitting to the one-phase association kinetics equations (Appendix B). To determine virtual concentrations of the ligand that match experimental data, several concentrations were used in simulations (black points in Fig. 2f), and the resulting data points were fitted to the association kinetics curves (black lines).

3.4   microPK/PD Predictions of Improved Drug Efficacy

While initially the *microPK/PD* model was calibrated to reproduce particular experimental data, we further explored the effects of various combinations of agent properties and different delivery schemes on agent efficacy. First, we used the association
kinetics fitted for a fast release of ligand particles and tested a wide range of diffusion values that covered a spectrum from small, rapidly diffusing to larger and less
soluble molecules, as well as diverse binding affinities (Fig. 2g). The results indicated that ligand affinity plays a significant role for small, rapidly diffusing agents,
which become uniformly distributed within the tumor tissue, thus enabling uniform
access to the ligand for every cell membrane receptor. However, in certain cases,
this led to incomplete saturation on the single-cell level. Strikingly, we observed
that, for the fast release scheme, the agents with moderate affinity bound to the cell-
surface receptors with similar efficacy to that of the high-affinity molecules released
at a slower rate (Fig. 2h). These predictions of *microPK/PD* may help the drug
development community in designing chemical compounds of preferable properties
that ensure the maximum effect in patient-specific extracellular matrix environments, tumor topologies, and receptor expression levels [18, 19].

4   In Silico Organoid Models for Personalized Medicine

Most cancers are diagnosed by inspecting patients' biopsy samples stained with
various immunohistochemical (IHC) markers. This allows a pathologist to recog-
nize the patterns of normal, tumor, and stromal cells within the tissue and to assess
the level of their distortion as compared to non-tumorigenic tissues. However, the
current histologic system does not enable further predictions of how the patient will
respond to available therapies and of the probabilities that the treated tumors will
recur. Being able to predict early, such as at the time of the tumor pre-treatment
biopsy, how the patient will respond to the available therapies would provide an
opportunity for more personalized medical care.

Mathematical modeling and computational simulations based on patients' individual tumor samples can provide the means to test various combination therapies
in silico before any treatment is administered to the patient. With a validated model,
an extensive series of simulations can be undertaken to test various dosing, timing,
and order of drugs. Therefore, for each patient's data, a virtual clinical trial can be
designed that will provide an optimized anti-cancer therapy customized for that
patient. Moreover, such virtual trials can be performed during therapy to test how
treatment can be adapted in order to benefit the patient the most.

We envision that the patient will follow the schematics presented in Fig. 3. The
patient will undergo a routine biopsy procedure to collect a tissue sample for further
diagnosis (Fig. 3a). Following current clinical practice, the tissue will be stained
with hematoxylin and eosin (H&E) to identify the tumor cells and their nuclei.

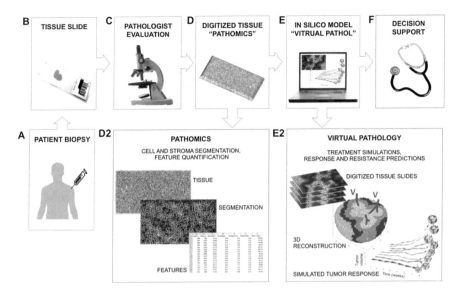

Fig. 3 Virtual Clinical Trials model—in silico analog of patient's tumor. Patient's biopsy tissue (**a**) sliced and fixed on a glass slide (**b**) is used for evaluation by a pathologist (**c**). Digitized image of this tissue (**d**) is used for quantitative assessment (Pathomics) of cell and stroma individual features (**d2**). Digitized tissue slides are also used for in silico modeling (Virtual Pathology) of various anti-cancer therapies (**e**), based on the patient's individual 3D tissue reconstruction and computer simulations of tumor response to therapies (**e2**). This provides support for clinical decisions about the outcomes of various therapies (**f**)

Subsequently, it will be sliced and fixed on the glass slide (Fig. 3b) and then examined under the microscope by a pathologist (Fig. 3c). However, for the purpose of the virtual trials, it will also be scanned and digitized (Fig. 3d). The magnified, high-resolution images of various tissue sections will be subjected to advanced image analysis techniques (Pathomics—the omics techniques applied to pathology images, Fig. 3d2) to identify and quantify the morphological and immunochemical features of individual tumor cells. This will involve segmentation of individual cell nuclei and cell cytoplasm and extraction of both the physical and molecular features in each individual cell. The physical features may include morphological parameters, such as cell and nuclei size, shape, and compactness, and the cytoplasm to nucleus ratio. The molecular futures include cell and cytoplasm staining intensity for each individual tumor or stromal cell, as well as the localization of tumor tissue vasculature, and/or the extracellular matrix fibrous composition. The quantified features can be used to characterize the tumor tissue state, such as its metabolic landscape pathology [25, 26] or tissue microenvironmental habitats [8, 10]. These quantified features can also be utilized to define cellular phenotypes for in silico Virtual Pathology modeling (Fig. 3e).

To determine the likelihood of the tumor being either responsive to the therapy or resistant, we combine the models described in Section 2 and Section 3, leading to a Virtual Pathology model highlighted in Fig. 3e2 . The patient's digitized histology tissue will be used to simulate drug penetration following the *microPK/PD* model. The digitized consecutive tissue slices (the z-stack) will be used to reconstruct the whole 3D tumor tissue by quantifying spatial configuration of tumor vasculature, as well as tumor cell sizes, their spatial configuration, and packing density. This metric will be used to reconstruct the tumor spheroid using the *IBCell* approach. With this model, the tumor response to a given treatment protocol will be simulated, and the tumor growth curves representing tumor dynamic response to the given therapy schedule will be recorded. By systematically varying the order of drugs, their timing (the length of the vacation periods between consecutive drug administrations), and dosage, we will be able to identify the optimal treatment schedules for a particular patient's tumor. Since tumors are very heterogeneous and can differ significantly between individual patients, the virtual clinical trials concept will provide support for clinical decisions (Fig. 3f), and can be tailored for each patient independently, providing a way of devising personalized treatment protocols.

5 Discussion

Mathematical modeling, when based on biological or clinical data and validated either in laboratory experiments or by using retrospective patient data, can be an invaluable tool for hypothesis testing. It offers the opportunity to run simulations with numerous parameters modified simultaneously, in order to predict the most favorable outcomes, whether that means suggesting new in vitro experiments or optimal drug treatment schedules. In this chapter, we described three different approaches to build in silico organoids or organotypic culture models and how they can be integrated with experimental or clinical data. For each of the models, we proposed a protocol indicating how these models can be used to generate testable hypotheses or predictions.

The *IBCell* model, an in silico analog of an organotypic culture of tumor spheroids, permitted examination of the intimate interactions between individual epithelial cells and testing how certain modifications in cell responses to extrinsic cues led to the development of distorted acinar morphologies. An interesting extension of this model would be to incorporate in it the mechanisms of drug action and to investigate how acinar morphology can change in response to different anti-cancer drugs.

The *microPK/PD* model, which is an in silico analog of tumor tissue organoid, allowed testing of how to design imaging agent properties and delivery schedules to achieve the most efficient cellular uptake. While our application dealt with a non-therapeutic fluorescent imaging agent, it would be interesting to extend this model by including the cytotoxic drugs and larger vascularized tumors. In particular, it could take advantage of the properties of clinically approved targeted agents and patients' biopsy samples that are routinely collected in clinic, and can provide a cost-effective tool for personalized drug delivery protocols.

We also proposed the Virtual Clinical Trials model, in which patient tumor-specific data quantified from initial diagnostic biopsies will be used to predict the most effective treatment protocols. Whereas in this chapter we provided only a general idea of such a model application, a bona fide example of the Virtual Clinical Trial model for osteosarcomas (VirtuOso) that predicts tumor chemoresistance to the standard-of-care therapy has been recently published [42]. In this work, we described in detail how the model can be validated in the so-called learning phase, using the retrospectively collected patient data and survival information. After validation, the model may be used for prospectively collected data (the so-called translational phase of the model) in a way similar to that described in the current chapter.

Although much bench effort devoted to testing how tumor cells respond to therapies has been acquired using conventional 2D culture systems, it is now evident that they do not fully replicate the complexity of cancers. In fact, cell gene expression patterns, cell–cell interactions and cell response to therapeutic insults vary greatly between 2D and 3D cultures [15, 30]. We have shown previously, using a 3D in silico model of multicellular spheroids, that, when cells are organized into tight 3D cell clusters, their response to cell cycle inhibitor drugs is altered when compared to more dispersed colonies [23]. In fact, numerous cells were growth-arrested in the G1 phase of the cell cycle, owing to contact inhibition with the neighboring tightly packed cells, and did not respond to the G2/M checkpoint inhibitors at all. However, small perturbations in this growth-arrested system resulted in tumor rapid outgrowth, despite the application of drugs.

Recently, there has been growing interest in investigating how the heterogeneous and dynamically changing tumor microenvironment influences the development of drug resistance in tumor cells [9, 29]. Particular attention is paid to the role of regions with unevenly distributed or low levels of nutrients or drugs. In these deregulated regions, the treatment often fails because of unsuccessful delivery or already disrupted cellular processes and signaling pathways. We have focused previously on two such regions: hypoxic niches containing low levels of both oxygen and drug; and pharmacological sanctuaries in which there is a normoxic level of oxygen but a very low concentration of drugs. Using an in silico analog of tumor organoid consisting of a vascularized tissue with micrometastatic tumor growth, we investigated whether these regions play a role in the emergence of resistance to DNA-damaging drugs [11, 32]. Our simulations revealed that tumor cells located in the regions with distorted levels of oxygen and/or drug may remain in a dormant, non-proliferative state, which allows them to overcome the drug-induced damage. As a result, these cells become resistant, implying that the drug-limited hypoxic niches and pharmacological sanctuaries play a significant role in altering cell response to treatments. Understanding the strategies pursued by tumor cells in order to survive under extreme microenvironmental conditions is another critical factor in the targeting of cell–ECM interactions and the development of new treatments.

Predictive models such as those described in this chapter can help researchers in the initial screening of a broad range of experimental conditions, before deciding which should be followed up in the laboratory. They can also assist pathologists and clinicians in assessing patients' risk for tumor recurrence or metastasis. Furthermore, they can improve the development of clinical trials by providing more objective means for patient selection and stratification. Ultimately, our goal is to develop computational systems that may be incorporated into the pathologist's and clinician's decision-supporting toolboxes.

Acknowledgements This work was supported in part by the U01-CA20229-01 grant from the National Institute of Health (NIH) via the National Cancer Institute—Physical Science Oncology Network (NCI-PSON). Data collection and analysis were supported by the Cancer Center Support Grant P30-CA-076292 from NIH to H. Lee Moffitt Cancer Center & Research Institute, an NCI-designated Comprehensive Cancer Center.

Appendix A: Mathematical Framework of the *IBCell* Model

The *IBCell* model belongs to the class of fluid-structure interaction models, and utilizes the immersed boundary method framework [33, 38]. The boundaries of all cells Γ are discretized, and every material point $X(l,t)$ represents a cell pseudo-receptor (l is a position along the boundary, t denotes time). The forces $F(l,t)$ defined at each boundary point (Eq. A1) arise from combining the elastic properties of cell boundaries, from cell-to-cell adhesion, and from contractile forces splitting a cell during its division. In this equation, G denotes spring stiffness, and L denotes spring resting length. These forces are applied to the surrounding fluid, as described in Eq. A2. The source points Y_k and sink points Z_m are placed in the cell local microenvironment, and the source and sink values $S^+(Y_k,t)$ and $S^-(Z_m,t)$ are chosen such that they balance around each cell separately (Eq. A3). They assume the non-zero values only during cell growth (proliferation) or cell shrinkage (apoptosis). The transitions between the material points on cell boundaries and the Cartesian grid $x = (x_1,x_2)$ in the domain Ω (Eqs. A3 and A7) are defined using the two dimensional Dirac delta function δ (Eq. A4). The fluid flow is described using the incompressible Navier-Stokes equation (Eq. A5), where p is the fluid pressure, μ is the fluid viscosity, ρ is the fluid density, s is the local fluid expansion, and f is the external force density. Eq. A6 is the law of mass balance. All material boundary points are carried along with the fluid (Eq. A7). The kinetics of ECM proteins $\gamma(x,t)$ is defined along the cell boundaries and includes: constant secretion of ECM (at a rate κ_1) along the cells' basal domains and ECM decay (at a rate κ_2) around all the cells' boundaries (Eq. A8). More details on the mathematical formulation of *IBCell* and the implementation of cell life processes can be found in [38, 40, 44].

$$F(l,t) = G\frac{\|X(k,t)-X(l,t)\|-L}{\|X(k,t)-X(l,t)\|}\left(X(k,t)-X(l,t)\right), \tag{A1}$$

$$f(x,t) = \int_{\Gamma} F(l,t)\delta\left(x-X(l,t)\right)dl, \tag{A2}$$

$$s(x,t) = \sum_{k \in \Xi +} S_+(Y_k,t)\delta(x - Y_k(t)) + \sum_{m \in \Xi -} S_-(Z_m,t)\delta(x - Z_m(t)), \quad \text{(A3)}$$

$$\delta_h(r) = \begin{cases} \dfrac{1}{4h}\left(1 + \cos\left(\dfrac{\pi r}{2h}\right)\right) & \text{if } |r| < 2h \\ 0 & \text{if } |r| \geq 2h \end{cases} \quad r = \| x - X(l,t) \|, \quad \text{(A4)}$$

$$\rho\left(\frac{\partial u(x,t)}{\partial t} + (u(x,t)\cdot\nabla)u(x,t)\right) = -\nabla p(x,t) + \mu\Delta u(x,t)$$

$$+ \frac{\mu}{3\rho}\nabla s(x,t) + f(x,t), \quad \text{(A5)}$$

$$\rho\nabla \cdot u(x,t) = s(x,t), \quad \text{(A6)}$$

$$\frac{\partial X}{\partial t} = u(X(t),t) = \int_\Omega u(x,t)\delta(x - X(t))dx, \quad \text{(A7)}$$

$$\frac{\partial\gamma(X(l,t))}{\partial t} = \kappa_1 X(l,t) - \kappa_2\gamma(X(l,t)). \quad \text{(A8)}$$

Appendix B: Mathematical Framework of the *microPK/PD* Model

The *microPK/PD* model is a discrete Brownian diffusion model, defined on an irregular domain and coupled with binding kinetics equations. In this model, the explicitly defined tumor cells $\{C^l\}_{l=1,...,N}$ (l is a cell index) are assumed to be non-motile and non-proliferative. The individual cell C^l is identified by a set of membrane virtual receptors $C^l = \{(X_i, Y_i)^l, A_i^l, B_i^l\}_{i=1...M^l}$, where $(X_i,Y_i)^l$ are the coordinates of the ith receptor, A_i^l is affinity to the receptor, and B_i^l is a receptor saturation level. Initially, the model was calibrated to the experiment-based values for moderate diffusion coefficient ($D = 2.5 \times 10^{-5}$ mm²/s), high binding affinity ($K_A = 100$), and a slow release scheme (as if during intravenous injection). Subsequently, it was used to explore the parameter space beyond the experimental boundaries. The transport of particles is modeled as Brownian motion with an effective diffusion coefficient D that was varied between 10^{-4} and 10^{-6} mm/s². Receptor binding affinity is defined as the probability with which a ligand molecule binds to the receptor after successful recognition. Therefore, three conditions for the binding probability are used: strong (100%), moderate (10%), or weak (1%). This results in three values of the pseudo-association constant (K_A): 100, 10, and 1, respectively.

The motion of a ligand particle (x,y) at the $n+1$ time point is defined by Eq. (B1). The cell membranes are non-penetrable for the ligand particles, unless they are successfully recognized by receptors (Eq. B1a). The successful ligand–receptor binding condition (BC) requires that the agent particle is in close proximity to the receptor, i.e., $\|(x_j,y_j)_n - (X_i,Y_i)^l\| < r_{min}$, where $(x_j,y_j)_n$ are coordinates of a jth ligand particle at n^{th} simulation step, $(X_i,Y_i)^l$ are coordinates of the ith receptor of the lth cell, and r_{min} is the criterion for a minimum distance. In addition, the receptor may not be saturated (number of already bound particles is below B_i^l), and the probability of binding meets the affinity criterion. Otherwise, if the new position will result in a particle crossing the cell boundary without satisfying the BC, the particle's position will remain unmodified (Eq. B1b) or continue to move through the tissue space with Brownian motion, as in Eq. (B1c), where Δt is a time step, ϖ a randomly chosen direction of motion. The effective diffusion coefficient D is defined in Eq. (B2), with k_B being the Boltzmann constant, R the ligand molecule radius, and η the tissue viscosity. The receptor–ligand binding is quantified by fitting the association kinetics to simulated data that represent the averaged saturation per tissue area as a function of time (Eq. B3), where B corresponds to the receptor saturation parameter describing ligand–receptor complex formation $[RL]$, with values between initial saturation and the maximum saturation B_0 and B_{max}, respectively; k is a reaction rate constant; t is time. Equation (B4) gives the logarithmic formula used to generate specific binding curves from multiple ligand concentrations, where B, B_0, and B_{max} are saturation parameters, K_D is a dissociation constant, h is the Hill slope defining the steepness of the fitting curve, and $[L]$ is ligand concentration.

$$(x,y)_{n+1} = \begin{cases} (X_i,Y_i)^l & {}^{(a)}\text{if the binding condition is satisfied} \\ (x,y)_n & {}^{(b)}\text{if the particle crosses cell boundary} \\ (x,y)_n + \sqrt{2D\Delta t}\,\varpi_n & {}^{(c)}\text{otherwise,} \end{cases} \tag{B1}$$

$$D = \frac{k_B T}{6\pi R\eta} \tag{B2}$$

$$B = B_0 + (B_{max} - B_0)/(1 - e^{-kT}) \tag{B3}$$

$$B = B_0 + (B_{max} - B_0)/(1 + 10^{([L]-\log K_D)}) \tag{B4}$$

References

1. Chauhan VP, Stylianopoulos T, Boucher Y, Jain RK (2011) Delivery of molecular and nanoscale medicine to tumors: transport barriers and strategies. Annu Rev Chem Biomol Eng 2:281–298. doi:10.1146/annurev-chembioeng-061010-114300
2. Chin LK, Xia Y, Discher DE, Janmey PA (2016) Mechanotransduction in cancer. Curr Opin Chem Eng 11:77–84

3. Debnath J, Brugge JS (2005) Modelling glandular epithelial cancers in three-dimensional cultures. Nat Rev Cancer 5(9):675–688. doi:10.1038/nrc1695
4. Debnath J, Mills KR, Collins NL, Reginato MJ, Muthuswamy SK, Brugge JS (2002) The role of apoptosis in creating and maintaining luminal space within normal and oncogene-expressing mammary acini. Cell 111(1):29–40
5. Debnath J, Muthuswamy SK, Brugge JS (2003) Morphogenesis and oncogenesis of MCF-10A mammary epithelial acini grown in three-dimensional basement membrane cultures. Methods 30(3):256–268
6. Dow LE, Elsum IA, King CL, Kinross KM, Richardson HE, Humbert PO (2008) Loss of human Scribble cooperates with H-Ras to promote cell invasion through deregulation of MAPK signalling. Oncogene 27(46):5988–6001. doi:10.1038/onc.2008.219
7. Fessart D, Begueret H, Delom F (2013) Three-dimensional culture model to distinguish normal from malignant human bronchial epithelial cells. Eur Respir J 42(5):1345–1356. doi:10.1183/09031936.00118812
8. Foroutan P, Kreahling JM, Morse DL, Grove O, Lloyd MC, Reed D, Raghavan M, Altiok S, Martinez GV, Gillies RJ (2013) Diffusion MRI and novel texture analysis in osteosarcoma xenotransplants predicts response to anti-checkpoint therapy. PLoS One 8(12):e82875. doi:10.1371/journal.pone.0082875
9. Fu F, Nowak MA, Bonhoeffer S (2015) Spatial heterogeneity in drug concentrations can facilitate the emergence of resistance to cancer therapy. PLoS Comput Biol 11(3):e1004142. doi:10.1371/journal.pcbi.1004142
10. Gatenby RA, Grove O, Gillies RJ (2013) Quantitative imaging in cancer evolution and ecology. Radiology 269(1):8–15. doi:10.1148/radiol.13122697
11. Gevertz JL, Aminzare Z, Norton KA, Perez-Velazquez J, Volkening A, Rejniak KA (2015) Emergence of anti-cancer drug resistance: exploring the importance of the microenvironmental niche via a spatial model. In: Radunskaya A, Jackson T (eds) Applications of dynamical systems in biology and medicine vol IMA volumes in mathematics and its applications. Springer, New York, NY pp 1–34
12. Hagios C, Lochter A, Bissell MJ (1998) Tissue architecture: the ultimate regulator of epithelial function? Philosophical transactions of the Royal Society of London Series B. Biological sciences 353(1370):857–870. doi:10.1098/rstb.1998.0250
13. Han J, Chang H, Giricz O, Lee GY, Baehner FL, Gray JW, Bissell MJ, Kenny PA, Parvin B (2010) Molecular predictors of 3D morphogenesis by breast cancer cell lines in 3D culture. PLoS Comput Biol 6(2):e1000684. doi:10.1371/journal.pcbi.1000684
14. Huang L, Holtzinger A, Jagan I, BeGora M, Lohse I, Ngai N, Nostro C, Wang R, Muthuswamy LB, Crawford HC, Arrowsmith C, Kalloger SE, Renouf DJ, Connor AA, Cleary S, Schaeffer DF, Roehrl M, Tsao MS, Gallinger S, Keller G, Muthuswamy SK (2015) Ductal pancreatic cancer modeling and drug screening using human pluripotent stem cell- and patient-derived tumor organoids. Nat Med 21(11):1364–1371. doi:10.1038/nm.3973
15. Imamura Y, Mukohara T, Shimono Y, Funakoshi Y, Chayahara N, Toyoda M, Kiyota N, Takao S, Kono S, Nakatsura T, Minami H (2015) Comparison of 2D- and 3D-culture models as drug-testing platforms in breast cancer. Oncol Rep 33(4):1837–1843. doi:10.3892/or.2015.3767
16. Jaalouk DE, Lammerding J (2009) Mechanotransduction gone awry. Nat Rev Mol Cell Biol 10(1):63–73. doi:10.1038/nrm2597
17. Jackson EL, Lu H (2016) Three-dimensional models for studying development and disease: moving on from organisms to organs-on-a-chip and organoids. Integr Biol (Quantitative Biosciences from Nano to Macro) 8(6):672–683. doi:10.1039/c6ib00039h
18. Karolak A, Estrella V, Chen T, Huynh A, Morse DL, Rejniak KA (2016) Using computational modeling to quantify targeted agent binding and internalization in pancreatic cancers. Cancer Res 76(Suppl 3):B21
19. Karolak A, Estrella V, Chen T, Huynh A, Morse DL, Rejniak KA (2017) Imaged-based computational predictions of imaging agent efficacy in pancreatic tumors expressing TLR2. Cancer Res 77(Suppl 2):A28

20. Kass L, Erler JT, Dembo M, Weaver VM (2007) Mammary epithelial cell: influence of extra-cellular matrix composition and organization during development and tumorigenesis. Int J Biochem Cell Biol 39(11):1987–1994. doi:10.1016/j.biocel.2007.06.025

21. Kenny PA, Bissell MJ (2003) Tumor reversion: correction of malignant behavior by microen-vironmental cues. Int J Cancer 107(5):688–695. doi:10.1002/ijc.11491

22. Kim M, Gillies RJ, Rejniak KA (2013) Current advances in mathematical modeling of anti-cancer drug penetration into tumor tissues. Front Oncol 3:278. doi:10.3389/fonc.2013.00278

23. Kim M, Reed D, Rejniak KA (2014) The formation of tight tumor clusters affects the effi-cacy of cell cycle inhibitors: a hybrid model study. J Theor Biol 352:31–50. doi:10.1016/j.jtbi.2014.02.027

24. Kolahi KS, Mofrad MR (2010) Mechanotransduction: a major regulator of homeostasis and development. Wiley Interdiscip Rev Syst Biol Med 2(6):625–639. doi:10.1002/wsbm.79

25. Lloyd MC, Rejniak KA, Brown JS, Gatenby RA, Minor ES, Bui MM (2015) Pathology to enhance precision medicine in oncology: lessons from landscape ecology. Adv Anat Pathol 22(4):267–272. doi:10.1097/PAP.0000000000000078

26. Lloyd MC, Rejniak KA, Johnson JO, Gillies R, Gatenby R, Bui MM (2012) Quantitative eval-uation of the morphological heterogeneity in breast cancer progression. Mod Pathol 25:392A

27. Martin-Belmonte F, Yu W, Rodriguez-Fraticelli AE, Ewald AJ, Werb Z, Alonso MA, Mostov K (2008) Cell-polarity dynamics controls the mechanism of lumen formation in epithelial morphogenesis. Curr Biol (CB) 18(7):507–513. doi:10.1016/j.cub.2008.02.076

28. Minchinton AI, Tannock IF (2006) Drug penetration in solid tumours. Nat Rev Cancer 6(8):583–592. doi:10.1038/nrc1893

29. Mumenthaler SM, Foo J, Choi NC, Heise N, Leder K, Agus DB, Pao W, Michor F, Mallick P (2015) The impact of microenvironmental heterogeneity on the evolution of drug resistance in cancer cells. Cancer Informat 14(Suppl 4):19–31. doi:10.4137/CIN.S19338

30. Pampaloni F, Reynaud EG, Stelzer EH (2007) The third dimension bridges the gap between cell culture and live tissue. Nat Rev Mol Cell Biol 8(10):839–845. doi:10.1038/nrm2236

31. Paszek MJ, Zahir N, Johnson KR, Lakins JN, Rozenberg GI, Gefen A, Reinhart-King CA, Margulies SS, Dembo M, Boettiger D, Hammer DA, Weaver VM (2005) Tensional homeosta-sis and the malignant phenotype. Cancer Cell 8(3):241–254. doi:10.1016/j.ccr.2005.08.010

32. Perez-Velazquez J, Gevertz JL, Karolak A, Rejniak KA (2016) Microenvironmental niches and sanctuaries: a route to acquired resistance. In: Rejniak KA (ed) Systems biology of tumor microenvironment: quantitative models and simulations. Springer, Switzerland

33. Peskin CS (2002) The immersed boundary method. Acta Numerica:479–527

34. Picollet-D'hahan N, Dolega ME, Liguori L, Marquette C, Le Gac S, Gidrol X, Martin DK (2016) A 3D toolbox to enhance physiological relevance of human tissue models. Trends Biotechnol 34(9):757–769. doi:10.1016/j.tibtech.2016.06.012

35. Plachot C, Chaboub LS, Adissu HA, Wang L, Urazaev A, Sturgis J, Asem EK, Lelievre SA (2009) Factors necessary to produce basoapical polarity in human glandular epithelium formed in conventional and high-throughput three-dimensional culture: example of the breast epithelium. BMC Biol 7:77. doi:10.1186/1741-7007-7-77

36. Radisky D, Hagios C, Bissell MJ (2001) Tumors are unique organs defined by abnormal sig-naling and context. Semin Cancer Biol 11(2):87–95. doi:10.1006/scbi.2000.0360

37. Reginato MJ, Muthuswamy SK (2006) Illuminating the center: mechanisms regulating lumen formation and maintenance in mammary morphogenesis. J Mammary Gland Biol Neoplasia 11(3–4):205–211. doi:10.1007/s10911-006-9030-4

38. Rejniak KA (2007) An immersed boundary framework for modelling the growth of indi-vidual cells: an application to the early tumour development. J Theor Biol 247(1):186–204. doi:10.1016/j.jtbi.2007.02.019

39. Rejniak KA (2014) IBCell Morphocharts: a computational model for linking cell molecular activity with emerging tissue morphology. In: Jonoska N, Saito M (eds) Discrete and toplogi-cal models in molecular biology. Natural Computing Series. Springer, Berlin

40. Rejniak KA, Anderson AR (2008) A computational study of the development of epithelial acini: I. Sufficient conditions for the formation of a hollow structure. Bull Math Biol 70(3):677–712. doi:10.1007/s11538-007-9274-1
41. Rejniak KA, Estrella V, Chen T, Cohen AS, Lloyd MC, Morse DL (2013) The role of tumor tissue architecture in treatment penetration and efficacy: an integrative study. Front Oncol 3:111. doi:10.3389/fonc.2013.00111
42. Rejniak KA, Lloyd MC, Reed DR, Bui MM (2015) Diagnostic assessment of osteosarcoma chemoresistance based on Virtual Clinical Trials. Med Hypotheses 85(3):348–354. doi:10.1016/j.mehy.2015.06.015
43. Rejniak KA, Quaranta V, Anderson AR (2012) Computational investigation of intrinsic and extrinsic mechanisms underlying the formation of carcinoma. Math Med Biol (A Journal of the IMA) 29(1):67–84. doi:10.1093/imammb/dqq021
44. Rejniak KA, Wang SE, Bryce NS, Chang H, Parvin B, Jourquin J, Estrada L, Gray JW, Arteaga CL, Weaver AM, Quaranta V, Anderson AR (2010) Linking changes in epithelial morphogenesis to cancer mutations using computational modeling. PLoS Comput Biol 6(8). doi:10.1371/journal.pcbi.1000900
45. Rizki A, Weaver VM, Lee SY, Rozenberg GI, Chin K, Myers CA, Bascom JL, Mott JD, Semeiks JR, Grate LR, Mian IS, Borowsky AD, Jensen RA, Idowu MO, Chen F, Chen DJ, Petersen OW, Gray JW, Bissell MJ (2008) A human breast cell model of preinvasive to invasive transition. Cancer Res 68(5):1378–1387. doi:10.1158/0008-5472.CAN-07-2225
46. Santner SJ, Dawson PJ, Tait L, Soule HD, Eliason J, Mohamed AN, Wolman SR, Heppner GH, Miller FR (2001) Malignant MCF10CA1 cell lines derived from premalignant human breast epithelial MCF10AT cells. Breast Cancer Res Treat 65(2):101–110
47. Saunders NA, Simpson F, Thompson EW, Hill MM, Endo-Munoz L, Leggatt G, Minchin RF, Guminski A (2012) Role of intratumoural heterogeneity in cancer drug resistance: molecular and clinical perspectives. EMBO Mol Med 4(8):675–684. doi:10.1002/emmm.201101131
48. Shamir ER, Ewald AJ (2014) Three-dimensional organotypic culture: experimental models of mammalian biology and disease. Nat Rev Mol Cell Biol 15(10):647–664. doi:10.1038/nrm3873
49. Thoma CR, Zimmermann M, Agarkova I, Kelm JM, Krek W (2014) 3D cell culture systems modeling tumor growth determinants in cancer target discovery. Adv Drug Deliv Rev 69-70:29–41. doi:10.1016/j.addr.2014.03.001
50. Tyson DR, Inokuchi J, Tsunoda T, Lau A, Ornstein DK (2007) Culture requirements of prostatic epithelial cell lines for acinar morphogenesis and lumen formation in vitro: role of extracellular calcium. Prostate 67(15):1601–1613. doi:10.1002/pros.20628
51. Weigelt B, Bissell MJ (2008) Unraveling the microenvironmental influences on the normal mammary gland and breast cancer. Semin Cancer Biol 18(5):311–321. doi:10.1016/j.semcancer.2008.03.013

Printed in the United States
By Bookmasters